MW01234736

online and in-print Internet
directories in medicine

ONCOLOGY & HEMATOLOGY 2000

AN INTERNET RESOURCE GUIDE

CONSULTING EDITOR
Martin D. Abeloff, M.D.

Director
The Johns Hopkins Oncology Center

Professor of Oncology and Medicine
The Johns Hopkins University School of Medicine

Oncologist-in-Chief of the
Johns Hopkins Hospital and Health Systems

Visit
Oncology &
Hematology at
www.eMedguides.com

Access code:
4596

eMedguides.com, Inc., Princeton, New Jersey

For electronic browsing of this book, see
http://www.eMedguides.com

The publisher offers discounts on the eMedguides series of
books. For more information, contact

Sales Department
eMedguides.com, Inc.
P.O. Box 2331
Princeton, NJ 08543
tel   800-230-1481
fax   609-520-2023
e-mail sales@eMedguides.com

This book is set in Avenir, Gill Sans, and Sabon typefaces
and was printed and bound in the United States of America.

10 9 8 7 6 5 4 3 2 1

ISBN 0-9676811-0-3

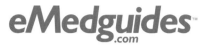

eMedguides.com

ONCOLOGY & HEMATOLOGY 2000
AN INTERNET RESOURCE GUIDE

Daniel R. Goldenson
Editor-in-Chief

Martin D. Abeloff, M.D.
Consulting Editor,
Director, The Johns Hopkins Oncology Center

Karen M. Albert, MLS
Consulting Medical Librarian,
Director of Library Services, Fox Chase Cancer Center

Adam T. Bromwich
Managing Editor

Rebecca L. Crane, MPH
Development Editor

Kristina Hasselbring
Alysa M. Wilson
Senior Research Editors

Rishi Bakshi
Senior Researcher

Sue Bannon
Designer

eMEDGUIDES.COM

Raymond C. Egan
Chairman of the Board

Daniel R. Goldenson
President

Adam T. Bromwich
Chief Operating Officer

Raymond Egan, Jr.
Marketing Director

P.O. Box 2331
Princeton, NJ 08543-2331
Book orders 800.230.1481
Facsimile 609.520.2023
E-mail oncology@eMedguides.com

2000 ANNUAL EDITION

Anesthesiology & Pain Management

Arthritis & Rheumatology

Cardiology

Dental Medicine

Dermatology

Diet & Nutrition

Emergency Medicine

Endocrinology & Metabolism

Family Medicine

Gastroenterology

General Surgery

Infectious Diseases & Immunology

Internal Medicine

Neurology & Neuroscience

Obstetrics & Gynecology

Oncology & Hematology

Ophthalmology

Orthopedics & Sports Medicine

Otolaryngology

Pathology & Laboratory Medicine

Pediatrics

Physical Medicine & Rehabilitation

Plastic Surgery

Psychiatry

Radiology

Respiratory & Pulmonary Medicine

Urology & Nephrology

Veterinary Medicine

| File | Edit | View | Favorites | Tools | Help |

| ← Back | → Forward | ⊗ Stop | ⟳ Refresh | ⌂ Home | 🔍 Search | History | 🖨 Print |

Address | http://www.eMedguides.com | ⌄ | ⤳ Go

VISIT US ON THE INTERNET

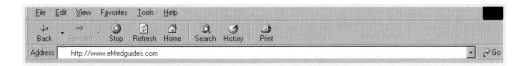

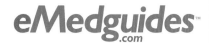

www.eMedguides.com

Instant access to all of our selected Web sites

Each print edition is online, *in its entirety*, so you can browse with your mouse, never typing in a single Web address. Simply visit www.eMedguides.com, click the appropriate specialty, enter your access code (printed in a circle on the title page), and you are presented with every site, listed by topic. Browse through the book online, or enter a keyword term to search the entire specialty.

Visit us often—our staff is continually adding new and interesting sites to each medical specialty database!

✺ Read the latest medical headlines each day in *your* specialty, as well as the top news in the medical field in general.

✺ Select a forthcoming conference, meeting, or CME program with a click of the mouse.

✺ Check out the latest issue of up to 100 medical journals in your field, and review abstracts and tables of contents without any charge.

✺ Review the newest drugs in your field, and the journal articles that discuss them.

✺ Use over 50 medical search engines to find any information in any field, just by typing in a keyword.

✺ Review the current bibliography of new books published in your field, organized topically for your convenience.

✺ Open up the world of the Internet. Find new and useful sites. Become Internet savvy!

The Art and Science of Oncology

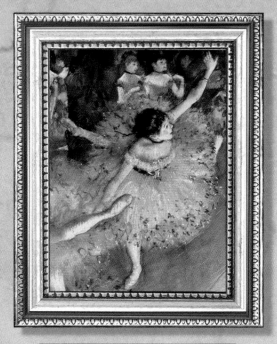

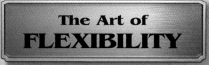

The Art of
FLEXIBILITY

Flexible Dosing*

SEMISYNTHETIC
TAXOL®†
(paclitaxel) Injection
Clearly Versatile

In general, TAXOL is well tolerated. The most common adverse events associated with TAXOL are neutropenia, peripheral neuropathy, arthralgia/myalgia, and alopecia.

*Please see Appendix A at the end of this book for brief summary of prescribing information including indications, dosing, and administration.

†TAXOL is a registered trademark of Bristol-Myers Squibb Company.

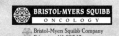

Bristol-Myers Squibb Company
Princeton, NJ 08543
U.S.A.

www.bms.com. Click on cancer.

©1999, Bristol-Myers Squibb Company
Princeton, New Jersey 08543, U.S.A.

K4-K030R   11/99

Table of Contents

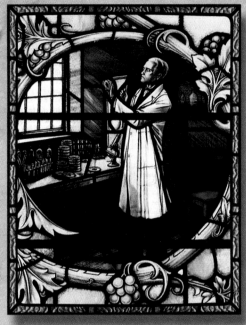
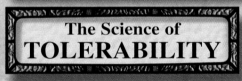
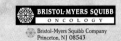

The Art and Science of Oncology

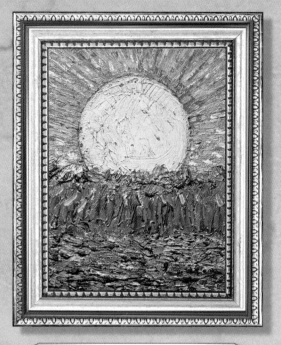

The Art of
ACTIVITY

SEMISYNTHETIC
TAXOL®*
(paclitaxel) Injection
Clearly Versatile

In general, TAXOL is well tolerated. The most common adverse events associated with TAXOL are neutropenia, peripheral neuropathy, arthralgia/myalgia, and alopecia.

Please see Appendix A at the end of this book for brief summary of prescribing information including indications, dosing, and administration.

*TAXOL is a registered trademark of Bristol-Myers Squibb Company.

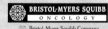

Bristol-Myers Squibb Company
Princeton, NJ 08543
U.S.A.

www.bms.com. Click on cancer.

The Art and Science of Oncology

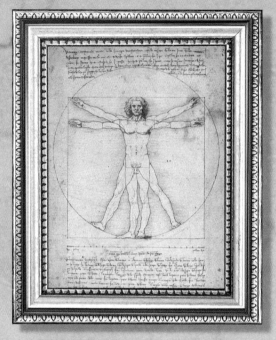

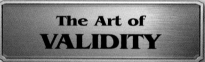

The Art of
VALIDITY

**Validated Continually as a
Single Agent and in Combination
Within Cooperative Group Trials*†**

SEMISYNTHETIC
TAXOL®‡
(paclitaxel) Injection
Clearly Versatile

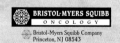
ONCOLOGY
Bristol-Myers Squibb Company
Princeton, NJ 08543
U.S.A.

Scala/Art Resource, NY. Leonardo da Vinci (1492-1519). Vitruvian Man, ca. 1492. Accademia, Venice, Italy.

In general, TAXOL is well tolerated. The most common adverse events associated with TAXOL are neutropenia, peripheral neuropathy, arthralgia/myalgia, and alopecia.

*As of 1999.

†Please see Appendix A at the end of this book for brief summary of prescribing information including indications, dosing, and administration.

‡TAXOL is a registered trademark of Bristol-Myers Squibb Company.

www.bms.com. Click on cancer.

©1999, Bristol-Myers Squibb Company
Princeton, New Jersey 08543, U.S.A.

K4-K029   11/99

**PART TWO   GENERAL MEDICAL
                      WEB RESOURCES**

**10.   REFERENCE
        INFORMATION
        AND NEWS SOURCES . . 335**

Foreword

Physicians play an essential role in their patient's health. They are a primary source of information. In the fast-paced and ever changing world of oncology treatments, oncologists strive to remain up-to-date on the latest trends, cutting-edge treatment options, and clinical trials in order to ensure that their patients receive the best possible care. With the recent emergence of health and cancer sites on the Internet, research information is being published at a more rapid pace than ever before.

In fact, there are nearly 25,000 Web sites now available on health and medical conditions. With millions of people logging onto Internet health sites every year, physicians are now faced with the overwhelming task of determining which sites actually offer credible medical information that will not only be of value to patients but also to physicians.

Towards this end, this guide has been formatted to provide clinicians with a comprehensive reference of available Web sites and a concise review of individual content. Clinicians, in turn, can direct patients and families to sites of greatest merit, thereby educating themselves with credible resources. With the avalanche of, at times unsubstantiated, information it is critical that patients have the most accurate and timely data. A patient clearly educated on viable treatment options is a better partner overall with the healthcare provider.

> — Diane Blum, ACSW
> Executive Director, Cancer Care, Inc.

I. INTRODUCTION

1.1 **Welcome to eMedguides**

Welcome to eMedguides, the newest and largest online and in-print Internet directories for physicians and other healthcare professionals, covering every major field in medicine!

As a user of this book, you now have a gateway to an extraordinary amount of information to help you find every possible, useful resource in your field, from electronic journals to selected Web sites on dozens of common and uncommon diseases and disorders.

We would like to thank our Consulting Medical Editor, Martin D. Abeloff, M.D., Director, The Johns Hopkins Oncology Center, for his valued assistance in this new project, and for his many organizational and topical suggestions. In addition, we wish to thank our Consulting Medical Librarian, Karen Albert, Director of Library Services for the Fox Chase Cancer Center, for her assistance in the development of this volume.

The focus of this volume is Oncology, including hematological aspects of the field. We have approached the compilation of this directory from the point of view of the professional practitioner and researcher, by organizing and heavily indexing topics and disorders, and associations and government agencies, so that we lead you directly to the right destination on the Internet. Our medical compilers are trained professionals, and have written and rated Web sites in every category to let you know ahead of time what you can expect to find.

This book has been divided into sections, providing ease of access to material. The first part this book is devoted solely to oncology resources, including clinical information, disorder profiles, glossaries, current news sources, electronic journals, latest books, statistics, clinical studies, "supersites," therapies, and numerous topical resources.

The second part of the book is focused on the broad fields of medicine reference, clinical practice, and patient education. We have listed online databases and general medical resources, sources of current news and legislation, library access sites, government agencies in the health field, pharmaceutical data, student resources, and patient planning information.

Through the cooperation of the National Organization for Rare Disorders, Inc. (NORD), we have been able to obtain descriptive abstracts and synonyms for rare oncology and hematology disorders, which are included in part three of this volume. We include links to NORD's site where support organizations can be obtained and in-depth reports can be purchased for a modest sum.

Finally, a very extensive index is included, covering every topic, disorder, association, and Web site title, to make the fact-finding mission as efficient as possible.

How to Benefit Most from this Book

We realize that many physicians and other healthcare professionals may be overwhelmed by the extraordinary number of search engines to choose from, and the difficulty in finding very specific information that may only appear in a few locations on the Web. Our aim, therefore, has been to organize this book logically, topic by topic, giving descriptions of Web sites that we feel our readers will want to visit. To access a Web site, the user can type in the provided Web address (URL), or go straight to http://www.eMedguides.com where sites are listed just as they are in the book—but with "hot" links that merely require a mouse click. *The access code included on the title page of this volume provides access to our Web site.*

Physicians and researchers may want to examine several of the unique resources in this volume. We have provided a list of the most recent books published in the past year in the specialty, which are all available at http://www.amazon.com. Those readers who are interested in research can browse through our comprehensive journal section for access to thousands of articles and article abstracts every month. A further exploration can lead to medical libraries, university and nonprofit centers for research across the country, clinical studies currently underway in every phase, FDA trials of the latest drugs, and instant news sources for the latest breakthroughs.

Although much of the material in this book is intended for a professional, medical audience, key patient Web resources are also provided. Physicians may wish to refer patients to these sites. Many patient sites include up-to-date news and research and clear descriptions of diseases and their treatments.

Oncology & Hematology 2000: An Internet Resource Guide is an annual volume, since so much information on the Web keeps changing, better sites and sources are assembled, hundreds of new books are published, new conferences are constantly scheduled, and major research progress is made every day.

The Benefits of Both Print and Online Editions

We feel that both the print and online editions of eMedguides can play an important role in the information gathering process, depending on the needs of the physician or health professional. The *print* edition is a "hands on" tool, enabling the reader to thumb through a comprehensive directory, finding Web information and topical sources that are totally new and unexpected. Each page can provide discoveries of resources previously unknown to the reader that may never have been the subject of an online search. Without knowing what to expect, the reader can be introduced to useful Web site information just by glancing at the book at different times, looking through the detailed Table of Contents, or examining the extensive Index. This type of browsing is difficult to achieve online.

The *online* edition serves a different purpose. It provides "hot links" for each Web site, so the user can click on a topic and visit the destination instantaneously, without having to type the Web address into a browser. In addition, there are search features in this edition that can be used to find specific information quickly, and then the user can print out only what he or she wishes to use. The online edition will also have more frequent updates during the year. Articles are posted daily, giving recent news and updates on each specialty, allowing the user to stay up-to-date.

Accessing the Online Edition

We encourage our readers to to visit our Web site, through which readers can access any of the included sites with a simple click of the mouse. Our Web address is http://www.eMedguides.com. You will need a special access code that is included on the title page of this volume. By simply clicking on a specialty and typing in this code, the entire contents of the book can be browsed and then used as an online Internet guide. We will continually update the information in this volume on our Web site. Information will be posted on new books published in the field, newly announced conferences, and of course additional Web resources that become available and are of interest to physicians. You can also submit the names of other Web sites that you have discovered by e-mailing us at oncology@eMedguides.com.

We hope you will find the print and online versions of this volume to be useful Internet companions, always on hand to consult.

Ratings Guide and Abbreviations

Abbreviations
See "Medical Abbreviations and Acronyms" under "Reference Information and News Sources" in Part 2 for Web sites that provide acronym translation. Below are a few acronyms you will find throughout this volume:

ACS   American Cancer Society
BMT   Bone Marrow Transplant
CME   Continuing Medical Education
FAQ   Frequently-Asked Questions
NCI   National Cancer Institute
NIH   National Institutes of Health
PDQ   Physician Data Query
URL   Uniform Resource Locator (the address of a Web site on the Internet)

Ratings

Each site is listed by category with its title, address, rating, description, and type.

We have rated each Internet Web site for content. Three stars (✦ ✦ ✦) is outstanding; one star (✦) is good. We assess the quality of content of a site as well at its overall usefulness to physicians.

If a site requires a fee or only free registration, we have indicated this next to the rating.

1.2 Getting Online

The Internet is growing at a fantastic rate, but the vast majority of individuals are not yet online. What is preventing people from jumping on the "information highway"? There are many factors, but probably the most common factor is a general confusion about what the Internet is, how it works, and how to access it.

The following few pages are designed to clear up any confusion for readers who have not yet accessed the Internet. We will look at the process of getting onto and using the Internet, step by step. It is also helpful to consult other resources, such as the technical support department of the manufacturer or store where you bought your computer. Although assistance varies widely, most organizations provide startup assistance for new users and are experienced with guiding individuals onto the Internet. Books can also be of great assistance, as they provide a simple and clear view of how computers and the Internet work, and can be studied at your own pace.

What is the Internet?

The Internet is a large network of computers that are all connected to one another. A good analogy is to envision a neighborhood, with houses and storefronts, all connected to one another by streets and highways. Often the Internet is referred to as the "information superhighway" because of the vastness of this neighborhood.

The Internet was initially developed to allow people to share computers, that is, sublet part of their "house" to others. The ability to connect to so many other computers quickly and easily made this feasible. As computers proliferated, people used the Internet for sending information quickly from one computer to another.

For example, the most popular feature of the Internet is electronic mail (e-mail). Each computer has a mailbox, and an electronic letter can be sent instantly. People also use the Internet to post bulletins, or other information, for others to see. The process of sending e-mail or viewing this information is simple. A computer and a connection to the Internet are all you need to begin.

How is an Internet connection provided?

The Internet is accessed either through a "direct" connection, which is sometimes found in businesses and educational institutions, or through a phone line. Phone line connections are commonly used in small businesses and at home (although direct connections are becoming available for home use via cable and special phone lines). There are many complex options in this area; for the new user it is simplest to use an existing phone line to experience the Internet for the first time. After connecting a computer to a common phone jack, the computer can access the Internet. It will dial the number of an Internet provider, ask you for a user name and password, and give you access to the Internet. Keep in mind that while you are using the Internet, your phone line is tied up, and callers will hear a busy signal. Also, call waiting can sometimes interrupt an Internet connection and disconnect you from your provider.

Who provides an Internet connection?

There are many providers at both the local and national levels. One of the easiest ways to get online is with America Online (AOL). They provide software and a user-friendly environment through which to access the Internet. Because AOL manages both this environment and the actual connection, they can be of great assistance when you are starting out. America Online takes you to a menu of choices when you log in, and while using their software you can read and send e-mail, view Web pages, and chat with others.

Many other similar services exist, and most of them also provide an environment using Microsoft or Netscape products. These companies, such as the Microsoft Network (MSN), Mindspring, and Earthlink, also provide simple, easy-to-use access to the Internet. Their environment is more standard and not limited to the choices America Online provides.

Internet connections generally run from $10–$20 per month (depending on the length of commitment) in addition to telephone costs. Most national providers have local phone numbers all over the country that should eliminate any telephone charges. The monthly provider fee is the only charge for accessing the Internet.

How do I get on the Internet?

Once you've signed up with a provider and installed their software (often only a matter of answering basic questions), your computer will be set up to access the Internet. By simply double-clicking on an icon, your computer will dial the phone number, log you in, and present you with a Web page (a "home" page).

What are some of the Internet's features?

From the initial Web page there are almost limitless possibilities of where you can go. The address at the top of the screen (identified by an "http://" in front) tells you where you are. You can also type the address of where you would like to go next. When typing a new address, you do not need to add the "http://". The computer adds this prefix automatically after you type in an address and press return. Once you press return, the Web site will appear in the browser window.

You can also navigate the Web by "surfing" from one site to another using links on a page. A Web page might say "Click here for weather." If you click on this underlined phrase, you will be taken to a different address, where weather information is provided.

The Internet has several other useful features. E-mail is an extremely popular and important service. It is free and messages are delivered instantly. Although you can access e-mail through a Web browser (AOL has this feature), many Internet services provide a separate e-mail program for reading, writing, and organizing your correspondence. These programs send and retrieve messages from the Internet.

Another area of the Internet offers chat rooms where users can hold round table discussions. In a chat room you can type messages and see the replies of other users around the world. There are chat rooms on virtually every topic, although the dialog certainly varies in this free-for-all forum. There are also newsgroups on the Internet, some of which we list in this book. A newsgroup is similar to a chat room but each message is a separate item and can be viewed in sequence at any time. For example, a user might post a question about Lyme disease. In the newsgroup you can read the question, and then read the answers that others have provided. You can also post your own comments. This forum is usually not managed or edited, particularly in the medical field. Do not take the advice of a chat room or newsgroup source without first consulting your physician.

How can I find things on the Internet?

Surfing the Internet, from site to site, is a popular activity. But if you have a focused mission, you will want to use a search engine. A search engine can scan lists of Web sites to look for a particular site. We provide a long list of medical search engines in this book.

Because the Internet is so large and unregulated, sites are often hard to find. In the physical world it is difficult to find good services, but you can turn to the yellow pages or other resources to get a comprehensive list. Physical proximity is also a major factor. On the Internet, none of this applies. Finding a reliable site takes time and patience, and can require sifting through hundreds of similar, yet irrelevant sites.

The most common way to find information on the Internet is to use a search engine. When you go to the Web page of a search engine, you will be presented with two distinct methods of searching: using links to topics, or using a keyword search. The links often represent the Web site staff's best effort to find quality sites. This method of searching is the core of the Yahoo! search engine (www.yahoo.com). By clicking on Healthcare, then Disorders, then Lung Cancer, you are provided with a list of sites the staff has found on the topic.

The keyword approach is definitely more daring. By typing in search terms, the engine looks through its list of Web sites for a match and returns the results. These engines typically only cover 15% of the Internet, so it is not a comprehensive process. They also usually return far too many choices. Typing lung cancer into a search engine box will return thousands of sites, including one entry for every site where someone used the words lung cancer on a personal Web page.

Where do eMedguides come in?

eMedguides are organized sources of information in each major medical specialty. Our team of editors continually scour the Net, searching for quality Web sites that relate to specific specialties, disorders, and research topics. More importantly, of the sites we find, we only include those that provide professional and useful content. eMedguides fill a critical gap in the Internet research process. Each guide provides more than 500 Web sites that focus on every aspect of a single medical discipline.

Other Internet companies that lack our medical and physician focus have teams of "surfers" who can only cover a subject on its surface. Search engines, even medical search engines, return far too many choices, requiring hours of time and patience to sift through. With an eMedguide in hand, you can quickly identify the sites worth visiting on the Internet and jump right to them. At our site, www.eMedguides.com, you can access the same listings as in this book, and can simply click on a site to go straight to it. In addition, we provide continual updates to the book through the site and annually in print. Our editors do the surfing for you, and do it professionally, making your Internet experience efficient and fulfilling.

Taking medical action must involve a physician

As interesting as the Internet is, the information that you will find is both objective and subjective. Our goal is to expose our readers to Web sites on hundreds of topics—for informational purposes only. If you are not a physician and become interested in the ideas, guidelines, recommendations, or experiences discussed online, bring these findings to a physician for personal evaluation. Medical needs vary considerably, and a medical approach or therapy for one individual could be entirely misguided for another. Final medical advice and a plan of action must come only from a physician.

PART ONE

ONCOLOGY & HEMATOLOGY WEB RESOURCES

2. QUICK REFERENCE

2.1 **Cancer Disease Profiles**

American Cancer Society (ACS): Cancer Types ◎ ◎ ◎
http://www2.cancer.org/crcGateway/index.cfm

Fifty-five (55) forms of cancer can be reviewed through profiles at this site. Just select or enter the type of cancer for which information is desired, and the database provides a description, incidence information, causes, tests and diagnostic data, treatment options, staging information, and other relevant material.

CancerNet Cancer Disorder Profiles: Alphabetical Listing ◎ ◎ ◎
http://cancernet.nci.nih.gov/alphalist.html

More than 100 types of cancer are profiled in PDQ, the National Cancer Institute's comprehensive cancer database. Each profile contains an extensive general description of the disorder, cell classification, stages of the disease, treatment options, sub-classifications of the disease, and bibliographic references.

CancerNet Cancer Disorder Profiles: By Body Location/System ◎ ◎ ◎
http://cancernet.nci.nih.gov/location.html

The National Cancer Institute (NCI) organizes the disorder profiles in its CancerNet database by body location/system. Numerous cancers are listed under 20 categories such as brain, breast, leukemia, lung, and skin. Clicking on a particular cancer takes the user to the PDQ database entry, which provides descriptive information and numerous links.

Disease-Oriented Menus for Oncology from OncoLink ◎ ◎ ◎
http://www.oncolink.upenn.edu/disease

The University of Pennsylvania Cancer Center has provided comprehensive disease-oriented menus for adult and pediatric cancers, including pathology images, technical articles, and case studies. Adult cancers covered include bone cancers, brain tumors, breast cancer, endocrine system cancers, gastrointestinal cancers, genitourinary (male) cancers, gynecologic cancers, head and neck cancers, adult leukemia, lung cancers, lymphomas, metastases, myelomas, sarcomas, skin cancers, and urinary tract cancers. Pediatric cancers covered include pediatric brain tumors, pediatric leukemias and lymphomas, pediatric liver cancer, neuroblastoma, retinoblastoma, rhabdomyosarcoma and other sarcomas, other pediatric cancers, and Wilms' tumor.

2.2 **Cancer Glossaries**

ACOR Cancer Glossary ⊙ ⊙ ⊙

http://www.acor.org/glossary/index.html

The Association of Cancer Online Resources has provided a glossary of more than 1,000 terms at this very useful site. There is an alphabetical scroll-down menu, and definition finder link for immediate answers.

Cancer Dictionary ⊙ ⊙ ⊙

http://www.cancer.ab.ca/overview/diction.htm

This comprehensive glossary covers several hundred terms, including procedures, disorders, therapies and treatments, types of drugs, parts of the body, devices, bodily processes, hormones, genes, and other subjects.

Cancer Glossary ⊙ ⊙ ⊙

http://rex.nci.nih.gov/INFO_CANCER/CANCER_DEFS/DEFS_AB.htm

Hundreds of cancer-related terms are succinctly defined in this useful Cancer Glossary compiled by the National Cancer Institute at the National Institutes of Health.

Dictionary of Cancer Terms ⊙ ⊙ ⊙

http://cancernet.nci.nih.gov/dictionary.html

An excellent, extensive dictionary of cancer terms is provided at this section of the CancerNet site, including hundreds of technical as well as less technical terms for the cancer patient seeking a better understanding of Oncology.

Medicine Online: Cancer Glossary ⊙ ⊙ ⊙

http://www.meds.com/glossary.html

Developed by the Nursing Advisory Board of Pharmacia and the Upjohn corporation, this cancer glossary offers succinct definitions of a large number of key terms, diseases, tumor names, glandular terms, conditions, types of drugs, bodily substances, drug agents, and other key subjects that would be encountered in a serious review of cancer literature and research. The definitions are clear and succinct and appropriate for general, medical student, and professional audiences.

Oncology Abbreviations and Acronyms ⊙ ⊙ ⊙

http://www.staff.ncl.ac.uk/s.j.cotterill/medtm15.htm

This site provides a detailed, technical reference list of abbreviations and acronyms for the field of oncology, a resource of interest to clinical practitioners. A list of abbreviations for cancer drugs, conditions, therapies, and other oncology topics are provided, along with a set of acronyms of cancer organizations.

2.3 Cancer News

Cancer and General Medical News at Medscape ◎ ◎ ◎
http://www.medscape.com

Daily stories in the medical field, research developments, drug testing, and cancer-specific news are provided at this free Web site for physicians and patients.

Cancer and Trials News from the National Cancer Institute (NCI) ◎ ◎ ◎
http://mednav10.vh.shore.net/NCI_CANCER_TRIALS/zones/TrialInfo/News

This site provides current news articles on both clinical trials underway and news developments for different forms of cancer, cancer research, new therapies, and current legislation affecting the cancer field.

Cancer News on the Net ◎ ◎ ◎
http://www.cancernews.com

Cancer News is a comprehensive source for up-to-date information concerning oncology. The site is linked to various sources and organizations that post news regarding cancer. Links to recent cancer news sites offer the user an opportunity to visit cancer information sections of search engines, major media news services, and drug review sites. Similar links exist for most major forms of cancer. In addition, there are updated resources that list meetings, seminars, and other related events.

Daily Apple Cancer Center ◎ ◎ ◎
http://www.thedailyapple.com

Click on "Cancer" under the "Quick Find" pull-down menu at this site to access cancer-related news for professionals and the public. There are news pages for individual types of cancers as well as general topics in oncology. Some topics covered are chemotherapy, pharmaceuticals, diet and nutrition, and radiation therapy.

Doctor's Guide Oncology and Hematology News ◎ ◎ ◎
http://www.pslgroup.com/dg/haematonews.htm

Dozens of daily articles on new developments in Oncology and Hematology are provided at this very useful Web site. For a review of other medical news developments in different fields, the user can navigate to any topic of interest through www.pslgroup.com/dg and click on Medical News and Alerts, a category that is further broken down by date and individual medical field.

2.4 **Conferences in Oncology and Hematology**

Introduction

The following Web sites provide access to listings of forthcoming conferences and meetings in the fields of Oncology and Hematology.

**Forward Conference Calendar
for Oncology and Hematology** ☺ ☺ ☺

http://www.pslgroup.com/dg/haemato.htm

This partial listing of conferences and meetings for the year 2000 is compiled by the Doctor's Guide to Medical Conferences and Meetings. Dates, places, and other details are located at the main Web site. Upon visiting this site, the reader can click on any conference listing for additional information. The conference list is continually updated and should be consulted frequently.

International Calendar of Cancer ☺ ☺ ☺

http://www.globalink.org/calendars

The International Union Against Cancer provides a conference schedule for cancer-related conferences worldwide. The search engine provided makes it easy to identify meetings of interest.

**Medical Conferences & Meetings:
Oncology, Hematology** ☺ ☺ ☺

http://www.medicalconferences.com/scripts/search_new.pl

Medical Conferences.com is an excellent source of information on forthcoming conferences and meetings in the fields of Oncology and Hematology. This site provides a search engine, enabling the visitor to type in "oncology," "hematology," or other topics into the keyword space in order to receive a lengthy listing of conferences to be held over the next 12 months or longer. Each conference is an active link in itself, further permitting the visitor to obtain more detailed information about the event. There are over 125 meetings in the database for oncology and hematology, and more are added on a regular basis.

**MediConf Online:
Oncology and Hematology Forthcoming Meetings** ☺ ☺ ☺

http://www.mediconf.com/online.html

MediConf online provides an excellent directory of forthcoming meetings and conferences in every major medical specialty. The menu at this site enables the visitor to select the field of choice, such as Oncology or Hematology, and this service produces a printout of meetings to be held in the near future. For each meeting there is a listing including the dates, the contact telephone number, the contact e-mail address, and a link to the city where the visitor can learn about accommodations, weather, and other information.

OncoLink: Meeting Announcements ⊙ ⊙ ⊙

http://www.oncolink.upenn.edu/conference

This site provides information on cancer-related meetings worldwide for both health-care professionals and cancer patients. Conferences are listed chronologically, giving locations of meetings, with links containing further details.

2.5 Topical Search Tools

OncoLink: Basic Search   ⊙ ⊙ ⊙

http://www.oncolink.upenn.edu:8083

Drawing on the extraordinarily extensive database of the University of Pennsylvania, this search engine produces hundreds of documents on subjects of interest. There is a choice of simple or advanced query, and the documents that are presented can be further examined individually.

Search at the National Cancer Society ⊙ ⊙ ⊙

http://www.cancer.org

At the top of the home page of the American Cancer Society is a very useful search feature that allows the visitor to select any topic of his or her interest. The search engine produces a listing of site resources, articles, and data in response to a query.

Search Options at CancerNet ⊙ ⊙ ⊙

http://cancernet.nci.nih.gov/searchoptions.html

The database at the National Cancer Institute is very extensive, but this Search section provides a quick method of locating general cancer information, clinical trials, cancer literature, and cancer genetic information. For each topic, the site gives instructions on how to search for desired information.

2.6 Cancer Statistics

American Cancer Society (ACS): Statistics ⊙ ⊙ ⊙

http://www.cancer.org/statistics/index.html

The ACS presents valuable statistical resources related to cancer rates by gender, age, race/ethnic group, and death rates from different forms of cancer in the 20th century. Breast cancer facts and figures are available, presenting statistics of occurrence, survival, and risk factors, and discussions of prevention, treatment, and current research. Risk factors and screening statistics are available by state. Users can also access data on other selected cancers, including childhood, colon and rectum, leukemia, lung and bronchus, lymphoma, oral cavity and pharynx, ovarian, pancreas, prostate, skin, urinary bladder, uterine cervix, and uterine corpus (endometrium). Tobacco use, nutrition and diet, and environmental risks in the United States are also outlined. A statistics archive is offered for data from 1995 to 1998.

Ask C/Net ☺ ☺ ☺

http://www.askcnet.org

This service allows the user to obtain customized data of various types. The Cancer Statistics on Demand section allows the user to retrieve cancer statistics of any kind from public files or from cancer registries. A list of cancer registries and their online reports is offered. There are links to online publications of the California Cancer Registry, and to the Breast Cancer Answers site. The latter provides a clinical trial matching system and other resources for patients. Information on obtaining software for health data registry operations is also provided. Free registration is required.

SEER: Cancer Statistics Review, National Cancer Institute ☺ ☺ ☺

http://www-seer.ims.nci.nih.gov/Publications/CSR7393/index.html

The National Cancer Institute provides statistical charts for 25 forms of cancer. This statistical data is from 1973 through 1993. The reports are also provided for 1973 through 1996, and a printed copy can be ordered.

2.7 Clinical Studies and Trials

All Trials

Centerwatch: Clinical Trials Listing Service (by disease) ☺ ☺ ☺

http://www.centerwatch.com/studies/listing.htm

Designed for both patients and healthcare professionals, this site provides an extensive listing of therapeutic clinical trials organized by disorder, sponsored by both industry and government. Over 50 forms of cancer are arranged alphabetically by type. It is international in scope and provides data on more than 5,200 clinical trials that are actively recruiting patients. Keyword search accessible, it also covers information on new FDA-approved drug therapies. Trials are listed by geographical region within each disorder.

NCI Clinical Trials

CancerTrials (by geographic location) ◎ ◎ ◎
http://mednav10.vh.shore.net/NCI_CANCER_TRIALS/zones/TrialInfo/Finding/centers

Covering important information for patients involved in or considering entering cancer clinical trials, this site also links to the PDQ search system for identifying trials available for many cancer types in a broad range of geographic areas. Over 1,700 clinical trials are active in this database. Produced by the National Cancer Institute, the site provides a wealth of valuable links to information on all aspects of cancer clinical trials and cancer in general. This site provides three critical links to find cancer clinical trials: (1) A Background Link that describes NCI-Designated Cancer Centers where trials are conducted; (2) A Check List of information you need to know before searching for clinical trials; and (3) A map of the United States which allows the user to click on a state or region in order to access the cancer trial centers in that region. Each center has its address and telephone number as well as information on trials being conducted at that location.

NIH Clinical Trials

Centerwatch: NIH Trials Listing (by disease) ◎ ◎ ◎
http://www.centerwatch.com/nih/index.htm

Centerwatch provides a convenient resource for accessing information on clinical trials at the National Institutes of Health (NIH). These are clinical trials publicized by the NIH, located at the Warren Grant Magnuson Clinical Center in Bethesda, Maryland. Trials are organized by disorder and have short descriptions.

2.8 Drug Pipeline: Approved and Developmental Drugs

Centerwatch: FDA Drug Approvals ◎ ◎ ◎
http://www.centerwatch.com/drugs/druglist.htm

This clinical trials listing service provides a listing and descriptive profile of each new drug approved by the FDA in the last five years. Drugs are organized by year and by specialty.

New Oncology and Hematology Drugs Under Development ◎ ◎ ◎
http://www.phrma.org/cancer/index.html

More than 350 new drugs are under development in all major oncology and hematology areas. This Web site is a detailed source providing the product names, pharmaceutical company developers, indications, and status.

3. JOURNALS, ARTICLES, AND 1999 BOOKS

3.1 **Abstract, Citation, and Full-text Search Tools**

CancerLit ⊙ ⊙ ⊙

http://cnetdb.nci.nih.gov/cancerlit.shtml

CancerLit is a bibliographic database that contains more than 1.3 million citations and abstracts from over 4,000 different sources including biomedical journals, proceedings, books, reports, and doctoral theses. The coverage period extends from 1963 to the present. Utilizing the Standard Search Form (accessible at the above URL), the user can perform rapid searches across all fields of cancer literature.

MEDLINE/PubMed at the National Library of Medicine (NLM) ⊙ ⊙ ⊙

http://www.ncbi.nlm.nih.gov/PubMed

PubMed is a free MEDLINE search service providing access to 11 million citations with links to the full text of articles of participating journals. Probably the most heavily used and reputable free MEDLINE site, PubMed permits advanced searching by subject, author, journal title, and many other fields. It includes an easy-to-use "citation matcher" for completing and identifying references, and its PreMEDLINE database provides journal citations before they are indexed, making this version of MEDLINE more up-to-date than most.

3.2 **Journals on the Internet: Oncology and Hematology**

Directories of Electronic Journals

OncoLink: Online Journal Access ⊙ ⊙ ⊙

http://ejo.univ-lyon1.fr/Oncolynx/Journals.html#journals

Maintained by the University of Pennsylvania, OncoLink is an excellent resource for online journal access. It provides links and descriptions of over 150 oncology journals accessible via the Internet. OncoLink also provides an extensive list of links to other online resources for physicians and patients alike.

Science Komm ⊙ ⊙ ⊙

http://www.sciencekomm.at

This is an extremely convenient, one stop site with direct link connections to over 160 different cardiology/hematology journals and over 100 oncology journals published around the world. The site user can click on a journal and usually gain access, without charge, to the current issue table of contents and to abstracts of articles in the current issue. Some publications offer access to the complete articles on a fee basis for journal subscribers by password, but certain others offer access to articles without charge. In either case, the reader is able to obtain a clear idea of the content of current journal issues and in most instances access back issues as well.

Individual Journal Web Sites

The following journals may be accessed on the Internet. Our table of information for each journal identifies content that is accessible free-of-charge or with a free registration, and also identifies content that requires a password and fee for access. We have also indicated if back issues are accessible. Journals are listed in alphabetical order by title.

Abstracts in Hematology and Oncology

http://oncology.medscape.com/SCP/AHO/public/AHO-journal.html

Publisher	SCP Communications, Inc.
Free resources	Table of Contents, Abstracts
Pay resources	Articles

Acta Haematologica

http://www.karger.com/journals/aha/aha_jh.htm

Publisher	Karger
Free resources	Table of Contents, Abstracts
Pay resources	Articles

Acta Oncologia

http://www.scup.no/journals/en/j-457.html

Publisher	Scandinavian University Press
Free resources	Table of Contents
Pay resources	Abstracts, Articles

American Journal of Hematology

http://www3.interscience.wiley.com/cgi-bin/jtoc?ID=35105

Publisher	Wiley
Free resources	Registration required; Table of Contents and Abstracts
Pay resources	Articles

Angiogenesis

http://www.wkap.nl/journalhome.htm/0969-6970

Publisher Kluwer

Free resources Table of Contents

Pay resources Abstracts, Articles

Annals of Hematology

http://link.springer.de/link/service/journals/00277/index.htm

Publisher Springer–Verlag

Free resources Table of Contents, Abstracts

Pay resources Articles

Annals of Oncology

http://www.wkap.nl/jrnltoc.htm/0923-7534

Publisher Kluwer

Free resources Table of Contents, Abstracts

Pay resources Articles

Anti-Cancer Drug Design

http://www3.oup.co.uk/antcan

Publisher Oxford University Press

Free resources Table of Contents, Abstracts

Pay resources Articles

Anti-Micrombial Agents and Chemotherapy

http://aac.asm.org

Publisher The American Society for Microbiology

Free resources Table of Contents, Abstracts

Pay resources Articles

Apoptosis

http://www.wkap.nl/journalhome.htm/1360-8185

Publisher Kluwer

Free resources Table of Contents

Pay resources Abstracts, Articles

Biochemica & Biophysical Acta (BBA): Reviews on Cancer Online
http://ejo.univ-lyon1.fr/Oncolynx/Journals.html#journals

Publisher	Elsevier Science
Free resources	Registration required; Table of Contents, Abstracts, and Articles
Pay resources	None

Blood
http://www.bloodjournal.org

Publisher	W. B. Saunders
Free resources	Table of Contents, Abstracts
Pay resources	Articles

Blood Cells, Molecules, and Diseases
http://seconde.scripps.edu

Publisher	Springer–Verlag
Free resources	Table of Contents, Abstracts, Articles
Pay resources	None

Blood Pressure
http://www.scup.no/journals/en/j-448.html

Publisher	Scandinavian University Press
Free resources	Table of Contents
Pay resources	Abstracts, Articles

Blood Purification
http://www.karger.com/journals/bpu/bpu_jh.htm

Publisher	Karger
Free resources	Table of Contents, Abstracts
Pay resources	Articles

Blood Weekly
http://www.homepage.holowww.com/x1b.htm

Publisher	C.W. Henderson
Free resources	Table of Contents, Abstracts
Pay resources	Articles

Bloodline
http://www.bloodline.net

Publisher	Carden Jennings Publishing Co., Ltd.
Free resources	Table of Contents, Abstracts, Articles
Pay resources	None

Bone Marrow Transplantation
http://www.stockton-press.co.uk/0268-3369/contents.html

Publisher	Stockton Press
Free resources	Table of Contents and Abstracts
Pay resources	Articles

Breast Cancer Research
http://breast-cancer-research.com/login.cfm?action=form&returnto=home_page.cfm

Publisher	Current Science Ltd.
Free resources	Registration required; Table of Contents, Abstracts, and Articles
Pay resources	None

Breast Cancer Research and Treatment
http://www.wkap.nl/journalhome.htm/0167-6806

Publisher	Kluwer
Free resources	Table of Contents
Pay resources	Abstracts, Articles

BreastCancer.net
http://www.breastcancer.net

Publisher	National Breast Cancer Centre
Free resources	Table of Contents, Abstracts, Articles
Pay resources	none

British Journal of Haematology
http://www.blackwell-science.com/products/journals/jnltitle.htm

Publisher	Blackwell Science
Free resources	Table of Contents
Pay resources	Abstracts, Articles

CA: A Cancer Journal for Clinicians
http://www.ca-journal.org

Publisher	American Cancer Society
Free resources	Table of Contents, Abstracts, Articles
Pay resources	None

Cancer and Metastasis Reviews
http://www.wkap.nl/journalhome.htm/0167-7659

Publisher	Kluwer
Free resources	Table of Contents
Pay resources	Abstracts, Articles

Cancer Causes and Controls
http://www.wkap.nl/journalhome.htm/0957-5243

Publisher	Kluwer
Free resources	Table of Contents
Pay resources	Abstracts, Articles

Cancer, Chemotherapy, and Pharmacology
http://link.springer.de/link/service/journals/00280/index.htm

Publisher	Springer–Verlag
Free resources	Table of Contents, Abstracts
Pay resources	Articles

Cancer Control
http://www.moffitt.usf.edu/pubs/ccj

Publisher	The Moffitt Cancer Center
Free resources	Table of Contents, Abstracts, Articles
Pay resources	None

Cancer Cytopathology
http://canceronline.wiley.com/cchome.html

Publisher	Wiley
Free resources	Table of Contents, Abstracts
Pay resources	Articles

Cancer Detection and Prevention

http://www.cancerprev.org

Publisher	International Society for Preventive Oncology
Free resources	Table of Contents, Abstracts
Pay resources	Articles

Cancer Epidemiolgy, Biomarkers, and Prevention

http://www.aacr.org/2000/2100/2130/2130.html

Publisher	American Association for Cancer Research
Free resources	Table of Contents, Abstracts
Pay resources	Articles

Cancer Genetics and Cytogenetics

http://www.elsevier.com

Publisher	Elsevier Science Inc.
Free resources	Table of Contents
Pay resources	Abstracts, Articles

Cancer Immunology Immunotherapy

http://link.springer.de/link/service/journals/00262/index.htm

Publisher	Springer–Verlag
Free resources	Table of Contents, Abstracts
Pay resources	Articles

Cancer Journal

http://www.tribunes.com/tribune/cancer-j.htm

Publisher	Association pour le Développement de la Communication Cancérologique
Free resources	Table of Contents, Abstracts, Articles
Pay resources	None

Cancer Online

http://www.acor.org

Publisher	American Cancer Society
Free resources	Table of Contents, Abstracts
Pay resources	Articles

Cancer Research

http://www.aacr.org/2000/2100/2110/2110.html

Publisher	American Association for Cancer Research
Free resources	Table of Contents, Abstracts
Pay resources	Articles

Cancer Treatment Reviews

http://journals.harcourt-international.com/wbs/ctr

Publisher	Academic Press
Free resources	Table of Contents, Abstracts
Pay resources	Articles

Cancer Weekly Plus

http://www.newsfile.com/x1c.htm

Publisher	C.W. Henderson
Free resources	Table of Contents, Abstracts
Pay resources	Articles

Carcinogenesis

http://carcin.oupjournals.org

Publisher	Oxford University Press
Free resources	Table of Contents, Abstracts
Pay resources	Articles

Cell Death and Differentiation

http://www.stockton-press.co.uk/cdd

Publisher	Stockton Press
Free resources	Table of Contents, Registration required to access Abstracts
Pay resources	Articles

Cell Growth and Differentiation

http://www.aacr.org/2000/2100/2120/2120.html

Publisher	The American Association for Cancer Research
Free resources	Table of Contents, Abstracts
Pay resources	Articles

Cellular Immunology
http://www.apnet.com/www/journal/ci.htm

Publisher   Academic Press

Free resources   Table of Contents, Abstracts

Pay resources   Articles

Chemotherapy
http://www.karger.ch/journals/che/che_jh.htm

Publisher   Karger

Free resources   Table of Contents, Abstracts

Pay resources   Articles

Clinical and Experimental Metastasis
http://www.wkap.nl/journalhome.htm/0262-0898

Publisher   Kluwer

Free resources   Table Of Contents

Pay resources   Abstracts, Articles

Clinical and Laboratory Haematology
http://www.blacksci.co.uk/~cgilib/jnlpage.bin?Journal=CLH&File=CLH&Page=aims

Publisher   Blackwell Science

Free resources   Table of Contents

Pay resources   Abstracts, Articles

Clinical Cancer Research
http://www.aacr.org/2000/2100/2140/2140.html

Publisher   American Association for Cancer Research

Free resources   Table of Contents, Abstracts

Pay resources   Articles

Critical Reviews in Oncology/Hematology
http://www.elsevier.com

Publisher   Elsevier Science Inc.

Free resources   Table of Contents

Pay resources   Abstracts, Articles

Current Issues in Transfusion Medicine
http://www.mdacc.tmc.edu:80/~citm

Publisher	The University of Texas M. D. Anderson Cancer Center
Free resources	Table of Contents, Abstracts, Articles
Pay resources	None

Current Opinions in Hematology
http://www.biomednet.com/cgi-bin/members1/shwtoc.pl?J:hem

Publisher	Lippincott, Williams, and Wilkins
Free resources	Table of Contents, Abstracts
Pay resources	Articles

Current Problems in Cancer
http://www1.mosby.com/scripts/om.dll/serve?action=home

Publisher	Mosby
Free resources	Table of Contents, Abstracts
Pay resources	Articles

Cytokine
http://www.academicpress.com/cytokine

Publisher	Academic Press
Free resources	Table of Contents, Abstracts
Pay resources	Articles

Developments in Supportive Cancer Care
http://www.meniscus.com/dscc/index.html

Publisher	Meniscus Limited
Free resources	Table of Contents, Abstracts
Pay resources	Articles

Doctor's Guide Haematology and Oncology News
http://www.pslgroup.com/dg/haematonews.htm

Publisher	P\S\L NuMedia
Free resources	Table of Contents, Abstracts, Articles
Pay resources	None

Drug Resistance Updates

http://www.churchillmed.com/Journals/DRU/jhome.html

Publisher	Churchill Livingstone
Free resources	Table of Contents
Pay resources	Abstracts, Articles

Electronic Journal of Oncology

http://ejo.univ-lyon1.fr

Publisher	Fédèration Nationale des Centres de Lutte Contre le Cancer
Free resources	Table of Contents, Articles, Abstracts
Pay resources	None

Endocrine-Related Cancer

http://journals.endocrinology.org/ERC/erc.htm

Publisher	Society for Endocrinology
Free resources	Table of Contents, Abstracts, Articles
Pay resources	None

Environmental and Molecular Mutagenesis

http://www3.interscience.wiley.com/cgi-bin/jtoc?ID=10009058

Publisher	Wiley
Free resources	Registration required; Table of Contents and Abstracts
Pay resources	Articles

Epidemiology

http://www.wwilkins.com/EDE/index.html

Publisher	Lippincott, Williams and Wilkins
Free resources	Table of Contents, Abstracts
Pay resources	Articles

European Journal of Cancer

http://www.elsevier.com

Publisher	Elsevier Science Inc.
Free resources	Table of Contents
Pay resources	Abstracts, Articles

European Journal of Cancer Care

http://www.blacksci.co.uk/~cgilib/jnlpage.bin?Journal=EJCC&File=EJCC&Page=aims

Publisher	Blackwell Science
Free resources	Table of Contents
Pay resources	Abstracts, Articles

European Journal of Surgical Oncology

http://journals.harcourt-international.com/wbs/jso

Publisher	W. B. Saunders
Free resources	Table of Contents, Abstracts
Pay resources	Articles

Experimental Cell Research

http://www.academicpress.com/ecr

Publisher	Academic Press
Free resources	Table of Contents, Abstracts
Pay resources	Articles

Frontiers

http://www.acs.ohio-state.edu/units/cancer/frontier.htm

Publisher	The Ohio State University
Free resources	Table of Contents, Abstracts, Articles
Pay resources	None

Gastric Cancer

http://link.springer.de/link/service/journals/10120/index.htm

Publisher	Springer–Verlag
Free resources	Table of Contents, Abstracts
Pay resources	Articles

Genes, Chromosomes, and Cancer

http://www.interscience.wiley.com/jpages/1045-2257

Publisher	Wiley
Free resources	Table of Contents, Abstracts
Pay resources	Articles

Gynecologic Oncology

http://www.apnet.com/www/journal/go.htm

Publisher	Academic Press
Free resources	Table of Contents, Abstracts
Pay resources	Articles

Haema

http://www.mednet.gr/eae/haema/top.htm

Publisher	Hellenic Society of Haematology
Free resources	Table of Contents, Abstracts, Articles
Pay resources	None

Haematologica

http://www.haematologica.it

Publisher	European Haematology Association
Free resources	Table of Contents, Abstracts
Pay resources	Articles

Haemophilia

http://www.blacksci.co.uk/~cgilib/jnlpage.bin?Journal=HAEM&File=HAEM&Page=aims

Publisher	Blackwell Science
Free resources	Table of Contents
Pay resources	Abstracts, Articles

Haemostasis

http://www.karger.com/journals/hae/hae_jh.htm

Publisher	Karger
Free resources	Table of Contents, Abstracts
Pay resources	Articles

Hematological Oncology

http://www3.interscience.wiley.com/cgi-bin/jtoc?ID=3182

Publisher	Wiley
Free resources	Registration required; Table of Contents and Abstracts
Pay resources	Articles

Hematology and Cell Therapy
http://link.springer.de/link/service/journals/00282/index.htm

Publisher	Springer–Verlag
Free resources	Table of Contents, Abstracts
Pay resources	Articles

Hematology Newspage
http://www.individual.com/browse/topic.shtml?level1=46610&level2=46618&level3=586

Publisher	News Edge
Free resources	Table of Contents, Abstracts, Articles
Pay resources	None

Hemoglobin
http://www.dekker.com/e/p.pl/0363-0269

Publisher	Marcel Dekker Inc
Free resources	Table of Contents, Abstracts
Pay resources	Articles

Hemotopathology and Molecular Hematology
http://www.dekker.com/e/p.pl/1082-8893

Publisher	Marcel Dekker Inc
Free resources	Table of Contents, Abstracts
Pay resources	Articles

Highlights in Oncology Practice
http://www.meniscus.com/hl/index.html

Publisher	Meniscus
Free resources	Table of Contents, Abstracts, Articles
Pay resources	None

Immunohematology
http://www.redcross.org/biomed/pubs/immuno/index.html

Publisher	American Red Cross
Free resources	Table of Contents, Abstracts
Pay resources	Articles

Infusion Therapy and Transfusion Medicine
http://www.karger.com/journals/iut/iut_jh.htm

Publisher	Karger
Free resources	Table of Contents, Abstracts
Pay resources	Articles

International Journal of Cancer
http://www.interscience.wiley.com/jpages/0020-7136

Publisher	Wiley
Free resources	Registration required; Table of Contents and Abstracts
Pay resources	Articles

International Journal of Gynecological Cancer
http://www.blackwell-science.com/products/journals/jnltitle.htm

Publisher	Blackwell Science
Free resources	Table of Contents
Pay resources	Abstracts, Articles

International Journal of Radiation Oncology
http://www.elsevier.com

Publisher	Elsevier Science Inc.
Free resources	Table of Contents
Pay resources	Abstracts, Articles

Invasion and Metastasis
http://www.karger.ch/journals/iam/iam_jh.htm

Publisher	Karger
Free resources	Table of Contents, Abstracts
Pay resources	Articles

Investigational New Drugs
http://www.wkap.nl/journalhome.htm/0167-6997

Publisher	Kluwer
Free resources	Table of Contents
Pay resources	Abstracts, Articles

Japanese Journal of Cancer Research

http://www.bcasj.or.jp/jjcr/index.htm

Publisher	Japanese Cancer Association
Free resources	Table of Contents, Abstracts, Articles
Pay resources	None

Japanese Journal of Clinical Oncology

http://wwwinfo.ncc.go.jp/jjco/index.html

Publisher	Oxford University Press
Free resources	Table of Contents, Abstracts, Articles
Pay resources	None

Journal of Cancer Research and Clinical Oncology

http://link.springer.de/link/service/journals/00432/index.htm

Publisher	Springer–Verlag
Free resources	Table of Contents, Abstracts
Pay resources	Articles

Journal of Clinical Apheresis

http://www.interscience.wiley.com/jpages/0733-2459

Publisher	Wiley
Free resources	Registration required; Table of Contents and Abstracts
Pay resources	Articles

Journal of Clinical Oncology

http://www.jco.org

Publisher	American Society of Clinical Oncology
Free resources	Table of Contents, Abstracts, Articles
Pay resources	None

Journal of Neuro-Oncology

http://www.wkap.nl/journalhome.htm/0167-594X

Publisher	Kluwer
Free resources	Table of Contents
Pay resources	Abstracts, Articles

Journal of Pain and Symptom Management
http://www.elsevier.com

Publisher	Elsevier Science Inc.
Free resources	Table of Contents
Pay resources	Abstracts, Articles

Journal of Surgical Oncology
http://www3.interscience.wiley.com/cgi-bin/jtoc?ID=31873

Publisher	Wiley
Free resources	Registration required; Table of Contents and Abstracts
Pay resources	Articles

Journal of the National Cancer Institute Online
http://www3.oup.co.uk/jnls/list/jnci/contents

Publisher	Oxford University Press
Free resources	Table of Contents, Abstracts
Pay resources	Articles

Journal of Thrombosis and Thrombolysis
http://www.wkap.nl/journalhome.htm/0929-5305

Publisher	Kluwer
Free resources	Table Of Contents
Pay resources	Abstracts, Articles

Leukemia
http://www.stockton-press.co.uk/leu

Publisher	Stockton Press
Free resources	Table of Contents
Pay resources	Abstracts, Articles

Leukemia Research
http://www.elsevier.com

Publisher	Elsevier Science Inc.
Free resources	Table of Contents
Pay resources	Abstracts, Articles

Lung Cancer
http://www.elsevier.com

Publisher	Elsevier Science Inc.
Free resources	Table of Contents
Pay resources	Abstracts, Articles

M. D. Anderson Oncology
http://www.mdacc.tmc.edu:80/~oncolog

Publisher	The University of Texas M. D. Anderson Cancer Center
Free resources	Table of Contents, Abstracts, Articles
Pay resources	None

Medical and Pediatric Oncology
http://www3.interscience.wiley.com/cgi-bin/jtoc?ID=32390

Publisher	Wiley
Free resources	Registration required; Table of Contents and Abstracts
Pay resources	Articles

Medical Oncology
http://www.stockton-press.co.uk/mo

Publisher	Stockton Press
Free resources	Table of Contents, Abstracts
Pay resources	Articles

Medscape Oncology
http://oncology.medscape.com/Medscape/oncology/journal/public/onc.journal.html

Publisher	Medscape
Free resources	Table of Contents, Abstracts, Articles
Pay resources	None

Medscape Oncology Issues
http://www.medscape.com/ACCC/OncIssues/public/journal.OncIssues.html

Publisher	Medscape
Free resources	Table of Contents, Abstracts, Articles
Pay resources	None

Molecular Carcinogenesis

http://www.interscience.wiley.com/jpages/0899-1987

Publisher	Wiley
Free resources	Registration required; Table of Contents and Abstracts
Pay resources	Articles

Mutagenesis

http://mutage.oupjournals.org

Publisher	Oxford University Press
Free resources	Table of Contents, Abstracts
Pay resources	Articles

Myeloma Today

http://myeloma.org/MyelomaToday.html

Publisher	International Myeloma Foundation
Free resources	Table of Contents, Abstracts
Pay resources	Articles

Neoplasia

http://www.neoplasia.org/contents.html

Publisher	Stockton Press
Free resources	Table of Contents, Abstracts
Pay resources	Articles

New Perspectives in Cancer Diagnosis and Treatment

http://www.meniscus.com/np/index.html

Publisher	Meniscus
Free resources	Table of Contents, Abstracts, Articles
Pay resources	None

Oncogene

http://www.stockton-press.co.uk/onc

Publisher	Stockton Press
Free resources	Table of Contents, Registration required to access Abstracts
Pay resources	Articles

OncoLink: Cancer News

http://www.oncolink.upenn.edu/cancer_news

Publisher	University of Pennsylvania
Free resources	Table of Contents, Abstracts, Articles
Pay resources	None

OncoLink: CancerLit Information

http://www.oncolink.upenn.edu/cancernet

Publisher	National Cancer Institute
Free resources	Table of Contents, Abstracts
Pay resources	Articles

Oncology

http://www.karger.ch/journals/ocl/ocl_jh.htm

Publisher	Karger
Free resources	Table of Contents, Abstracts
Pay resources	Articles

Oncology Issues

http://gort.ucsd.edu/newjour/o/msg02317.html

Publisher	Medscape
Free resources	Table of Contents, Abstracts, Articles
Pay resources	None

Oral Oncology

http://www.elsevier.nl/inca/publications/store/1/0/5/index.htt

Publisher	Elsevier Science Inc.
Free resources	Table of Contents
Pay resources	Abstracts, Articles

Ovarian Cancer Research Notebook

http://www.slip.net/~mcdavis/ovarian.html

Publisher	National Ovarian Cancer Association
Free resources	Table of Contents, Abstracts, Articles
Pay resources	None

Pain

http://www.elsevier.com

Publisher	Elsevier Science Inc.
Free resources	Table of Contents
Pay resources	Abstracts, Articles

Pathology Oncology Research

http://journals.harcourt-international.com/wbs/por.htm#online

Publisher	Arányi Lajos Foundation, W. B. Saunders
Free resources	Table of Contents, Abstracts
Pay resources	Articles

Prostate Cancer

http://www.stockton-press.co.uk/pcan/contents.html

Publisher	Stockton Press
Free resources	Table of Contents, Registration required to access Abstracts
Pay resources	Articles

Psycho-Oncology

http://www3.interscience.wiley.com/cgi-bin/jtoc?ID=5807

Publisher	Wiley
Free resources	Registration required; Table of Contents and Abstracts
Pay resources	Articles

Radiation and Environmental Biophysics

http://link.springer-ny.com/link/service/journals/00411/tocs.htm

Publisher	Springer–Verlag
Free resources	Table of Contents, Abstracts
Pay resources	Articles

Radiation Oncology Investigations

http://www3.interscience.wiley.com/cgi-bin/jtoc?ID=38729

Publisher	Wiley
Free resources	Registration required; Table of Contents and Abstracts
Pay resources	Articles

Radiotherapy & Oncology

http://www.elsevier.com

Publisher	Elsevier Science Inc.
Free resources	Table of Contents
Pay resources	Abstracts, Articles

Reviews of Cancer Online

http://www1.elsevier.com/journals/roco/Menu.html

Publisher	Elsevier
Free resources	Table of Contents
Pay resources	Abstracts, Articles

Sarcoma

http://www.tandf.co.uk/journals/carfax/1357714X.html

Publisher	Carfax
Free resources	Table of Contents
Pay resources	Abstracts, Articles

Seminars in Cancer Biology

http://www.academicpress.com/semcancer

Publisher	Academic Press
Free resources	Table of Contents, Abstracts
Pay resources	Articles

Seminars in Radiation Oncology

http://www.wbsaunders.com/SemRadOnc

Publisher	W.B.Saunders
Free resources	Table of Contents, Abstracts
Pay resources	Articles

Seminars in Surgical Oncology

http://www3.interscience.wiley.com/cgi-bin/jtoc?ID=39350

Publisher	Wiley
Free resources	Registration required; Table of Contents and Abstracts
Pay resources	Articles

Supportive Care in Cancer

http://link.springer.de/link/service/journals/00520

Publisher	Springer–Verlag
Free resources	Table of Contents, Abstracts
Pay resources	Articles

Transfusion Medicine

http://www.blacksci.co.uk/~cgilib/jnlpage.bin?Journal=TRANS&File=TRANS&Page=aims

Publisher	Blackwell Science
Free resources	Table of Contents
Pay resources	Abstracts, Articles

Tumor Biology

http://www.karger.ch/journals/tbi/tbi_jh.htm

Publisher	Karger
Free resources	Table of Contents, Abstracts
Pay resources	Articles

Tumor Targeting

http://www.stockton-press.co.uk/tt

Publisher	Stockton Press
Free resources	Table of Contents, Registration required to access Abstracts
Pay resources	Articles

Tumori-Experimental and Clinical Oncology

http://www.cilea.it/tumori

Publisher	Il Pensiero Scientifico Editore
Free resources	Table of Contents, Abstracts
Pay resources	Articles

Urologic Oncology

http://www.elsevier.com

Publisher	Elsevier Science Inc.
Free resources	Table of Contents
Pay resources	Abstracts, Articles

Vox Sanguinis

http://www.karger.com/journals/vox/vox_jh.htm

Publisher	Karger
Free resources	Table of Contents, Abstracts
Pay resources	Articles

3.3 Books on Oncology and Hematology Published in 1999

Introduction

The following listing contains books published during the past 12 months in the fields of Oncology and Hematology. We have categorized books under major topics, although many of the books contain material that extends beyond the highlighted subject. All of these books may be purchased through Amazon at the URL: http://www.amazon.com.

AIDS/HIV

HIV Homecare Handbook (Jones and Bartlett Series in Oncology), Barbara Daigle, Kathryn E. Lasch, Christine McCluskey, Beverly Wancho. Jones & Bartlett Pub., 1999, ISBN: 0763707031.

Bladder Cancer

Advances in Bladder Research (Advances in Experimental Medicine and Biology, V. 462), Laurence S. Baskin (Editor), Simon W. Hayward (Editor). Plenum Pub. Corp., 1999, ISBN: 0306461129.

Bladder Cancer: Biology, Diagnosis, and Management (Oxford Medical Publications), Konstantinos N. Syrigos (Editor), Donald G. Skinner (Editor). Oxford University Press, 1999, ISBN: 0192630385.

Comprehensive Textbook of Genitourinary Oncology, Nicholas Vogelzang (Editor). Lippincott Williams & Wilkins Publishers, 1999, ISBN: 0683306456.

Neurology of Bladder, Bowel and Sexual Dysfunction (Blue Books of Practical Neurology, 23), Clare J. Fowler (Editor). Butterworth–Heinemann, 1999, ISBN: 0750699590.

Renal, Bladder and Prostate Cancer: An Update, Fritz H. Schroder (Editor), K. H. Kurth (Editor), G. H. Mickisch (Editor). Parthenon Pub. Group, 1999, ISBN: 1850700818.

Breast Cancer

A Darker Ribbon: A Twentieth-Century Story of Breast Cancer, Women and Their Doctors, Ellen Leopold. Beacon Press, 1999, ISBN: 0632052422.

A Safe Place: A Journal for Women With Breast Cancer, Jennifer Pike. Crown Pub., 1999, ISBN: 0609603213.

A Step-By-Step Guide to Dealing With Your Breast Cancer: Revised and Updated, Rebecca Y. Robinson, Jeanne A. Petrek. Scribner, 1999, ISBN: 0684822644.

Atlas of Breast Imaging, Daniel B. Kopans. Springer–Verlag, 1999, ISBN: 0387986707.

Bosom Buddies: Learn, Laugh and Live Through Breast Cancer, Rosie O'Donnell, Deborah Axelrod, M.D., Tracy Chutorian Semier (Contributor). Lippincott–Raven Publishers, 1999, ISBN: 0781717205.

Breast Cancer, Daniel F. Roses (Editor). Lippincott, Williams & Wilkins, 1999, ISBN: 0683307703.

Breast Cancer: A Guide For Fellows, O. E. Silva (Editor). Nova Kroshka Books, 1999, ISBN: 156072322X.

Breast Cancer: A Patient Guide, 2nd Edition, Patricia J. Anderson, R.N., M.N.. Creative Health Services, 1999, ISBN: 1881915026.

Breast Cancer: Can You Prevent It?, James Lawson M.D., Amelia Lawson M.D.. W. B. Saunders Company, 1999, ISBN: 0443055815.

Breast Cancer: Molecular Genetics, Pathogenesis, and Therapeutics (Contemporary Cancer Research), Anne M. Bowcock (Editor). McGraw Hill Text, 1999, ISBN: 007470723X.

Breast Cancer: Molecular Genetics, Pathogenesis, and Therapeutics (Contemporary Cancer Research), Anne M. Bowcock (Editor). Humana Press, 1999, ISBN: 0896035603.

Breast Cancer: Sharing the Decision (Oxford Medical Publications), Anna M. Maslin (Editor), Trevor J. Powles (Editor). Oxford University Press, 1999, ISBN: 0192629670.

Breast Cancer: The Fight of Your Life, Robert P. Lenk. Little Brown & Company, 1999, ISBN: 0316051098.

Breast (Guides to Clinical Aspiration Biopsy), Tilde S. Kline, Irwin K. Kline, Lydia Pleotis Howell. Warner Books, 1999, ISBN: 0446676209.

Breast Pathology: Diagnosis by Needle-Core Biopsy, Paul Peter Rosen, D. David Dershaw, Laura Liberman. La Leche League Intl., 1999, ISBN: 0912500506.

Breast Ultrasound: A Systematic Approach to Technique and Image Interpretation, Christof Sohn, Jens-U. Blohmer, Ulrike M. Hamper. Lowell House, 1999, ISBN: 0737302496.

Cancer Sourcebook for Women (Health Reference Series), Edward J. Prucha (Editor). Thieme Medical Pub., 1999, ISBN: 0865777225.

Challenges in Breast Cancer, Ian S. Fentiman (Editor). Omnigraphics, Inc., 1999, ISBN: 0780802268.

Diseases of the Breast, Jay R. Harris (Editor). Beacon Press, 1999, ISBN: 0807065129.

Early Breast Cancer: From Screening of Multidisciplinary Management, M. W. E. Morgan (Editor), R. Warren (Editor), G. Querci Della Rovere (Editor). 1999, ISBN: 0781718392.

Endocrinology of Breast Cancer (Contemporary Endocrinology, Vol 11), Andrea Manni (Editor). Humana Press, 1999, ISBN: 0896035913.

Expert Consultations in Breast Cancer: Critical Pathways and Clinical Decision Making (Basic and Clinical Oncology, 17), William N. Hait (Editor), David A. August (Editor), Bruce G. Haffty (Editor). Marcel Dekker, 1999, ISBN: 0824719549.

Handbook of Breast Surgery, Adrian Shervington Ball, Peter M. Arnstein. Edward Arnold, 1999, ISBN: 0340741619.

Handbook of Chemotherapy for Gynecologic Cancers, Maurie Markman. Hunter House, 1999, ISBN: 0897932692.

History of Breast Cancer, Olson. Precept Press, 1999, ISBN: 0944496628.

Information Systems in Breast Cancer Detection, Melvyn Greberman (Editor). Free Press, 1999, ISBN: 0684828065.

Living on the Margins: Women Writers on Breast Cancer, Hilda Raz (Editor). Hogrefe & Huber Pub., 1999, ISBN: 0889370362.

Lymphatic Drainage of the Skin and Breast: Locating the Sentinel Nodes, Roger Uren, John Thompson, Robert Howman-Giles. Persea Books, 1999, ISBN: 0892552441.

Lymphedema: A Breast Cancer Patient's Guide to Prevention and Healing, Mark Rucker, Peter Bjarkman, Jeannie Burt, Gwen White, Judith R. Casley-Smith. Harwood Academic Pub., 1999, ISBN: 9057024101.

Mammographic Image Analysis: Computational Imaging and Vision (Computational Imaging and Vision, V. 14), Ralph Highnam, Michael Brady. Hunter House, 1999, ISBN: 089793265X.

My Mother's Breast; Daughters Face Their Mothers' Cancer, Laurie Tarkan. Marcel Dekker, 1999, ISBN: 0824719549.

Pathology of the Breast, Fattaneh A. Tavassoli. McGraw-Hill Professional Publishing, 1999, ISBN: 0838577040.

Prognostic Variables in Node-Negative and Node-Positive Breast Cancer, Giampietro Gasparini (Editor). Harvard Common Press, 1999, ISBN: 1558321527.

Radioguided Surgery, Eric D. Whitman (Editor), Douglas Scott Reintgen (Editor). Appleton & Lange, 1999, ISBN: 0838577040.

Rainbow of Hope; Seventy Women and Their Journey with Breast Cancer, Marie Eckess. R. G. Landes Company, 1999, ISBN: 1570595690.

Red Devil: To Hell With Cancer—And Back, Katherine Russell Rich. Kluwer Academic Pub., 1999, ISBN: 0792384474.

She Came to Live Out Loud: An Inspiring Family Journey Through Illness, Loss, and Grief, Myra MacPherson, Kenneth J. Doka (Introduction). Scribner, 1999, ISBN: 0684822644.

Speak the Language of Healing: A New Approach to Breast Cancer, Susan Kuner, Carol Orsborn, Robert Romanyshyn, Linda Quigley, Karen Leigh Stroup. Chronicle Books, 1999, ISBN: 0811822672.

Talking About Treatment: Recommendations for Breast Cancer Adjuvant Therapy (Oxford Studies in Sociolinguistics), Felicia D. Roberts. Conari Press, 1999, ISBN: 1573241687.

Tamoxifen and Breast Cancer, Michael W. DeGregorio, Valerie J. Wiebe. Oxford University Press, 1999, ISBN: 0195121910.

Tamoxifen for the Treatment and Prevention of Breast Cancer, V. Craig Jordan Ph.D., D.S.C. (Introduction), Nancy Brinker, V. Craig Ph.D, D.S.C.. Publisher Research & Representation, Inc., 1999, ISBN: 1891483005.

Tamoxifen: New Hope in the Fight Against Breast Cancer, John F. Kessler M.D., Greg A. Annussek. Citadel Press, 1999, ISBN: 0806521066.

The Artistry of Breast Reconstruction With Autologous Tissue, Stephen S. Kroll. Sumerel Enterprises, 1999, ISBN: 0967123607.

The Artistry of Breast Reconstruction With Autologous Tissue, Stephen S. Kroll. Springer–Verlag, 1999, ISBN: 0387986707.

The Breast Cancer Prevention Diet: The Powerful Foods, Supplements, and Drugs That Can Save Your Life, Robert Arnot M.D., Jim Arnosky. Humana Press, 1999, ISBN: 0896035603.

The Breast Sourcebook: Everything You Need to Know About Cancer Detection, Treatment, and Prevention, M. Sara Rosenthal. Lippincott–Raven Publishers, 1999, ISBN: 0397587902.

The Feisty Woman's Breast Cancer Book, Warren Grossman, Mary Kelsey, Elaine Ratner. Benedet Publishing, 1999, ISBN: 0963791729.

The Feisty Woman's Breast Cancer Book, Bruce Hyman, Cherry Pedrick, Elaine Ratner. Hunter House, 1999, ISBN: 0897932706.

Total Breast Health, Robin Keuncke. Parthenon Pub. Group, 1999, ISBN: 1850708266.

Traditional Chinese Medicine: A Woman's Guide to Healing from Breast Cancer, Nan Lu, Ellen Schaplowsky (Contributor). Kensington Pub. Corp. (Trd), 1999, ISBN: 1575664593.

Victory Through Breast Cancer, Glenda B. Sumerel. Wholecare, 1999, ISBN: 038081028X.

Woman to Woman: A Handbook for Women Newly Diagnosed With Breast Cancer, Hester Hill Schnipper, Joan Feinberg, Ph.D. Wholecare, 1999, ISBN: 0380809028.

Cancer Cell Biology

Basic Science of Cancer, Gary Kruh (Editor), Kenneth D. Tew (Editor). Current Medicine, 1999, ISBN: 1573401439.

Developmental Biology Protocols (Methods in Molecular Biology, 137), Rocky S. Tuan (Editor), Cecilia W. Lo (Editor). Humana Press, 1999, ISBN: 089603576X.

Electrically Mediated Delivery of Molecules to Cells (Methods in Molecular Medicine, 37), Mark J. Jaroszeski (Editor), Richard Heller (Editor), Richard Gilbert. Humana Press, 1999, ISBN: 0896036065.

Hematopoiesis and Gene Therapy (Blood Cell Biochemistry, 8), Leslie J. Fairbairn (Editor), Nydia G. Testa (Editor). Kluwer Academic Pub., 1999, ISBN: 0306459620.

Hematopoietic Cell Transplantation, E, Donnall Thomas (Editor), Karl G. Blume (Editor), Stephen J. Forman. Blackwell Science Inc., 1999, ISBN: 0632043717.

Hematopoietic Stem Cells: Biology and Transplantation (Annals of the New York Academy of Sciences, Vol. 872), Donald Orlic (Editor), Thomas A. Bock (Editor), Lothar Kanz (Editor). New York Academy of Sciences, 1999, ISBN: 157331188X.

Introduction to Tumor Biology (Surgical Oncology), I. De Wever (Editor). Leuven University Press, 1999, ISBN: 9061869501.

Natural Obsessions: Striving to Unlock the Deepest Secrets of the Cancer Cell, Natalie Angier, Laura Van Dam (Editor), Lewis Thomas. Mariner Books, 1999, ISBN: 0395924723.

One Renegade Cell: How Cancer Begins, Robert A. Weinberg. Basic Books, 1999, ISBN: 0465072763.

Perspectives on Biologically Based Cancer Risk Assessment (NATO Challenges of Modern Society, V. 23), Vincent James Cogliano (Editor), E. Georg Luebeck (Editor), Giova Zapponi. Plenum Pub. Corp., 1999, ISBN: 0306461080.

Primary Hematopoietic Cells (Human Cell Culture, V. 4), Manfred R. Koller (Editor), Bernhard Palsson (Editor), J. R. W. Masters. Kluwer Academic Pub., 1999, ISBN: 079235821X.

Clinical Oncology

Biophosphonates in Clinical Oncology: The Development in Pamidronate (Recent Results in Cancer Research, 149), B. Thurlimann (Editor). Springer–Verlag, 1999, ISBN: 3540636897.

Cancer Clinical Trials: Experimental Treatments & How They Can Help You (Patient-Centered Guides), Robert Finn, Linda Lamb (Editor). O'Reilly & Associates, 1999, ISBN: 1565925661.

Cancer Genetics for the Clinician, Gail L. Shaw (Editor). Plenum Pub. Corp., 1999, ISBN: 0306461943.

Cancer Screening: Theory and Practice (Basic and Clinical Oncology, 18), Barnett S. Kramer (Editor), John Kenneth Gohagan (Editor), P. C. Prorok. Natl. Cancer Center, 1999, ISBN: 082470200X.

Clinical Applications of Cytokines and Growth Factors (Developments in Oncology, No. 80), John R. Wingard (Editor), George D. Demetri (Editor). Kluwer Academic Pub., 1999, ISBN: 0792384865.

Clinical Oncology, Martin D. Abeloff (Editor). 1999, ISBN: 044307545X.

Clinical Radiation Oncology: Indications, Techniques, and Results, C. C. Wang (Editor). John Wiley & Son Ltd., 1999, ISBN: 0471238031.

Communication Disorders in Childhood Cancer, Bruce E. Murdoch. Whurr Pub. Ltd., 1999, ISBN: 1861561156.

Current Practice & Therapy in Surgical Oncology, J. Vetto. Lippincott–Raven Publishers, 1999, ISBN: 041207771X.

Fluorescence Probes in Oncology, Elli Kohen. Imperial College Press, 1999, ISBN: 1860941508.

Hepatocellular Carcinoma: Diagnosis, Investigation, and Management, Anthony S. Leong (Editor), C. T. Liew, J. W. Y. Lau. Edward Arnold, 1999, ISBN: 0340740965.

M. D. Anderson Approach to Surgical Oncology, Mark Roh. Quality Medical Pub.,1999, ISBN: 1576260143.

Manual of Clinical Oncology, Raphael E. Pollock. Wiley–Liss, 1999, ISBN: 0471238287.

Neurofibromatosis: Phenotype, Natural History, and Pathogenesis, J. M., Md Friedman, J. M. Friedman, M.D., Ph.D. (Editor), David H. Gutmann M.D., Ph.D. (Editor), Vincent M. Riccardi (Editor), Mia MacCollin (Editor). Johns Hopkins University Press, 1999, ISBN: 080186285X.

Regional Chemotherapy: Clinical Research and Practice (Current Clinical Oncology), Maurie Markman (Editor). Humana Press, 1999, ISBN: 0896037290.

The Sentinel Node in Surgical Oncology, M. R. S. Keshtgar (Editor), Waddingtom. W. A., S. R. Lakhani, P.J. Ell.. Springer–Verlag, 1999, ISBN: 3540651764.

The Unequal Burden of Cancer: An Assessment of NIH Research and Programs for Ethnic Minorities and the Medically Underserved, M. Alfred Haynes (Editor), Brian D. Smediey (Editor), Brian D. Smedley (Editor). National Academy Press, 1999, ISBN: 0309071542.

Understanding Cancer: A Scientific and Clinical Guide for the Lay Person, Peter A. Dervan. McFarland & Company, 1999, ISBN: 0786406283.

Vaccines for Human Papillomavirus Infection and Disease (Medical Intelligence Unit), Robert W. Tindle (Editor). R. G. Landes Company, 1999, ISBN: 1570595895.

WHO Laboratory Manual for the Examination of Human Semen and Sperm-Cervical Mucus Interaction, World Health Organization. Cambridge University Press (Short), 1999, ISBN: 0521645999.

Colon Cancer

Colon and Rectal Cancer: A Comprehensive Guide for Patients and Families, Lorraine Johnston. O'Reilly & Associates, 1999, ISBN: 1565926331.

Laparoscopic Colorectal Surgery (Protocols in General Surgery), Steven D. Wexner (Editor), Jonathan M. Sackier (Editor). Wiley–Liss, 1999, ISBN: 0471240303.

Recent Advances in Coloproctology, J. Beynon (Editor), Nicholas David Carr (Editor). 1999, ISBN: 1852331690.

The American Cancer Society: Colorectal Cancer, Bernard, Levin, M.D.. Random House (Paper), 1999, ISBN: 0679778136.

General Oncology

American Cancer Society: Women and Cancer: A Thorough and Compassionate Resource for Patients and Their Families, Carolyn D. Runowicz, M.D., Jeanne A. Petrek, M.D., Ted S. Gansler, M.D. Carolyn Runowitz, Jeanne Petrick. Villard Books, 1999, ISBN: 0679778144.

Cancer (Diseases and People), Steven I. Benowitz. Enslow Publishers, Inc., 1999, ISBN: 076601181X.

Cancer Facts: A Concise Oncology Text, James F. Bishop. Harwood Academic Pub., 1999, ISBN: 9057024705.

Cancer: Increasing Your Odds for Survival: A Resource Guide for Integrating Mainstream, Alternative and Complementary Therapies, David Bognar. Hunter House, 1999, ISBN: 089793248X.

Cancer Management: A Multidisciplinary Approach, Compilation. Research & Representation, Inc., 1999, ISBN: 1891483013.

Cancer Sourcebook (Health Reference Series), Edward J. Prucha (Editor). Omnigraphics, Inc., 1999, ISBN: 0780802276.

Cancer Symptom Management (Jones and Bartlett Series in Oncology), Connie Henke Yarbro (Editor), Margaret Hansen Frogge (Editor), Michelle Goodman. Jones & Bartlett Pub., 1999, ISBN: 076370864X.

Curing Cancer: The Story of Men and Women Unlocking the Secrets of Our Deadliest Illness, Michael Waldholz. Touchstone Books, 1999, ISBN: 0684848023.

Everything You Need to Know About Cancer (Need to Know Library), Francesca Massari. Rosen Publishing Group, 1999, ISBN: 0823931641.

Fatigue in Cancer: The Art and Science, Margaret Barton Burke, Maryl Lynne Winningham. Jones & Bartlett Pub., 1999, ISBN: 0763706302.

Hematology/Oncology Secrets (The Secrets Series), Marie E. Wood (Editor). Hanley & Belfus, 1999, ISBN: 1560533137.

Integrated Cancer Management: Surgery, Medical Oncology, and Radiation Oncology (Basic and Clinical Oncology, 20), Michael Torosian (Editor). Marcel Dekker, 1999, ISBN: 0824771958.

Now Breathe: A Journal of Life After a Cancer Diagnosis, Claudia Sternbach. Taylor Pub., 1999, ISBN: 0878332278.

Oncology: A Case-Based Manual, Paul Harnett (Editor), John Cartmill (Editor), Paul Glare (Editor). Oxford University Press, 1999, ISBN: 0192629786.

Oncology Nursing Review, Connie Henke Yarbro, Margaret Hansen Frogge, Michelle Goodman. Jones & Bartlett Pub., 1999, ISBN: 0763711268.

Study Guide for the Core Curriculum for Oncology Nursing, Claudette G. Varricchio. W B Saunders Company, 1999, ISBN: 0721671578.

The Cancer Dictionary, Roberta Altman, Michael J. Sarg, M.D.. Facts on File, Inc., 1999, ISBN: 0816039542.

Understanding Cancer: A Patient's Guide to Diagnosis, Prognosis, and Treatment, Norman C. Coleman, Ellen L. Stovall. Johns Hopkins University Press, 1999, ISBN: 0801860202.

Genetics

A Practical Guide to Human Cancer Genetics, Shirley V. Hodgson, Eamonn R. Maher. Cambridge University Press, 1999, ISBN: 0521649617.

Catalog of Human Cancer Genes: McKusick's Mendelian Inheritance in Man for Clinical and Research Oncologists (Onco-Mim), John J. Mulvihill, Kimberly V. Talley. Johns Hopkins University Press, 1999, ISBN: 0801847990.

Progress in Oncology (Progress in Anti-Cancer Chemotherapy), David Khayat (Editor), Gabriel N. Hortobagyi (Editor). Springer–Verlag, 1999, ISBN: 3540596666.

Gynecologic Oncology

Cancer Obstetrics and Gynecology, Edward L. Trimble (Editor), Cornelia Liu Trimble (Editor). Lippincott Williams & Wilkins Publishers, 1999, ISBN: 0781714109.

Laparoscopic Surgery in Gynecological Oncology, Denis Querleu (Editor), Joel M. Childers (Editor), D. Dargent (Editor). Blackwell Science Inc., 1999, ISBN: 0865426929.

Head and Neck

Diagnosis and Treatment of Cancer of the Glottis and Subglottis (Continuing Education Program (American Academy of Otolaryngology), Steven D. Schaefer, Joseph Leach. Lippincott Williams & Wilkins Publishers, 1999, ISBN: 1567720722.

Iowa Head and Neck Protocols: Surgery, Nursing, and Speech-Language Pathology, Henry T. Hoffman, M.D. (Editor), Gerry F. Funk, M.D. (Editor), Cind Dawson. Singular Pub. Group, 1999, ISBN: 0769300618.

Hematology

A Guide to Blood and Marrow Transplation, H. J. Deeg (Editor), G.L. Philips, G.V. Zant. Springer–Verlag, 1999, ISBN: 3540625402.

Blood Feuds: AIDS, Blood, and the Politics of Medical Disaster, Eric Feldman (Editor), Ronald Bayer (Editor). Oxford University Press, 1999, ISBN: 0195131606.

Clinical Hematology, A. Victor Hoffbrand. Mosby-Year Book, 1999, ISBN: 0723431159.

Clinical Management of Bleeding and Thrombosis, Edward R. Burns. 1999, ISBN: 086542036X.

Clinical Transfusion Medicine (Vademecum), Joseph Sweeney, Yvonne Rizk. Landes Bioscience, 1999, ISBN: 1570594945.

Critical Limb Ischemia, Alain Branchereau (Editor), Michael Jacobs (Editor), European Vascular cou. Futura Pub. Company, 1999, ISBN: 0879934123.

E-Z Abgeez: Arterial Blood Gases, Gregory L. Culver. Vantage Press, 1999, ISBN: 0533126975.

Exercise and Circulation in Health and Disease, Bengt Saltin (Editor). 1999, ISBN: 0880116323.

Haematology at a Glance, A. V. Hoffbrand, Atul Mehta. Blackwell Science Inc., 1999, ISBN: 0632047933.

Haematology (Biomedical Sciences Explained Series.), Chris Pallister. Butterworth–Heinemann, 1999, ISBN: 0750624574.

Hematology: Basic Principles and Practice, Ronald Hoffman (Editor), Edward J. Banz, Jr., Sanford J. Shattil (Editor). Churchill Livingstone, 1999, ISBN: 0443079544.

Hematology (Colour Guide; Picture Tests), Barbara J. Bain. Churchill Livingstone, 1999, ISBN: 0443059438.

Hematology/Oncology Secrets (The Secrets Series), Marie E. Wood (Editor). Hanley & Belfus, 1999, ISBN: 1560533137.

Hemostasis and Thrombosis Protocols (Methods in Molecular Medicine), David J. Perry (Editor), K. John Pasi (Editor). Humana Press, 1999, ISBN: 0896034194.

Hodgkin's Disease, Peter M. Mauch (Editor). Lippincott Williams & Wilkins Publishers, 1999, ISBN: 0781715024.

Human Blood Cells: Consequences of Genetic Polymorphisms and Variations, Mary-Jean King (Editor). World Scientific Pub. Company, 1999, ISBN: 9810239378.

Lipoproteins in Health and Disease, John Betteridge (Editor), D. R. Illingworth (Editor), J. Shepherd (Editor). Oxford University Press, 1999, ISBN: 0340552697.

Living With Haemophilia, Peter Jones. Oxford University Press, 1999, ISBN: 0192629611.

McQs for the Mrcp Part 1: Clinical Chemistry, Haematology, and Infectious Disease, David W. Galvani (Editor). Saunders College Pub., 1999, ISBN: 070202306X.

Platelet Protocols: Research and Clinical Laboratory Procedures, Melanie McCabe White, Lisa K. Jennings. Academic Press, 1999, ISBN: 0123842603.

Scientific Basis of Transfusion Medicine: Implications for Clinical Practice, Kenneth C. Anderson (Editor), Paul M. Ness (Editor). W B Saunders Company, 1999, ISBN: 0721676847.

Standard Haematology Practice/3, Keith Wood (Editor), British Committee for Standards in Haematology. Blackwell Science Inc., 1999, ISBN: 0632053224.

T-Cell Lymphoproliferative Disorders: Classification, Clinical and Laboratory Aspects (Advances in Blood Disorders, Vol 4), Estella Matutes. Harwood Academic Pub., 1999, ISBN: 9057023520.

Textbook of Malignant Haematology, Degos, Laurent Degos. Dunitz Martin Ltd., 1999, ISBN: 1853173223.

Vascular Disease: Molecular Biology and Gene Therapy Protocols (Methods in Molecular Medicine, 30), Andrew H. Baker (Editor). Humana Press, 1999, ISBN: 0896037312.

Imaging

Antibody Tumor Imaging (Nuclear Medicine Self-Study Program IV Nuclear Medicine Oncology, Unit 3), H. Abdel Nabi. Society of Nuclear Medicine, 1999, ISBN: 093200461X.

Molecular Imaging in Oncology: PET, MRI, and MRS, E. Edmund Kim, E. F. Jackson. Springer–Verlag, 1999, ISBN: 3540641017.

Leukemia

Childhood Leukemias, Ching-Hon Pui (Editor). Cambridge University Press (Short), 1999, ISBN: 0521581761.

Drug Resistance in Leukemia and Lymphoma III (Advances in Experimental Medicine and Biology, V. 457), G. J. L. Kaspers (Editor), R. Pieters (Editor). Plenum Press, 1999, ISBN: 0306460556.

Leukemia and Related Disorders, J. A. Whittaker (Editor), J. A. Holmes (Editor). Blackwell Science Inc., 1999, ISBN: 0865426074.

Leukemia Diagnosis, Barbara J. Bain. Blackwell Science Inc., 1999, ISBN: 0632051655.

Living With Leukemia (Living With Series). Raintree/Steck Vaughn,1999, ISBN: 0817257438.

Methods in Hematologic Malignancies (Methods in Molecular Medicine), Guy B. Faguet (Editor). Humana Press, 1999, ISBN: 0896035433.

Surviving Leukemia: Practical Guide, Robert Patenaude. Firefly Books, 1999, ISBN: 1552093549.

Understanding Leukemia and Related Cancers, Mughal. Blackwell Science Inc., 1999, ISBN: 0632053461.

Liver Cancer

Ascites and Renal Dysfunction in Liver Disease: Pathogenesis, Diagnosis, and Treatment, Vincente Arroyo (Editor), Pere Gines (Editor), Juan Rodes (Editor), Schrier. Blackwell Science Inc., 1999, ISBN: 0632043423.

Biopsy Interpretation of the Liver (Biopsy Interpretation Series), Stephen A. Geller, Lidija, M. Petrovic. Raven Press, 1999, ISBN: 039751784X.

Hepatotoxicity: The Adverse Effects of Drugs and Other Chemicals on the Liver, Hyman J. Zimmerman. Lippincott–Raven Publishers, 1999, ISBN: 0781719526.

Liver Disorders in Childhood, Alex P. Mowat. Butterworth–Heinemann, 1999, ISBN: 0750642009.

Liver Malignancies: Diagnostic and Interventional Radiology (Medical Radiology), C. Bartolozzi (Editor), R. Lencioni (Editor). 1999, ISBN: 3540647562.

Malignant Liver Tumors: Current and Emerging Therapies, Pierre-Alain Clavien (Editor). Blackwell Science Inc., 1999, ISBN: 0632044063.

The Function and Regulation of Nucleotide Pyrophosphates/Phosphodiesterases in Rat Liver, Christina Stefan-Bodea. Leuven University Press, 1999, ISBN: 9061869471.

Lung Cancer

Analysis of Panels and Limited Dependent Variable Models, Cheng Hsiao (Editor), Kajal Lahiri (Editor), Lung-Fei Lee, Hashem Pesaran. Cambridge University Press (Short), 1999, ISBN: 0521631696.

Histological Typing of Lung and Pleural Tumours (International Histological Classification of Tumours, No. 1, 1999), William D. Travis (Editor), L. H. Sobin (Editor). Springer–Verlag, 1999, ISBN: 3540652191.

Management of Heart & Lung Transplant Patients, Schofield (Editor), Corris, P. M. Schofield. B M J Books, 1999, ISBN: 0727913654.

Molecular Biology of the Lung: Asthma and Cancer (Respiratory Pharmacology and Pharmacotheraphy, Vol. 2), R. A. Stockley. Birkhauser, 1999, ISBN: 3764359684.

Myths & Facts About Lung Cancer, John C. Ruckdeschel. P. R. R., Incorporated, 1999, ISBN: 1891483048.

Occupational Lung Disease: An International Perspective, John R. Parker (Editor), Daniel E. Banks (Editor). Lippincott–Raven Publishers, 1999, ISBN: 0412736306.

Progress and Perspectives in the Treatment of Lung Cancer (Medical Radiology), P. Van Houtte (Editor), J. Klastersky (Editor), P. Rocmans (Editor). Springer–Verlag, 1999, ISBN: 3540625488.

Pulmonary Disorders (Managing Major Diseases). Mosby-Year Book, 1999, ISBN: 0323008550.

Lymphoma

Drug Resistance in Leukemia and Lymphoma III (Advances in Experimental Medicine and Biology, V. 457), G. J. L. Kaspers (Editor), R. Pieters (Editor). Plenum Press, 1999, ISBN: 0306460556.

Non-Hodgkin's Lymphomas: Making Sense of Diagnosis, Treatment, and Options, Lorraine Johnston, Linda Lamb (Editor). O'Reilly & Associates, 1999, ISBN: 1565924444.

Melanoma

Coping With Melanoma and Other Skin Cancers (Coping), Wendy Long. Rosen Publishing Group, 1999, ISBN: 0823928527.

Neuro-Oncology

Controversies in Neuro-Oncology (Frontiers of Radiation Therapy and Oncology, Vol. 33), International Symposium on Special Aspects of Radiotherapy 1998 berli. S. Karger Publishing, 1999, ISBN: 3805568347.

Nutrition

Oncology Nutrition Handbook, Karen Kulakowski, Laura Molseed. Skidmore-Roth Pub., 1999, ISBN: 1569300631.

Other Cancers

Disorders of the Spleen (Major Problems in Pathology, Vol 38), Richard S. Neiman, Attillo Orazi, Barbara C. d Wolf. W B Saunders Company, 1999, ISBN: 0721675514.

Environmental Cancer: A Political Disease?, S. Robert Lichter, Stanley Rothman. Yale University Press, 1999, ISBN: 0300076347.

Medical and Surgical Management of Adrenal Diseases, Joseph C. Cerny (Editor), Jay Knipstein (Illustrator). Lippincott, Williams & Wilkins, 1999, ISBN: 0683303449.

Multiple Primary Cancers, Alfred I. Neugut (Editor), Eliezer Robinson (Editor), Anna T. Meadows. Lippincott Williams & Wilkins Publishers, 1999, ISBN: 0683301241.

Textbook of Uncommon Cancer, D. Raghavan (Editor), M. L. Brecher (Editor), D. H. Johnson (Editor). John Wiley & Son Ltd., 1999, ISBN: 0471929212.

Ovarian Cancer

A Feather in My Wig: Ovarian Cancer Cured: Twelve Years and Going Strong!, Barbara Van Billiard. Peter Randall Publisher, 1999, ISBN: 0914339699.

Histological Typing of Ovarian Tumours (Histological Classification of Tumours), Robert E. Scully, L. H. Sobin, S. F. Histological Typing of Serov. Springer–Verlag, 1999, ISBN: 3540640592.

No Time to Die: Living With Ovarian Cancer, Liz Tilberis, Aimee Lee Ball (Contributor). Avon, 1999, ISBN: 0380732262.

Pancreatic Disease

Cell and Molecular Biology of Pancreatic Carcinoma: Recent Developments in Research and Experimental Therapy (Annals of the New York Academy of Science, J.-Matthias Lohr (Editor). New York Academy of Sciences, 1999, ISBN: 1573312207.

Pancreatic Disease: State of the Art and Future Aspects of Research, Paul Georg Lankisch (Editor), E. P. Dimagno (Editor). 1999, ISBN: 3540653570.

Radiology of the Pancreas (Medical Radiology), A. L. Baert (Editor), G. Delorme (Editor), L. Van Hoe (Editor). Springer–Verlag, 1999, ISBN: 3540634797.

Pediatric Oncology

Challenges & Opportunities in Pediatric Oncology (Annals of the New York Academy of Sciences, Vol 824), Frederick F. Holmes (Editor), John J. Kepes (Editor), Tribhawan S. Vats. New York Academy of Sciences, 1999, ISBN: 0801862116.

Childhood Leukemias, Ching-Hon Pui (Editor). Cambridge University Press (Short), 1999, ISBN: 0521581761.

Conquering Kids Cancer: Triumphs and Tragedies of a Childrens Cancer Doctor, Kenneth H. Lazarus. Emerald Ink Pub., 1999, ISBN: 1885373228.

International Incidence of Childhood Cancer (Iarc Scientific Publications, 144), D. M. Parkin (Editor), E. Kramarova (Editor), G. J. Draper (Editor), Masuyer. Oxford University Press, 1999, ISBN: 9283221443.

Pediatric Cancer Sourcebook: Basic Consumer Health Information About Leukemias, Brain Tumors, Sarcomas (Health Reference Series), Edward J. Prucha (Editor). Omnigraphics, Inc., 1999, ISBN: 0780802454.

Pediatric Radiation Oncology, Edward C. Halperin, Louis S. Constine, Nancy J. Tarbell, Larry Kun. Lippincott–Raven Publishers, 1999, ISBN: 0781715008.

Speech and Language Disorders in Childhood Cancer, Bruce Murdoch. Whurr Publishers, 1999, ISBN: 1861561156.

Supportive Care of Children With Cancer: Current Therapy and Guidelines from the Children's Cancer Group, Arthur R. Ablin (Editor), W. Archie Bleyer. Johns Hopkins University Press, 1999, ISBN: 0801857260.

Prevention

Dr. Gaynor's Cancer Prevention Program, Mitchell L. Gaynor, Jerry Hickey, William Fryer (Contributor), Gerard P. Hickey. Kensington Pub. Corp. (Trd), 1999, ISBN: 1575663821.

Familial Cancer and Prevention: Molecular Epidemiology: A New Strategy Toward Cancer Control, Joji Utsunomiya (Editor), John J. Mulvihill (Editor), Walter Weber (Editor). Wiley–Liss, 1999, ISBN: 0471249378.

Preventing and Controlling Cancer in North America: A Cross-Cultural Perspective, Diane Weiner (Editor). Praeger Pub. Text, 1999, ISBN: 027596180X.

Stopping Cancer Before It Starts: The American Institute for Cancer Research's Program for Cancer Prevention, American Institute for Cancer Research (Editor). Golden Books Pub. Company (Adult), 1999, ISBN: 1582380007.

Prostate Cancer

ABC's of Advanced Prostate Cancer, Mark A. Moyad, Kenneth J. Pienta. Sleeping Bear Press, 1999, ISBN: 1886947686.

ABC's of Nutrition and Supplements for Prostate Cancer, Mark A. Moyad. Sleeping Bear Press, 1999, ISBN: 1886947694.

Advances in the Radiotherapeutic Management of Adenocarcinoma of the Prostate, A. V. D'Amico, G. E. H. Hanks. Edward Arnold, 1999, ISBN: 0340741104.

Best Options for Treating and Diagnosing Prostate Cancer: Based on Research, Clinical Trials, and Scientific and Investigational Studies, James Lewis. Health Education Literary Pub., 1999, ISBN: 1883257042.

Management of Prostate Cancer (Current Clinical Urology), Eric A. Klein (Editor). Humana Press, 1999, ISBN: 0896037975.

Men's Cancers: How to Prevent Them, How to Treat Them, How to Beat Them, Pamela J. Haylock (Editor). Hunter House, 1999, ISBN: 0897932676.

Prostate Cancer: A Doctor's Personal Triumph, Robert Fine, Saralee Fine. P. S. Eriksson, 1999, ISBN: 0839768087.

Prostate & Cancer: A Family Guide to Diagnosis, Treatment & Survival, Sheldon Marks, M.D., Judd Moul. Fisher Books, 1999, ISBN: 1555612067.

Prostate Cancer: Portraits of Empowerment, Nadine Jelsing (Editor), Paul Georgeades (Editor). Westview Press, 1999, ISBN: 0813366577.

Renal, Bladder and Prostate Cancer: An Update, Fritz H. Schroder (Editor), K. H. Kurth (Editor), G. H. Mickisch (Editor). Parthenon Pub. Group, 1999, ISBN: 1850700818.

The American Cancer Society: Prostate Cancer, revised edition, David G. Bostwick M.D., Gregory T. MacLennan M.D., Thayne R. Larson. Villard Books, 1999, ISBN: 0375753192.

The Herbal Remedy for Prostate Cancer: Based on a Clinical Trial, an Investigational Study, and a Survey of an International Support Group, James Lewis. Health Education Literary Pub., 1999, ISBN: 1883257026.

Under the Fig Leaf: A Comprehensive Guide to the Care and Maintenance of the Penis, Prostate and Related Organs, Angelo S. Paola. Health Information Press, 1999, ISBN: 1885987153.

Understanding Prostate Disease, Charles B. Inlander. Macmillan General Reference, 1999, ISBN: 002862436X.

Psychosocial

Cancer and Emotion: A Practical Guide to Psycho-Oncology, Jennifer Barracloug. John Wiley & Son Ltd., 1999, ISBN: 047198597X.

Cutting Edge Medicine and Liaison Psychiatry: Psychiatric Problems of Organ Transplantation, Cancer, HIV/AIDS, and Genetic Therapy, Japan, Tokyo Institute of Psychiatry International Symposium 1998 Tokyo. Elsevier Science Ltd., 1999, ISBN: 0444502203.

Experiencing Cancer: Quality of Life in Treatment (Facing Death), Kirsten Costain Schou, Jenny Hewison. Open University Press, 1999, ISBN: 0335198929.

Radiology

Modern Technology of Radiation Oncology, J. Van Dyk (Editor). Medical Physics Pub. Corp., 1999, ISBN: 0944838227.

Radiation Injury (Frontiers of Radiation Therapy and Oncology, Vol. 32), John San Francisco Cancer Symposium 1997 Meyer. S. Karger Publishing, 1999, ISBN: 3805568029.

Shielding Techniques for Radiation Oncology Facilities, Patton H. McGinley. Medical Physics Pub. Corp., 1999, ISBN: 0944838820.

Stedman's Radiology & Oncology Words, Lippincott. Williams & Wilkins, 1999, ISBN: 0683307789.

Research

Advances in Cancer Research (Advances in Cancer Research, Vol 76), George F. Vande Woude, George Klein. Academic Press, 1999, ISBN: 0120066769.

Animal Models of Cancer Predisposition Syndromes (Progress in Experimental Tumor Research, Vol. 35), Hiroshi Hiai (Editor), Okio Hino (Editor). S. Karger Publishing, 1999, ISBN: 3805567197.

Skin Cancer

Atlas of Cancer of the Skin, Gunter Burg (Editor). Churchill Livingstone, 1999, ISBN: 0443058210.

The Skin Cancer Answer, Willian I. Lane, Linda Comac. Avery Pub. Group, 1999, ISBN: 0895298651.

Stomach Cancer

Multimodality Therapy for Gastric Cancer, Toshifusa Nakajima (Editor), T. Yamaguchi (Editor). 1999, ISBN: 4431702555.

Supportive Care

Palliative Care and Rehabilitation of Cancer Patients (Cancer Treatment and Research, V. 100), Charles F. Von Gunten. Kluwer Academic Pub., 1999, ISBN: 079238525X.

Palliative Medicine: Symptomatic and Supportive Care for Patients With Advanced Cancer and AIDS, Roger Woodruff. Oxford University Press, 1999, ISBN: 0195506472.

Supportive Care in Cancer: A Handbook for Oncologists (Basic and Clinical Oncology, 19), J. Klastersky (Editor), Stephen C. Schimpff (Editor), Hansjorg Senn (Editor). Marcel Dekker, 1999, ISBN: 0824719980.

Surgery

Organ Preservation Surgery of the Larynx, Gregory S. Weinstein (Editor), Ollivier Laccourreye, Daniel Brasnu. Singular Pub. Group, 1999, ISBN: 1565939034.

Therapies and Treatments

Apoptosis and Cancer Chemotherapy (Cancer Drug Discovery and Development), John A. Hickman (Editor), Caroline Dive (Editor). Humana Press, 1999, ISBN: 0896037436.

Cancer and the Search for Selective Biochemical Inhibitors, E. J. Hoffman. CRC Press, 1999, ISBN: 0849391180.

Cancer Salves: A Botanical Approach to Treatment, Ingrid Naiman. North Atlantic Books, 1999, ISBN: 1556432704.

Chemokines and Cancer (Contemporary Cancer Research), Barrett Rollins (Editor). Humana Press, 1999, ISBN: 089603562X.

Companion Handbook to the Chemotherapy Source Book, Michael C. Perry (Editor). Lippincott, Williams & Wilkins, 1999, ISBN: 0683302485.

Current Controversies in Bone Marrow Transplantation (Current Clinical Oncology), Brian J. Bolwell (Editor). Humana Press, 1999, ISBN: 0896037827.

Current Therapy in Cancer, John F. Foley (Editor), Julie M. Vose (Editor), James O. Armitage (Editor). W B Saunders Company, 1999, ISBN: 0721675484.

Cytotoxic Drug Resistance Mechanisms (Methods in Molecular Medicine, No. 28), Robert Brown (Editor), Uta Boger-Brown (Editor). Humana Press, 1999, ISBN: 0896036030.

Endosurgery for Cancer (Vademecum), Ricardo Victor Cohen (Editor). Landes Bioscience, 1999, ISBN: 1570595259.

Evaluating Alternative Cancer Therapies: A Guide to the Science and Politics of an Emerging Medical Field, David J. Hess (Editor). Rutgers University Press, 1999, ISBN: 0813525942.

Ex Vivo Cell Therapy, Klaus Schindhelm (Editor), Robert Nordon (Editor). Academic Press, 1999, ISBN: 0126249601.

Gene Therapy of Cancer: Methods and Protocols (Methods in Molecular Medicine, 35), Wolfgang Walther (Editor), Ulrike Stein (Editor). Humana Press, 1999, ISBN: 0896037142.

Handbook of Cancer Chemotherapy, Roland T. Skeel (Editor). Lippincott Williams & Wilkins Publishers, 1999, ISBN: 0781716179.

Herbal Medicine, Healing, and Cancer: A Comprehensive Program for Prevention and Treatment, Donald Yance, Arlene Valentine (Contributor). Keats Pub., 1999, ISBN: 0879839686.

High Dose Cancer Therapy: Pharmacology, Hematopoietins, Stem Cells, James O. Armitage (Editor), Karen Antman (Editor). Lippincott, Williams & Wilkins, 1999, ISBN: 0683306545.

Intraoperative Irradiation: Techniques and Results (Current Clinical Oncology, 1), Leonard L. Gunderson (Editor), Christopher G. Willet (Editor), Harrison. Humana Press, 1999, ISBN: 0896035239.

Levitt and Tapley's Technological Basis of Radiation Therapy: Clinical Applications, Seymour H. Levitt (Editor), Roger A. Potish (Editor), Faiz M. Kahn (Editor). Lippincott, Williams & Wilkins, 1999, ISBN: 0683301233.

Marrow Protection: Transduction of Hematopoietic Cells with Drug Resistance Genes, Joseph R. Bertino (Editor). S. Karger Publishing, 1999, ISBN: 3805568282.

Medicine Hands: Massage Therapy for People With Cancer, Gayle MacDonald. Findhorn Press, 1999, ISBN: 1899171770.

Metallopharmaceuticals: DNA Interactions (Topics in Biological Inorganic Chemistry), E. Alessio (Editor), M. J. Clarke (Editor), P. J. Sadler (Editor). Springer–Verlag, 1999, ISBN: 3540648895.

Multiple Drug Resistance in Cancer 2: Molecular, Cellular and Clinical Aspects, M. Clynes (Editor). Kluwer Academic Pub., 1999, ISBN: 0792352726.

Nuclear Oncology, C. Aktolun (Editor), W. Newlon Tauxe (Editor). Springer–Verlag, 1999, ISBN: 3540647600.

Oncologic Therapies, E. E. Vokes (Editor), H. M. Golomb (Editor). Springer–Verlag, 1999, ISBN: 3540640525.

Patient Positioning and Immobilization in Radiation Oncology, Gunilla Carleson Bentel. McGraw Hill Text, 1999, ISBN: 0071341587.

Peptides in Oncology: Somatostatin and Lh-Rh Analogues (Recent Results in Cancer Research, 153), K. Hoffken (Editor), R. Kath (Editor). Springer–Verlag, 1999, ISBN: 3540644296.

Prescribing, Recording, and Reporting Photon Beam Therapy, Icru Report, 50. Intl. Commission on Radiation, 1999, ISBN: 0913394610.

Radiation from Medical Procedures in the Pathogenesis of Cancer and Ischemic Heart Disease: Dose-Response Studies with Physicians per 100,000 Population, John W. Gofman. CNR Books, 1999, ISBN: 0932682979.

Radioguided Surgery, Eric D. Whitman (Editor), Douglas Scott Reintgen (Editor). R. G. Landes Company, 1999, ISBN: 1570595690.

Signal Transduction and Cell Cycle Inhibitors (Cancer Drug Discovery and Development, 5), J. Silvio Gutkind (Editor). Humana Press, 1999, ISBN: 089603710X.

Supportive Group Therapy With Cancer Patients, David Spiegel, Catherine Classen, David Classen. Basic Books, 1999, ISBN: 0465095658.

The Application of Problem-Solving Therapy to Psychosocial Oncology Care, Julia A. Bucher (Editor). Haworth Medical Press, 1999, ISBN: 0789007592.

The Society of Cells: Control of Cell Proliferation and Cancer, Carlos Sonnen-schein, Ana M. Soto. Bios Scientific Pub. Ltd., 1999, ISBN: 0387915834.

Transplantation in Hematology and Oncology, T. H. Buchner (Editor). Springer–Verlag, 1999, ISBN: 3540648984.

Thyroid Cancer

Radiation and Thyroid Cancer, G. Thomas (Editor), A. Karaoglou (Editor), E. D. Williams (Editor). World Scientific Pub. Company, 1999, ISBN: 9810238142.

Thyroid Cancer: Clinical Management, L. Wartofsky (Editor). Humana Press, 1999, ISBN: 0896034291.

4. CONTINUING MEDICAL EDUCATION (CME)

4.1 **Continuing Medical Education Resources**

Accredited Council for Continuing Medical Education (ACCME) ⚙ ⚙ ⚙

http://www.accme.org

The Accredited Council for Continuing Medical Education offers voluntary accreditation to providers of continuing medical education who are interested in being recognized further for their high standards and quality. At the ACCME Web site visitors will discover necessary information regarding all aspects of the accreditation process, as well as the current activities of the organization regarding communications and quality control protocols.

American Medical Association (AMA): CME Locator ⚙ ⚙ ⚙

http://www.ama-assn.org/iwcf/iwcfmgr206/cme

The AMA CME Locator is a database of over 2,000 AMA PRA Category 1 activities sponsored by CME providers accredited by the Accreditation Council for Continuing Medical Education or approved by the American Medical Association. This site also lists United States and Canadian conferences, seminars, workshops, international conferences, seminars, workshops, and home study.

American Medical Association (AMA): Online Continuing Medical Education ⚙ ⚙ ⚙

http://www.ama-assn.org/cmeselec/cmeselec.htm

This site provides online courses and the opportunity to earn credit by reviewing the available material and answering test questions. A CME certificate is mailed or faxed within three to four weeks after the completion of the course.

CMEWeb ⚙ ⚙ ⚙

http://www.cmeweb.com/#pdr

Through CMEWeb, physicians can register through an online process, take electronic Continuing Medical Education (CME) tests over the Internet, and receive feedback and credit. The questions on these tests are pulled from the American Health Consultants publications corresponding to the particular testing areas.

Continuing Education from the NIH Consensus Development Program ⚙ ⚙ ⚙

http://text.nlm.nih.gov/nih/upload-v3/Continuing_Education/cme.html

This continuing medical education activity, sponsored by the National Institutes of Health and the Foundation for Advanced Education in the Sciences, invites users to participate in an online experiment in distance learning. Continuing medical education credits may be earned upon successful completion of testing materials, and further offerings, assuming the activity has been successful in its efforts, will be added to the Web site, including past NIH Consensus Development Conference reviews.

Continuing Medical Education at Physician's Guide ⊚ ⊚ ⊚
http://www.physiciansguide.com/cme.html

The Physician's Guide to Internet offers links to Continuing Medical Education resources at this site. Examples include links to information on the MMWR Continuing Education Program and the AMA's CME Locator. A short description of each link is provided.

Continuing Medical Education
Courses Online from Medical Matrix ⊚ ⊚ ⊚ (some features fee-based)
http://www.medmatrix.org/reg/login.asp

Medical Matrix's CME Courses Online is a one-stop resource for excellence in continuing medical education on the World Wide Web, with 39 accessible CME credit listing sites. General learning modules are available via Virtual Lecture Hall Health Professionals CME, HealthGate CME Courses, and Medscape's Online Articles for CME Reviews. The Cleveland Clinic Foundation, the National Institutes of Health, and Virtual Hospital Online all provide opportunities to access Internet-based CME courses, often with immediate feedback on performance. A multitude of top-rated CME modules and interesting feature sites include The Interactive Patient, which provides users with the ability to view a simulated online patient, request history, perform exams, and review diagnostic data. Credit fees vary by organization site.

Continuing Medical Education Resources ⊚ ⊚ ⊚ (some features fee-based)
http://www.slis.ua.edu/cdlp/cme/UAB

From the University of Alabama comes this comprehensive listing of continuing medical education opportunities. Listings are available from a wide variety of sources including the American Medical Association, the American Academy of Family Physicians, the American College of Physicians, and other medical associations and CME conference Web pages. Registration and organization membership may be required for access to online course information and material.

Continuing Medical Education
Sites from Medical Computing Today ⊚ ⊚ ⊚ (some features fee-based)
http://www.medicalcomputingtoday.com/0listcme.html

This Web site of Medical Computing Today presents an alphabetical listing of currently available category I CME credit offerings listed by the Accredited Council for Continuing Medical Education (ACCME). Principal areas of specialty covered at each of 85 sites are listed and directions for searching the text via Netscape Navigator are viewable. Alphabetical navigation bars throughout the text also enable visitors the opportunity to successfully locate educational materials of their choosing. CME descriptions, credits, and associated costs are included in CME entries. Registration for CME credit may be done at the individual, online sites.

Continuing Medical Education Unlimited ⊚ ⊚ ⊚

http://www.landesslezak.com/cgi-bin/start.cgi/cmeu/index.htm

This nonprofit division of Audio-Digest Foundation, specializes in producing audio CME programs for delivery to physicians and allied healthcare professionals on a subscription basis, providing high-quality selection of over 6,000 continuing medical education products from medical associations, institutions, and societies via audio, video, and CD-ROM. The offerings at this Web site include 13 specialty series and two jointly sponsored activities, with audio materials of medical symposia, review courses, and specialty meetings readily available. Each course listing includes its description, sponsor, target audience, accreditation, objectives, and faculty in addition to a list of currently available formats.

Cyberounds ⊚ ⊚ ⊚

http://www.cyberounds.com/links/home.html

Cyberounds is an online, interactive forum moderated by distinguished professionals, and is available for use by physicians, medical students, and other selected healthcare professionals. All users must register to access resources at the site. Registration is free-of-charge but restricted to healthcare professionals. Continuing Medical Education opportunities, an online bookstore, links to quality sites relevant to a variety of specialties, and additional educational resources are available at the site.

Ed Credits ⊚ ⊚ ⊚

http://www.edcredits.com

Formerly CEUs On Line, Ed Credits offers opportunities for Continuing Education credits for medical and other professionals. Registration is available for an annual fee of US$55, and any number of courses can be taken within this time. Material for the courses is available for free on the Web site, but registration is necessary to take the tests and to receive certificates.

Newpromises.com ⊚ ⊚

http://www.caso.com/home/home.phtml

NewPromises.com, founded by Harvard University and MIT professors, is an online education program working closely with accredited institutions of higher learning to offer courses in a variety of fields including health topics. The site offers information on registration, financial aid, career advice, links to research material, textbook resources, and degree and certificate details.

5. ONCOLOGY AND HEMATOLOGY OVERVIEW SITES

5.1 **Supersites**

American Cancer Society (ACS)   ⚙ ⚙ ⚙

http://www.cancer.org

The ACS is one of the most important supersites for information on all aspects of cancer, primarily directed to the public. The site's home page includes headlines and brief stories on new cancer developments and treatments, as well as links to types of cancer, pediatric cancer, prevention, treatment options, therapies, research, statistics, and media resources. Details about the ACS itself are provided, including an annual report, financial statements, employment, meetings, and e-mail. There is a state-by-state scroll menu to link to state organizations, services, and support; an online directory of medical resources, including a hospital locator; information on legislative and public action issues; and extensive sublinks focusing on more than fifty (50) different forms of cancer. Each cancer description is quite thorough, and is augmented by additional links to other resources on the same topic, such as specialized glossaries, imaging, drugs, and alternative therapies.

Bloodline   ⚙ ⚙ ⚙ (free registration)

http://www.bloodline.net

This site serves as an extensive online resource for hematology education and news. Site content covers the subspecialties of BMT/Stem Cell Therapy/ Cord Blood, Thrombosis and Hemostasis, Lab Hematology, Malignant Hematology, Pediatric Hematology, Red Cell Disorders, Transfusion Medicine, and Veterinary Hematology. The site features case studies, meeting reports, lectures, book reviews, an image atlas, a newsletter, news, meetings calendar, classifieds, grant information, full-length articles, and more. A free, online registration is required to access all of these services. Professional and patient links are provided.

CancerBACUP   ⚙ ⚙ ⚙

http://www.cancerbacup.org.uk/index.shtml

An extensive cancer information resource of over 1,500 pages for patients, families, and health professionals, this site notes its recognition as the foremost provider of cancer information in the United Kingdom. Links to an online database of over 600 UK-wide support groups and organizations, UK hospice database, links to online journals, drug information, and information regarding international conferences are conveniently available. Also, the site provides a way for one to view and/or order by mail its information booklets free-of-charge. There are links to worldwide cancer organizations and information sources as well.

Cancerlinks ○ ○ ○

http://www.cancerlinks.org

This valuable site is a directory to other sites offering resources on many forms of cancer, with topics including bladder, brain, breast, cervical, colon, colorectal, endometrial, esophagus, eye, leukemia, liver, lung, lymphoma, melanoma, myelomas, ovarian, pancreatic, prostate, sarcoma, testicular, thyroid, vaginal, and vulvar cancers. Information on cancer drugs is also available. Resources on specific cancers include links to sites providing general medical information, clinical trials resources, genetics information, pain management tools, health insurance information, advocacy and legislation sites, alternative medicine information, journals and magazines, support groups, and resources for minority groups. Visitors can also access a tutorial on using the Internet.

CancerNet ○ ○ ○

http://cancernet.nci.nih.gov

CancerNet is truly a supersite for information on all aspects of cancer, operated by the National Cancer Institute (NCI). The main site is the starting place for exploring vast databases of information about cancer types, treatments, trials, genetics, prevention, testing, support, and literature. CancerNet provides patients, health professionals, and basic researchers with a wide range of accurate, credible cancer information, reviewed regularly by oncology experts and based on the latest research. Resources include access to PDQ (Physician Data Query), NCI's comprehensive cancer database, CancerLit, NCI's bibliographic database, fact sheets, glossary, news, and links to additional useful resources. Patients, the general public, and health professionals will find information on treatment, complementary and alternative medicine, screening and prevention, cancer genetics, supportive care, clinical trials, anti-angiogenesis, and information for specific ethnic/racial groups. Basic researchers will find links to databases and specimen resources, the NCI Cooperative Human Tissue Network and Family Registry for Breast Cancer Studies, cancer statistics, the Cancer Genome Anatomy Project, and genetics information.

Guide to Internet Resources for Cancer ○ ○ ○

http://www.ncl.ac.uk/child-health/guides/clinks1.htm

The University of Newcastle's Guide to Internet Resources for Cancer offers information for health professionals, researchers, patients, family, and the general public. The guide contains over 100 pages of links to cancer related information. The choices on the main menu include: Alphabetical Index of Diseases and Topics; Resources by Disease; Resources by Country; Treatments and Medical Specialties; National and International Cancer Organizations; Cancer Centers and Institutes; Childhood Cancer Resources; Online Journals and Bulletins; and Discussion Lists and News Groups.

Hardin Meta Directory
of Internet Health Services: Oncology, Hematology ⊙ ⊙ ⊙
http://www.lib.uiowa.edu/hardin/md/index.html

This site provides links to a variety of sources of Oncology and Hematology information. Links exist to journals, libraries, government sites, academic institutions, and to other resources concerning these fields.

Medicine Online ⊙ ⊙ ⊙
http://www.meds.com

Access to a tremendous amount of medical information and services concerning Oncology is available here. Links to major oncology and hematology societies are offered in addition to links to literature searches, software information, forums, and discussion groups. The site's own Cancer Information Libraries offer direct access to news, treatment information, medical reports from meetings, and more. There are also a number of links to other major Web sites.

Medmark: Hematology ⊙ ⊙ ⊙
http://www.medmark.org/hem/hem.html

A comprehensive directory of Internet resources on Hematology, Medmark provides listings of direct links to hundreds of associations and societies in the field; research centers, laboratories, and institutes; medical school and hospital departments of hematology; education and training resources; consumer information; images and atlases; professional journals; and other Web information related to hematology topics and disorders.

Medmark: Oncology ⊙ ⊙ ⊙
http://www.medmark.org/onco

A vast number of links to Internet oncology resources is provided, including associations, institutes/labs, departments, government sources, programs, and resources for individual disorders. Links are categorized by subject to help refine searches for information.

MedNets: Hematology, Oncology ⊙ ⊙ ⊙
http://www.Internets.com/mednets/hemeonco.htm

The site serves as a link that can point the user in a number of desired directions, including clinical information, news, and hospitals specializing in Oncology and Hematology. Thirty-four oncology databases are directly accessible from this site, under "Databases." In addition, the site has its own search engine where the user can search the databases for a topic.

MedWebPlus: Medical Oncology, Hematology ◎ ◎ ◎

http://www.medwebplus.com/subject/Medical_Oncology.html

Topics appropriate for professionals, patients, and others are listed alphabetically for user-friendly access. This site contains a tremendous body of information on hundreds of disorders, publications, associations, educational tools, support services, and other sources of information relating to oncology.

National Cancer Institute (NCI) ◎ ◎ ◎

http://www.nci.nih.gov

The National Cancer Institute is a U.S. federal government agency and a component of the National Institutes of Health in the Department of Health and Human Services. Resources for health professionals, patients, and the public are available at this site. Featured is specific information about NCI health initiatives, news releases about current clinical trials, information concerning NCI-supported/extramural research, and extensive information about every aspect of cancer. Information about available positions, training opportunities, and research funding is also available.

Network for Oncology
Communication and Research (NOCR) ◎ ◎ ◎

http://www.nocr.com

NOCR is an association that assists professionals with their cancer information requirements and provides a source for recent advances in the field of Oncology. The NOCR Web site features a fax news service, a list of news summaries, abstract lists, clinical updates and research information. The research section provides access to online journals, a reference bookshelf, statistical packages, resources for writers, search tools, and databases. Each section provides a number of excellent links to sites that provide services or information.

OncoLink ◎ ◎ ◎

http://www.oncolink.upenn.edu

Affiliated with the University of Pennsylvania Cancer Center (UPCC), OncoLink provides introductory and in-depth information regarding various types of cancer, cancer treatments, and research advances. It features a virtual classroom, links to databases of all open UPCC clinical trials, and other sources of information for both healthcare providers and patients. The comprehensive resources section includes information concerning medical specialties that deal with cancer, as well as much more information.

Oncology and Radiology Portal Site ⊙ ⊙ ⊙

http://www.intravsn.com

Both professionals and patients are served by this site. Various sections of the site are intended for physicians, managers, physicists, nurses, dosimetrists, medical imagers and radiation therapists. Information available includes articles, government standards, journals, vendors, billing information, and relevant books. There are lists of codes, standards, and policies for professionals as well as patient information sections containing abstracts and links. Links are also provided in every section for each type of profession.

OncologyChannel ⊙ ⊙ ⊙

http://www.oncologychannel.com

OncologyChannel provides a wealth of information and several useful tools for patients and physicians. Extensive descriptions of disorders and diseases are offered with data on stages, symptoms, and treatments. An "MD Locator" allows patients to find oncologists using a zip code, and a "HealthProfiler" provides PSA calculators. News, editorials, and several interactive forums (live chat with a physician, patient chat rooms, and discussions) provide a community for patient and physician communication.

5.2 General Resources for Oncology

About.com: Cancer Resources ⊙ ⊙ ⊙

http://cancer.miningco.com/health/cancer

Well-organized and varied, About.com contains links to general cancer information sources and to categorized subsections that offer more specific information. A listing of oncology resources includes links to articles, news, reviews, and relevant sites.

Alpha Oncology ⊙ ⊙

http://www.alphaoncology.com

Geared towards medical professionals, this educational resource for the Coalition of National Cancer Cooperative Groups offers a large number of educational tools such as CME Webcasts, the ability to ask other professionals questions, and a bookstore. Educational programs are organized into focus groups that offer latest developments, management, clinical trial summaries, and other information. Currently, major focus areas are lung, breast and colorectal cancers; more are added monthly.

Ask NOAH About: Cancer ⊙ ⊙ ⊙
http://noah.cuny.edu/cancer/cancer.html

New York Online Access to Health (NOAH) is a partnership consisting of The City University of New York, The Metropolitan New York Library Council, The New York Academy of Medicine, and The New York Public Library. The Web site provides health information on a variety of topics and seeks to answer frequently asked questions. The section devoted to cancer provides educational information for patients, links and PDQ information for healthcare professionals. There are links to information about each type of cancer, risk factors, cancer prevention and treatments available.

Canadian Oncology Society (COS) ⊙ ⊙ ⊙ (fee-based)
http://www.cos.ca

The COS Web site contains information for patients and physicians. Open to all are links to the COS newsletter, information about the organization, membership application materials, and numerous links to affiliated societies. A section of the Web site is restricted to members, and provides access to search engines, information about clinical trials, an events calendar, professional and educational opportunities, and a membership directory.

CancerGuide ⊙ ⊙
http://cancerguide.org

CancerGuide provides links to a set of resources on the Web grouped by user needs. Both patients and physicians can find useful information about specific diseases as well as possible treatments. The site is written informally, and is meant to collect a set of useful sites into a single cohesive starting point. Although the number of referenced sites is limited, CancerGuide links to many of the basic, important sources of cancer information on the net.

CancerResources ⊙ ⊙
http://www.cancerresources.com

For professionals, a number of links provide information about therapy, complimentary and alternative medicine, and pain management. For patients, helpful information comes in the form of online videos and links to both educational and support resources.

CancerWeb ⊙ ⊙ ⊙
http://www.graylab.ac.uk/cancerweb.html

Issues affecting patients and families, and clinicians and researchers are addressed here. There are links for clinicians to pages that cover patient management details, specific cancers, symptom management, alternative treatments, drug information, and clinical trials. For researchers, the site provides a reference tool with access to material on academic subjects such as biology, biochemistry, immunology, gene databases, molecular modeling, and pharmacology. For patients, resources available cover causes, risk factors, symptom management, and support.

European Society for Medical Oncology (ESMO) ◎
http://www.esmo.org

Information about the organization, its structure, activities, its journal, and news is offered at this site for professionals. There is an extensive listing of ESMO-organized courses and fellowships.

International Society for Prevention Oncology (ISPO) ◎ ◎
http://www.cancerprev.org/ISPO

ISPO is an organization that serves to study etiologic factors in the development of cancer for its primary and secondary prevention. The ISPO Web site offers information about its journal, *Cancer Detection and Prevention,* its international meetings and workshops, awards, membership, and news. The user can search abstracts and view the organization of past meetings. One can download a membership application and the membership fee includes a yearly subscription to the ISPO journal.

International Union Against Cancer (UICC) ◎ (fee-based)
http://www.uicc.org

UICC is an international, independent organization based in Geneva, Switzerland, and consists of medical, scientific, and other members who are devoted to the fight against cancer. The organization promotes the advancement of scientific research and prevention and treatment of cancer. Also emphasized is professional and public education. The site provides information regarding membership, fellowships available, and educational opportunities and materials provided by the UICC. There is a member section of the site that has restricted access to UICC members.

Oncology Nursing Society (ONS) Online ◎ (fee-based)
http://www.ons.org

The Web site of the ONS has sections for members, healthcare providers, and for patients/consumers. Access to each section requires a registration that can be completed online. Members receive access to journals, educational opportunities, employment information, and more. Details of membership and registration are provided.

Oncology Online ◎ ◎ ◎ (fee-based)
http://205.239.179.160:81

This is a resource site for physicians that provides news, research, and an online dialogue. Access to the Oncology Therapeutics Network (OTN) is offered. OTN is a service firm that aids in the management of Oncology practices. The research section offers access to Paper Chase, an online information search service; it also provides information on upcoming conferences and other online resources. Oncology Online is a free service that requires registration. A special section that allows for physicians to pose questions to a panel of experts requires a DEA number for entry. The links section is extensive and provides disease-specific and general oncology links.

Southern Association for Oncology ⊙

http://www.sma.org/sao

This association sponsors a quarterly newsletter and annual meeting. Its Web site offers information concerning the annual meeting, the Association, and membership. The Oncology Online section offers select abstracts and articles from recent journals.

5.3 General Resources for Hematology

American Association of Blood Banks (AABB) ⊙ ⊙ ⊙

http://www.aabb.org

The AABB is an international association of blood banks that seeks to implement high standards for patients and donors in all aspects of the process. The AABB Web site provides facts about blood, donation, receiving, subscription services, and news. Percentage testing reports, practice guidelines, statements on transfusion practices, reviews, and ISO reports are provided for medical professionals. Educational materials available include information on workshops, meetings, and certification information.

American Society for Histocompatibility and Immunogenetics (ASHI) ⊙ ⊙

http://www.swmed.edu/home_pages/ASHI/ashi.htm

The Society seeks to provide a forum for discussion of recent advances, to aid professionals, to maintain histocompatibility testing laboratory quality and fidelity, and to provide a voice for its members in governmental regulatory agencies. Its site provides detailed information about the Society, ASHI services, discussion, directories, employment updates, Histocompatibility and Immunogenetics archives, ASHI products and news, information, and meetings updates. There is also a restricted section for members that requires a password, and includes information about its members, committees, bylaws, and council.

American Society of Hematology (ASH) ⊙ ⊙

http://www.hematology.org

The ASH Web site provides information about the professional Society, ASH awards, the annual meeting, training programs, news, membership, and educational materials.

There is an extensive list of educational documents that are organized by topic. There is also a link to *Blood,* the journal of the American Society of Hematology.

American Society of Pediatric Hematology/Oncology (ASPH/O)
http://www.aspho.org

ASPH/O is a professional society of pediatric hematologists/oncologists. This Web site provides a forum for communication for medical professionals, and also serves the patients and families afflicted with these diseases by providing a source of current peer-reviewed scientific and clinical research drawn from ASPH/O's annual scientific meeting and journal. Further online resources and links are provided to aid in finding other related information through the Internet for both professionals and patients. The site also contains information on ASPH/O career awards.

British Society for Histocompatibility and Immunogenetics (BSHI)
http://www.umds.ac.uk/tissue/bshi1.html

A nonprofit society that provides a forum for the sharing of scientific information, new technology, and education, this site provides information about the BSHI annual scientific meeting, the Histocompatibility and Immunogenetics Group (HIG), and other internal groups, membership, a newsletter, relevant sites, and more. A listing of useful software, such as CD antigen files and sound files, can be downloaded directly from the site.

International Society for Hematotherapy and Graft Engineering (ISHAGE)
http://www.ishage.org

This professional organization for researchers and physicians serves as a forum for communication, education, training, research, and standardized technology, and as a representation vehicle. Symposia schedules, abstracts, news, FAQs, organization and director information, guidelines, and an information library are provided at the site. Discussion lounges are available for members that are password protected. There is also a link to the new official ISHAGE journal, *Cytotherapy.*

5.4 Awards and Honors

Introduction

Public recognition of important contributions to the fields of Oncology and Hematology is achieved through awards and honors from major scientific, nonprofit, and corporate organizations. We have included many such awards in this section. Awards and honors are subject to change at any time, however, and some awards may not be granted every year. Organizations periodically discontinue awards, change their terms and qualifications, or add new awards and honors. For these reasons, the reader should visit these Web sites directly to obtain the latest information on current awards and honors.

Awards for Research

American Association for Cancer Research (AACR): AFLAC Scholar Awards for Associate Members

http://www.aacr.org

AACR associate members who present outstanding abstracts at the AACR Annual Meeting or Special Conferences are granted this award. Presentations are automatically considered for the award and the award is partial support of meeting expenses.

American Association for Cancer Research (AACR): Career Development Awards in Cancer Research

http://www.aacr.org

There are two awards for junior, tenure-track scientists at the Assistant Professor level who are engaged in praiseworthy research. The AACR-Susan G. Komen Breast Cancer Foundation Career Development Award is for basic, clinical, or translational research related to breast cancer, and the AACR-National Foundation for Cancer Research Career Development Award is for basic research for any type of cancer. Awards are two-year international grants of $50,000 per year. Eligibility, selection, and application information is available at the AACR Web site.

American Association for Cancer Research (AACR): G.H.A. Clowes Award

http://www.aacr.org

Presented in recognition of outstanding research accomplishments, the award is for basic research, and AACR members must make nominations to the AACR Awards Committee. The award is presented at the AACR Annual Meeting.

American Association for Cancer Research (AACR): Gerald Grindey Memorial Young Investigator Award

http://www.aacr.org

This award is presented to a young investigator for an abstract in the area of preclinical science. The abstract is then presented at the AACR Annual Meeting. Abstract submission forms can be downloaded from the AACR site.

American Association for Cancer Research (AACR): Gertrude B. Elion Cancer Research Award

http://www.aacr.org

A one-year $30,000 grant is given to foster meritorious research in the U.S. or Canada for an assistant professor who is nontenured and tenure tracked. The award is supported by Glaxo Wellcome.

American Association for Cancer Research (AACR): Glaxo Wellcome Oncology Scholar Awards

http://www.aacr.org

Young scientists chosen to present abstracts in the areas of clinical/translational research at an AACR meeting compete for this award. Abstract submission forms can be downloaded from the AACR Web site.

American Association for Cancer Research (AACR): HBCU Faculty Award in Cancer Research

http://www.aacr.org

Full-time faculty of historically black colleges and universities who participate in AACR Special Conferences may apply for this award. Assistant professors or above must be engaged in meritorious basic, clinical, or translational research. The award is up to $1,500 for AACR conference participation. The AACR Web site provides details of requirements and application procedures.

American Association for Cancer Research (AACR): Joseph H. Burchenal Clinical Research Award

http://www.aacr.org

For outstanding achievement in clinical cancer research, the award was established by Bristol-Myers Squibb. There are no age or geographic restrictions on this award, and AACR members must nominate candidates. The award is presented at the AACR Annual Meeting.

American Association for Cancer Research (AACR): Pezcoller International Award for Cancer Research

http://www.aacr.org

An award for a cancer related major scientific discovery is given annually. A lecture at the AACR Annual Meeting will be given by the recipient. The recipient will receive a US $75,000 honorarium and a commemorative plaque. Nominations for the award are to be made by anyone affiliated with an institution of cancer research.

American Association for Cancer Research (AACR): Young Investigator Awards

http://www.aacr.org

Graduate and medical students, residents, and clinical and postdoctoral fellows who are abstract presenters are eligible for this particular award. Abstracts highly rated by the AACR Annual Meeting Program Committee are presented at sessions during the Annual Meeting and this committee selects recipients of the award. An abstract submission form must be filed and a request for award consideration must be noted.

American Cancer Society (ACS): Award for Research Excellence in Cancer Epidemiology and Prevention

http://www.aacr.org

This award recognizes research achievement in epidemiology, biomarkers, and prevention. AACR members may submit nominations to the Award Committee. There are no geographic or age limitations for this award.

American Society of Hematology (ASH): Merit Awards

http://www.hematology.org

These merit awards are for medical or graduate students, resident physicians, or postdoctoral fellows who are the first author/presenter of an abstract that receives the highest score in their category. The award is a U.S. $500 honorarium and travel reimbursement.

Brinker International Awards for Breast Cancer Research

http://www.komen.org

This award of honor is given for distinguished basic, clinical, and social-behavioral breast cancer research. Application materials are available online.

Bruce F. Cain Memorial Award

http://www.aacr.org

This memorial award seeks to "give recognition to an individual or research team for outstanding preclinical research that has implications for the improved care of cancer patients." Contributions in medicinal chemistry, biochemistry, or tumor biology that cover anticancer, antiviral, and antifungal agents will be recognized. The award is provided by the Warner-Lambert Company and has no geographical or age limitations.

Cornelius P. Rhoads Memorial Award

http://www.aacr.org

The annual Rhoads award serves to recognize an "individual on the basis of meritorious achievement in cancer research." The award recipient must be under the age of 41 years at the time of the award presentation. Nominations by AACR members must be directed to the Award Committee, and presentation occurs at the Annual Meeting.

Richard and Hinda Rosenthal Foundation Award

http://www.aacr.org

This award has been established to "recognize research which has made or gives the promise of soon making a notable contribution to improved clinical care in the field of cancer." The award is restricted to American investigators under 50 years of age, engaged in medical practice.

Awards for Service

American Cancer Society (ACS): Lane W. Adams Award

http://www.cancer.org

These awards are granted in recognition of individuals who provide direct care in the ACS "warm hand of service" concept. Roughly 15 awards are presented and recipients are recognized in a special ceremony with media coverage and a commemorative momento.

Fellowships and Research Grants

American Association for Cancer Research (AACR): Research Fellowships

http://www.aacr.org

Research fellowships in basic, clinical, translational, and prevention research are available to young scientists at the postdoctoral or clinical research fellow level. The fellowships are one-year grants and are renewable for a second year. A salary of $30,000 per year is provided along with a separate travel grant that supports AACR Annual Meeting participation. More information and eligibility requirements are available at the AACR Web site.

American Cancer Society (ACS): Health Professional Training Grants

http://www.cancer.org

The American Cancer Society provides awards in seven Health Professional Training Grant categories: Cancer Control Career Development Awards for Primary Care Physicians (CCCDA); Training Grants in Clinical Oncology Social Work (TGCOSW); Physician Training Awards in Preventative Medicine (PTAPM); Doctoral Degree Scholarships in Cancer Nursing (SCN); Master's Degree Scholarships in Cancer Nursing (MSCN); Professorship of Clinical Oncology (PCO); and Professorship in

Oncology Nursing (PON). Policies and grant application instructions are available online. Details of awards and criteria for each category are also available.

American Cancer Society (ACS): Research Grants

http://www.cancer.org

The American Cancer Society provides awards in nine Research Grant categories: Research Project Grants (RPG); Postdoctoral Fellowships (PF); Clinical Research Training Grants for Junior Faculty (CRTG); Institutional Research Grants (IRG); Research Opportunity Grants (ROG); Research Professorships (RP); Clinical Research Professorships (CRP); Targeted Grants (TG); and Targeted Intervention Opportunity Grants (TIOG). Policies and grant application instructions are available online. Details of awards and criteria for each category are also available.

American Institute for Cancer Research (AICR): Research Grant Programs

http://www.aicr.org

The American Institute for Cancer Research offers grants to promote research in the field of diet, nutrition, and cancer. Applications are accepted in the areas of cancer prevention and cancer treatment as they relate to diet, nutrition, and cancer. Funding is offered in four grant programs: Investigator-Initiated Grant Program; Postdoctoral Awards; AICR/NCTR Collaborative Research Grant Programs, and the Matching Grant Program.

American Society of Clinical Oncology (ASCO): Career Development Award

http://www.asco.org/prof/sh/f_sh.htm

This program provides funds to young clinical investigators to support research with a clinical focus. Applicants must be physicians (M.D. or D.O.) within the first three years of full-time, primary faculty appointment in a clinical department of an academic medical institution. More than 50% of an applicant's time must be spent in research. Award terms are available online.

American Society of Clinical Oncology (ASCO): Young Investigator Award

http://www.asco.org/prof/sh/f_sh.htm

This program offers funds to young investigators in order to promote clinical oncology research. The applicant must be a physician (M.D. or D.O.) and must be in the final year of a fellowship or first year of post fellowship. The grant is for a one-year period and funds are directed towards the sponsoring institution. Award terms are available online.

American Society of Hematology Summer Medical Student Program

http://www.hematology.org

ASH offers medical students an opportunity for an introduction to Hematology via summer project work with a hematologist. The medical school receives $2,500 and applications must come through a medical school.

Amy Strezler Manasevit Scholars Program for the Study of Post-Transplant Complications

http://www.marrow.org

This program is geared towards professionals who wish to study the events that occur after allogenic hematopoietic cell transplantation. Clinical investigations, translational research, or basic laboratory research may be included in the proposal, and applicants must have a doctoral degree i.e., M.D., Ph.D. or equivalent. Maximum support of $240,000 over two years is granted.

Basic, Clinical, and Translational Research

http://www.komen.org

Grants of up to $250,000 over two years are offered for these areas: Basic Science Studies; Clinical Studies for Improved Treatments; Translational Research; Complimentary Medicine; Diagnostic Methods; Environmental Factors; Genetic Epidemiology; Diet and Nutrition; Psychosocial Support; Prevention; and Survivorship Research.

Cancer Research Foundation of America (CRFA) Grant & Fellowship Programs

http://www.preventcancer.org

Consistent with its mission to prevent cancer, the CRFA offers grants and fellowships in three categories: Basic, Clinical, Translational and Applied Research Projects and Fellowships; Cancer Prevention Education Programs; and Early Detection Projects. Research and educational grants are awarded for a one-year period with opportunity for renewal. Research fellowships may be requested by a principal investigator and are typically awarded for a two-year period.

CaP CURE Competitive Awards

http://205.139.28.245/research/programs.html

Awards are distributed by the Association for the Cure of Cancer of the Prostate and are intended to promote searches for cures and controls of advanced prostate cancer. One year of funding is provided and research areas such as genomics, molecular biology, angiogenesis, nutrition, alternative therapies, and clinical medicine are considered appropriate. Guidelines and application materials are available online.

CaP CURE Young Investigator Awards

http://www.capcure.org

Conferred by the Association for the Cure of Cancer of the Prostate, these awards are intended to attract young investigators, both clinical and scientific, to prostate cancer research. Awards are allocated to cover direct costs only. Guidelines and application materials are available online.

Career Development Awards 2000

http://www.leukemia.org

Support for basic, clinical, or translational research is offered by the Leukemia Society of America for the study of leukemia, lymphoma, Hodgkin's disease, and myeloma. These awards offer three levels of support: Scholar, Special Fellow, and Fellow. Details of each support level, award guidelines, and application materials are available online.

International Fellowships for Beginning Investigators

http://www.cancer.org

These fellowships are funded by the American Cancer Society and subject to International Union Against Cancer (UICC) General Conditions for fellowships. Fellowship objectives are to promote the flow of information to and from the U.S. recipients are to be in the early stages of their career, and work is to be carried out abroad. The fellowships are awarded to enable researchers to carry out basic and clinical research to advance information in the areas of epidemiology, prevention, causation, detection, diagnosis, treatment, and psycho-oncology.

International Union Against Cancer Fellowships

http://fellows.uicc.org

The International Union Against Cancer offers fellowships in nine International Cancer Fellowship categories: Translational Cancer Research Fellowships; American Cancer Society International Fellowships for Beginning Investigators; Yamagiwa-Yoshida Memorial International Cancer Study Grants; ICRETT Fellowships for Bilateral Exchanges Between Indonesia and the Netherlands; International Oncology Nursing Fellowships; Asia-Pacific Cancer Society Training Grants; Latin America COPES Training and Education Fellowships; and Becas de Educacion y Entrenamiento COPES American Latin Fellowships. Award criteria, application forms, and guidelines are available online.

KCA Eugene P. Schonfield Young Researcher's Award for Basic Research in Renal Cancer

http://www.nkca.org/index.stm

This award from the Kidney Cancer Association is meant for a young M.D., D.O., or Ph.D. and is payable over two years. Submission guidelines are available online.

Patricia Manson Memorial Fellowship

http://www.lymphoma.ca

This fellowship is named in the memory of the founder of the Lymphoma Research Foundation of Canada. It provides a two-year stipend of $45,000 and an allocation of $5,000 for related expenses. The project must take place in a Canadian laboratory and it should contribute to the scientific understanding of malignant lymphoma.

Population Specific Research Projects

http://www.komen.org

Funding, in the form of grants, is presented to individuals conducting projects that focus on breast cancer epidemiology within at-risk populations. Such populations may be African American, Asian/Pacific Islander, Hispanic, Native American, lesbian, or low literacy. Two-year grants of up to $75,000 per year are available.

Postdoctoral Fellowships

http://www.komen.org

Offered by the Susan G. Komen Breast Cancer Foundation, fellowship support is available for basic, clinical, or translational research; public health or epidemiology. Grants extend over three years and are for $35,000 per year. The recipient's area of study must be breast cancer.

Translational Research Program

http://www.leukemia.org

The Leukemia Society of America offers early stage support for clinical research that seeks to uncover information for treatment, diagnosis, or prevention of leukemia, lymphoma, Hodgkin's disease or myeloma. Monetary support is offered for a three-year period, and the program is run in conjunction with the National Cancer Institute. Details of scope, eligibility requirements, funds available, and application procedures are available online.

General Awards

American Association for Cancer Research (AACR): Minority Scholar Awards

http://www.aacr.org

AACR provides travel funds for minority students to attend the AACR Annual Meeting and Special Conferences. Full time predoctoral students, postdoctoral fellows, physicians in training, and junior faculty scientists are eligible. The program applies to minority groups defined by the National Cancer Institute as being underrepresented in cancer research.

American Cancer Society (ACS): Clinical Research Professorship

http://www.cancer.org

This ACS grant is for mid-career clinician-scientists considered to be field leaders. Applicants who undertake clinical, epidemiological, or translational laboratory research may be considered as long as they are U.S. citizens or permanent residents and have at least ten years of experience past their receipt of the M.D. or other doctoral degree. The Professorship is awarded for a five-year period and the grant can be allocated towards salary and/or research. Recipients are required to be spokespeople for the ACS. Full award criteria are available online.

American Society of Hematology (ASH): Scholar Awards

http://www.hematology.org

Funding is awarded to beginning biomedical scientists in order to encourage a hematology career. Awards are $60,000 or $40,000 per year for two years. The competition is held each September, and application materials may be downloaded.

5.5 National Cancer Institute (NCI): A Comprehensive Profile

Introduction to the National Cancer Institute (NCI) ⊙ ⊙ ⊙

http://www.nci.nih.gov

The National Cancer Institute (NCI) is a component of the National Institutes of Health (NIH), one of eight agencies that compose the Public Health Service (PHS) in the Department of Health and Human Services (DHHS). The NCI, established under the National Cancer Act of 1937, is the federal government's principal agency for cancer research and training. The National Cancer Institute coordinates the National Cancer Program, which conducts and supports research, training, health information dissemination, and other programs with respect to the cause, diagnosis, prevention, and treatment of cancer, rehabilitation from cancer, and the continuing care of cancer patients and the families of cancer patients.

Important components of the Web site are summarized below.

Departments and Services

Budget Proposal for Fiscal Year 2000 ⊙ ⊙ ⊙

http://wwwosp.nci.nih.gov/newosp/spa/bypass/bypass2000/01_director/1index.htm

The Institute's Budget Proposal for Fiscal Year 2000 presents an itemized budget plan for the year, descriptions of current research programs funded by the National Cancer

Institute, narrative articles related to drug discovery, and stories from cancer survivors. The NCI's Infrastructure for Discovery is described in detail, including discussions of extramural and intramural research, clinical studies, training, education, career development, research support contracts, AIDS research, research management, and support. Investment opportunities in cancer genetics, preclinical models of cancer, imaging technologies, and defining cancer cell signatures are also presented. Research subjects highlighted at the site include investigations in cancer pain, monoclonal antibodies, lung cancer, angiogenesis, and cancer statistics. Visitors can also search the site by keyword, and access instructions for downloading documents from the site.

Cancer Genome Anatomy Project (CGAP) ◎ ◎ ◎

http://www.ncbi.nlm.nih.gov/CGAP

The Cancer Genome Anatomy Project (CGAP) is an interdisciplinary program to establish the information and technological tools needed to decipher the molecular anatomy of the cancer cell. The site offers a wide range of tools and information resources for investigators, including links to the Human Tumor Gene Index, Molecular Fingerprinting, Cancer Chromosome Aberration Project, Genetic Annotation Initiative, and Mouse Tumor Gene Index resources. Specific molecular resources include CGAP reagents information, a cDNA library browser, cDNA library source information, summary tables of libraries, genes, and sequences, a link to the IMAGE Consortium for obtaining cDNA clones, tumor suppression and oncogene directory, additional tools for searching cDNA libraries, and other technology resources. Frequently asked questions are answered regarding online molecular tools, and links to many genetic databases are available.

Cancer Information Service (CIS) ◎ ◎ ◎

http://cis.nci.nih.gov

The Cancer Information Service, a national information and education network, is a free public service of the National Cancer Institute (NCI), providing visitors with the latest, most accurate cancer information for patients, their families, the general public and health professionals. The Service interprets and explains research findings to the general public in a clear and understandable manner through a network of hotlines in 19 regional offices. The site offers links to NCI and other cancer resources, information on ordering publications, regional programs and research information, and contact details.

CancerNet ◎ ◎ ◎

http://cancernet.nci.nih.gov

CancerNet provides patients, health professionals, and basic researchers with a wide range of accurate, credible cancer information, reviewed regularly by oncology experts and based on the latest research. Resources include access to PDQ (Physician Data Query), NCI's comprehensive cancer database, CancerLit, NCI's bibliographic database, fact sheets, glossary, news, and links to additional useful resources. Patients, the general public, and health professionals will find information on treatment, complementary and alternative medicine, screening and prevention, cancer genetics, supportive care, clinical trials, anti-angiogenesis, and information for specific ethnic/racial groups. Basic researchers will find links to databases and specimen resources, the NCI Cooperative Human Tissue Network and Family Registry for Breast Cancer Studies, cancer statistics, the Cancer Genome Anatomy Project, and genetics information.

CancerTrials ◉ ◉ ◉

http://cancertrials.nci.nih.gov

CancerTrials offers patients and health professionals on understanding clinical trials, making the decision to participate in a trial, finding specific trials, news, contacts, and links for additional resources. Special features include informed consent documents, anti-angiogenesis information, and a link to details about a breast cancer risk disk software tool.

Developmental Therapeutics Program ◉ ◉ ◉

http://dtp.nci.nih.gov

The Developmental Therapeutics Program site offers public data from drug and natural product screenings, a catalog of compounds, and a chemical name table. The site also lists available research samples and services, current projects, resources for research in anti-angiogenesis, and a summary of published molecular target work.

Event Calendar ◉ ◉ ◉

http://spot.nci.nih.gov/internal

The National Cancer Institute (NCI) Calendar for Cancer-Related Scientific Meetings and Events permits users to view calendars by day, week, month, or year, search for specific events, and find links to cancer-related scientific meeting information and government sources for cancer information. The NCI Events Calendar at this site provides a centralized and easily accessible place to obtain information about meetings and events related to NCI Advisory Committees, NCI Planning and Oversight Groups, cancer-related scientific meetings, conferences, symposia, seminars, and workshops.

Frederick Research and Development Center ◉ ◉ ◉

http://Web.ncifcrf.gov

The Frederick Research and Development Center conducts research efforts exploring the causes of cancer and related diseases. The site offers detailed information on research programs and research support services, a campus directory and phonebook, bulletin board, technologies database, calendar of events, and library services.

Office of International Affairs ◎ ◎ ◎

http://cancernet.nci.nih.gov/oia/master.html

The National Cancer Institute (NCI) Office of International Affairs coordinates the Institute's worldwide activities in a number of arenas, including: liaison with foreign and international agencies; coordination of cancer research activities under agreements between the US and other countries; planning and implementation of international scientist exchange programs; sponsorship of international workshops; and dissemination of cancer information. A report summarizing international activities, information on scientist exchange programs, and links to additional cancer information at NCI are available at the site.

Patients, Public, and Mass Media ◎ ◎ ◎

http://rex.nci.nih.gov

Information for Patients, the Public, and Mass Media at the National Cancer Institute (NCI) provides a wealth of resources to each of these audiences. Patient information includes links to cancer sites by type, resources for coping with challenges during treatment, educational resources for adults and children, a clinical trials listing, medical explanations of diagnosis and treatment, resources for cancer survivors, publication index, cancer fact sheets, and a glossary of terms. Prevention, early detection, and genetic testing information, and DES publications are available for the general public. Press releases, ideas for articles, cancer fact sheets, science education resources, links to additional media resources, basic statistics, and photo archives, are provided for those involved in science reporting. One section publishes the results from a Study to Estimate Iodine (I-131) Doses from Nuclear Fallout, as a result of atmospheric nuclear tests in Nevada, and contains fact sheets on thyroid cancer, maps documenting exposure, and executive and technical summaries of the NCI report.

Press Releases ◎ ◎ ◎

http://rex.nci.nih.gov/massmedia/pressrelease.htm

Press releases include information on advances in basic research as well as in cancer prevention, detection and diagnosis, and treatment. Previous press releases are archived by year. All press releases are labeled with date of broadcast.

Technology Transfer ◎ ◎ ◎

http://www.nci.nih.gov/hpage/TTrans.htm

Technology Transfer resources include links to the Technology Development and Commercialization Branch, Public Health Service Technology Development Coordinators, and the National Institutes of Health (NIH) Extramural Invention Information Management System (Edison).

Research

Division of Basic Sciences ○ ○ ○

http://rex.nci.nih.gov/RESEARCH/basic/dbspage.htm

The Division of Basic Sciences is the largest basic science research enterprise in cancer, with the primary goal of providing the best environment to perform quality science and to develop programs that will define the cutting edge of biomedical cancer research. The site presents the Division's mission, principal investigators, research directories, available positions, and links to individual laboratories.

Division of Cancer Epidemiology and Genetics ○ ○ ○

http://www-dceg.ims.nci.nih.gov/index.html

The Division of Cancer Epidemiology and Genetics is the primary focus within the National Cancer Institute (NCI) for population-based research on environmental and genetic determinants of cancer. The site offers a mission statement, descriptions of individual branches, a searchable publications database, an online newsletter, fellowships and other position postings, and research resources.

Division of Clinical Sciences ○ ○ ○

http://www-dcs.nci.nih.gov

The Division of Clinical Sciences site offers news and events notices, a research directory, information on joining National Institutes of Health (NIH) clinical trials, and descriptions of internal branches. Visitors can also employ a search tool for keyword searches.

Extramural Research ○ ○ ○

http://www.nci.nih.gov/hpage/extra.htm

This site offers information about extramural research efforts (through grants, cooperative agreements, and contracts awarded to institutions of higher education, governmental organizations, nonprofit research organizations, for-profit organizations, and individuals). NCI-supported extramural research is represented by the following programs:

- Biometric Research Branch
- Cancer Diagnosis Program
- Cancer Therapy Evaluation Program
- Developmental Therapeutics Program
- Diagnostic Imaging Program
- Division of Cancer Biology
- Division of Cancer Control and Population Sciences
- Division of Cancer Prevention
- Cancer Centers Program
- Training/Cancer Education
- Division of Extramural Activities
- Biostatistics
- The National Five-A-Day for Better Health Program
- Surveillance, Epidemiology, and End Results Program (SEER)

Research at the National Cancer Institute (NCI) ◎ ◎ ◎

http://www.nci.nih.gov/intra/intra.htm

This site provides information about research at NCI, with links to the three research divisions within the Institute, including the Division of Basic Sciences, the Division of Cancer Epidemiology and Genetics, and the Division of Clinical Sciences. Links to specific Internet sites of interest to investigators are offered at the site, including biosciences resources, cytokine resources, electronic journals, immunology resources, laboratory animal resources, laboratory safety information, library resources, molecular biology and sequence analysis resources, molecular modeling resources, NIH intramural research news, NIH special interest groups, PCR resources, meeting information, and information on biomedical suppliers.

Research Awards and Grants

Funding Opportunities ◎ ◎ ◎

http://deainfo.nci.nih.gov/funding.htm

Funding Opportunities are presented at this site, including news items, special National Cancer Institute (NCI) initiatives, and a listing of advisory boards and groups. Researchers interested in grants and contracts resources will find extramural research notices, recently cleared concepts, grant guidelines and descriptions, suggestions for preparing grant applications, a description of the grants review process, a link to research contracts management, policies, research resources, National Insitutes of Health (NIH) guide for grants and contracts, and contact information. Requests for grants applications, program announcements, and requests for proposals are available. Links to additional funding resources are provided at the site.

6. BIOLOGICAL, DIAGNOSTIC, AND THERAPEUTIC ASPECTS OF ONCOLOGY

6.1 **Principles of Cancer Cell Biology**

Cell Biology Tutorials

Biology Project ◎ ◎ ◎
http://www.biology.arizona.edu

Produced by the University of Arizona, the Biology Project is an online interactive resource for learning biology. It includes tutorials on biochemistry, cell biology, chemicals and human health, developmental biology, human biology, immunology, Mendelian genetics, and molecular biology.

Cell and Molecular Biology Online ◎ ◎ ◎
http://www.cellbio.com

Cell and Molecular Biology Online is a valuable directory of Internet resources related to these sciences. Visitors will find links to recommended Web sites, online publications, protocols and methods sources, and laboratory home pages highlighting current research. Educational resources found through the site include general information sources, online courses and texts, images and videos, and miscellaneous interesting biology sites. Career resources, professional societies, conference information sources, and sites providing grant information are also accessible through this site.

General Biology ◎ ◎ ◎
http://schmidel.com/bionet/biology.htm

A guide to the best biology and chemistry educational resources on the Internet, this site provides links to tutorials on cell biology, microbiology, antibiotic-resistant microbes, vaccines, and virology.

MIT Biology Hypertextbook ◎ ◎ ◎
http://esg-www.mit.edu:8001/esgbio

Written by the experimental study group at Massachusetts Institute of Technology, this site is a virtual textbook on biology. The table of contents includes an introduction, textbook chapters, a searchable index, and practice problems. There are chapters on chemistry, large molecules, cell biology, enzyme biochemistry, glycolysis and the Krebs cycle, photosynthesis, Mendelian genetics, central dogma, prokaryotic genetics, recombinant DNA, and immunology.

Signal Transduction

Signal Transduction ⊙ ⊙ ⊙
http://www.med.unibs.it/~marchesi/signal.html

This very technical tutorial on signal transduction in cells is geared for researchers and medical professionals. It covers mechanisms of signal transduction and the different classifications of signal transducing receptors. Special sections cover Receptor and Nonreceptor Tyrosine Kinases; Receptor and Nonreceptor Serine/Threonine Kinases; Phospholipases and Phospholipids in Signal Transduction; G-Protein Coupled Receptors; G-Protein Regulators; Intercellular Hormone Receptors; and Phosphatases in Signal Transduction.

Signal Transduction ⊙ ⊙ ⊙
http://ncmi.bioch.bcm.tmc.edu/~twensel/glec99/sld001.htm

Through a presentation of 23 slides, the viewer will learn or review the process of how cells handle information about the outside world in the process of signal transduction. The tutorial is quite technical, with charts and explanations of each mechanism.

Signal Transduction in Cancer ⊙ ⊙ ⊙
http://intouch.cancernetwork.com/canmed/Ch004/004-0.htm

This excellent chapter from Yusuf Hannun's book, Cancer Medicine, provides a complete description of cellular signal transduction, the process of oncogenesis and signal transduction. The discussion includes anti-oncogenes and cell regulation, tumor promoters and signal transduction, viruses and oncogenesis, metastasis and signal transduction, and implications for treatments.

Cancer Biology Tutorials and Resources

Biomedical Research: Cancer and the Cell Cycle ⊙ ⊙
http://www.hhmi.org/communic/annrep/research/start.htm

The Chief Scientific Officer of the Howard Hughes Medical Institute has prepared a readable and useful description of cancer cell operations, including oncogenes and tumor suppressors, regulating the cell cycle, the Rb pathway, the P53 molecule, programmed cell death, and treatment/prevention.

Cancer Biology Lectures and Laboratory ⊙ ⊙ ⊙
http://www.pathology.pitt.edu/lectures/mjb/index02.html-ssi

Dr. Michael J. Becich of the Department of Pathology at the University of Pittsburgh Medical Center is responsible for the information on this valuable site. The cancer biology lectures deal with the following topics: basic structural histology; introduction to neoplasia and altered growth; carcinogenesis, progression, and detection of cancer; and a laboratory where slides are displayed online.

Cancer Cell Biology ☉ ☉ ☉
http://www.esb.utexas.edu/palmer/bio303/group7/CancerTwo.html

This educational site associated with an undergraduate biology course at the University of Texas, Structure and Function of Organisms, offers detailed information on cancer and cancer cell biology. Information covers risk factors and prevention, neoplastic conversion, clonal evolution, and metastasis. Nonprofessionals might find the site useful for minimally technical information on the mechanisms of cancer. A short glossary of terms, a bibliography of information sources, and many suggested site addresses for additional resources are available at this site.

Carcinogenesis: A Cancer Biology Lecture ☉ ☉ ☉
http://www.ooo.dent.umich.edu/ooo/neolecII/index.htm

In this 18-slide tutorial from the University of Michigan, Professor Peter Polverini explores the subject of cancer biology step by step, with the following topics: initiating agents, mutations of cancer cells, oncogenes, tumor-suppressor genes, protein products of tumor suppressor genes, and the consequences of oncogene activation and tumor suppressor gene inactivation in cancer.

Dr. Horowitz' Cancer Lectures ☉ ☉ ☉
http://134.197.54.100/teaching/cellbiology/cancer/index.htm

Authored by Dr. Burton Horowitz, this site contains the slides presented in his class. The user can either go through the slides from beginning to end or use the Table of Contents to choose a particular slide. The topics on the Table of Contents include: Squamous cell carcinoma; stages in tumor growth and metastasis; stages in the establishment of a cell culture; classes of oncogenes; autocrine induction of tumor-cell growth; creation of oncogenes from proto-oncogenes; checkpoints in the cell cycle; list of representative oncogenes; kinetics of tumor appearance in transgenic mice; response of permissive and nonpermissive cells to viral infection; genetic elements of a retroviral genome; the formation of a transducing retrovirus.

Kimball's Biology Pages: Table of Contents ☉ ☉ ☉
http://www.excited.com/~jkimball/BiologyPages/T/TOC.html

In-depth descriptions of terms related to cancer, cell biology, and other topics are offered. Full-page discussions of a concept are available in most cases, and links are offered to related terms. Terms include mutations, oncogenes, tumor suppressor genes, apoptosis, cell specific gene expression, intermediary metabolism, and other related concepts.

M. D. Anderson Cancer Center: Department of Cell Biology ◎ ◎ ◎

http://research.mdacc.tmc.edu/~resrep/2/08CellZ.html

A general discussion of the nature of cancer cell biology and immunology at this site is followed by a description of research interests within the Department and a faculty and staff listing. Specific research interests, biographies, and publications bibliographies of faculty members are also available.

Genetics of Cancer

Cancer Genetics Tutorial ◎ ◎ ◎

http://www.muc.edu/bi/bi102/CANCER/tsld002.htm

This is a basic tutorial on cancer genetics, covering the topics of tumors and cancers; predisposition to cancer; tumor suppressor genes; oncogenes; chromosome aberrations; and environmental factors and cancer. It is presented through the use of slides, headings, and explanations.

Cancer Genome Anatomy Project (CGAP) ◎ ◎ ◎

http://www.ncbi.nlm.nih.gov/CGAP

A technical research and study site, the Cancer Genome Anatomy Project presentation addresses efforts to decipher the molecular anatomy of the cancer cell. The Web site offers a menu of major links to cDNA Libraries, cDNA Clone Resources, a Tumor Suppressor and Oncogene Directory, Chromosome Breakpoint Map, and Gene Expression Profiles. The CGAP project is a major initiative of the National Institutes of Health (NIH).

Genetics of Cancer ◎ ◎ ◎

http://www.cancergenetics.org/sitemap.htm

The table of contents on this page directs the visitor to an excellent discussion of the genetics of cancer, including an overview, proto-oncogenes and oncogenes; tumor-suppressor genes; DNA repair genes; genes, cell-cycle clock and cancer; and environment-gene interactions. There is a second excellent tutorial on the Basics of Molecular Genetics, along with a useful section presenting Case Studies of different forms of cancer. Finally, there is a Genetic Counseling Section and Risk Management Section, as well as a site search engine for topics.

Oncogenesis

Cell Growth Control and Oncogenesis ⊙ ⊙ ⊙
http://dio.cnb.uam.es/Informacion/Ann_CNB_98/AR9819.htm

This series of eleven technical research reports examines tumor progression, molecular mechanisms in angiogenesis, regulation and function of specific tumor suppressors, and cell cycle control.

Genetic Basis for Oncogenesis ⊙ ⊙ ⊙
http://parasite.arf.ufl.edu/path/teach/vem5131/publish/ve00017.htm

Dr. David Allred in the Department of Pathobiology at the University of Florida has provided a very informative lecture outline, beginning with very basic definitions and explanations, and moving through the more complex elements of cancer biology, including mechanisms of transformation involving oncogenes, transformations involving tumor suppressor genes, and cell cycle control genes. There are also links to a glossary of molecular biology terms and other Internet sites related to cancer.

Oncogenes and Proto-Oncogenes ⊙ ⊙ ⊙
http://www.cancergenetics.org/onco.htm

Produced by the Robert H. Lurie Comprehensive Cancer Center of Northwestern University, this site is a tutorial on oncogenes and proto-oncogenes. The site provides a general overview and definitions of oncogenes and proto-oncogenes. There is a discussion of the signaling process, the activation of proto-oncogenes, functional characteristics, and examples of oncogenes. The text contains hyperlinks to detailed discussions of terms within the tutorial.

Oncogenes Tutorial ⊙ ⊙
http://views.vcu.edu/ana/OB/oncogenes

Utilizing 27 slides, this tutorial provides a detailed overview of the subjects of oncogenes, proto-oncogenes, mutational mechanisms, and growth factor signaling. It is technical in nature, designed for medical students or healthcare professionals who seek a greater understanding of cancer cell biology.

Oncogenesis ⊙ ⊙ ⊙
http://biology.indstate.edu/prentice/meded/biochem/Oncogenesis_files/slide0022.htm

Dr. David Prentice at Indiana State University has prepared an informative presentation exploring oncogenesis in 25 slides, with an outline and definition of terms, components, and processes. The slides cover cellular transformation, non-genetic and genetic causes, DNA and RNA tumor viruses, proto-oncogenes, signal transduction, tumor suppressors, cel lcycle control proteins, and the ultimate process of oncogenesis.

Oncogenesis and the Cell Cycle ⊗ ⊗ ⊗
http://testzygote.swarthmore.edu/cleave6.html

This Swarthmore College tutorial examines the cell cycle, mutations in its components, and different types of oncogenes. The discussion involves viral oncogenes, oncogenes that mimic growth factors, such as the v-sis oncogene, the oncogene that involves cytoplasmic signal transduction pathway proteins, and a fourth type that involves transcription factors. Additional information is provided on tumor suppressor factors.

Proto-oncogenes and Cancer ⊗ ⊗ ⊗
http://www.dentistry.leeds.ac.uk/biochem/thcme/oncogene.html

Provided by the Terre Haute Center for Medical Education, this site provides a tutorial on proto-oncogenes and cancer. There is an introduction and sections on viruses and cancer and classifications of proto-oncogenes, including growth factors, receptor tyrosine kinases, membrane associated non-receptor tyrosine kinases, g-protein coupled receptors, and membrane associated g-proteins.

Proto-oncogenes and Cancer ⊗ ⊗ ⊗
http://www-isu.indstate.edu/thcme/mwking/oncogene.html

This eight-page Indiana State tutorial was developed by Michael W. King, Ph.D. in the Medical Biochemistry Division of the Terre Haute Center for Medical Education. It explores cancer cell biology and genetics, including proto-oncogenes and oncogenes, viruses and cancer, classifications of proto-oncogenes, and hereditary cancer syndromes. The latter information is set forth in a useful chart of syndromes, cloned genes, function, chromosomal location, and tumor types.

Tumor Suppressor Genes

Oncogenes and Tumor Suppressor Genes ⊗ ⊗ ⊗
http://views.vcu.edu/ana/OB/cytology/sld001.htm

This slide presentation was written by Oliver Bogler, Ph.D. It discusses growth factor signaling and oncogenes, the cell cycle and tumor suppressor genes, p53, and cancer as a disease caused by multiple mutations. The slides provide graphic illustrations.

Oncogenes and Tumor Suppressor Genes ⊗ ⊗ ⊗
http://www.epsilon-assoc.com/~jkimball/BiologyPages/O/Oncogenes.html

Professor John Kimball provides a useful tutorial on the subjects of Oncogenes and Tumor-Suppressor Genes. He discusses the signals for normal mitosis, growth factors, the role of oncogenes in converting normal cells into cancer cells, and mutations that convert proto-oncogenes into oncogenes. The second part of the tutorial explores the role of tumor suppressor genes in inhibiting mitosis of cancer cells. In addition, there is a discussion of the process of mitosis.

Oncogenes, Suppressor Genes, and Cell Cycle Control ⊙ ⊙ ⊙

http://www.igm.cnrs-mop.fr/anglais/oncogenesandcell.html

This site provides links to current projects and research on topics related to oncogenes, suppressor genes, and cell cycle control. Topics include nuclear oncogenes and cell cycle effectors, intracellular signaling and gene regulation, recombinant retroviruses and oncogenes, and many others. The principal researcher is listed.

Tumor Suppressor Genes: Description and Examples ⊙ ⊙ ⊙

http://www.cancergenetics.org/tsg.htm

Addressing the genetics of cancer, this site provides an informative discussion of tumor suppressor genes, including their characteristics, along with examples of specific tumor suppressor genes, including DPC-4 (involved in pancreatic cancer); NF-1 (involved with the nervous system and myeloid leukemia); the NF-2 gene (involved in several nervous system cancers); as well as the RB, p53, WT1, BRCA1, and BRAC2 genes. Though technical in nature, the tutorial is very readable for all levels of readers.

Invasion and Metastasis

Cancer Invasion and Metastasis ⊙ ⊙ ⊙

http://www.path.sunysb.edu/courses/im/default.htm

This is a highly informative, 11-page tutorial covering steps in cancer metastasis, experimental models of cancer invasion, cell adhesion and migration, extracellular matric, proteolytic enzymes, plasminogen activators, MMMPs, tissue inhibitors, tumor angiogenesis, and metastatic genes. It is quite technical in nature, and is not appropriate for the general reader, but is a solid review for medical students and health professionals interested in cancer cell biology.

Invasion and Metastasis ⊙ ⊙ ⊙

http://www.vetmed.lsu.edu/oncology/inv,met/index.htm

From Louisiana State University, this informative tutorial by Antonio Correa covers this central theme of cancer cell biology, with slides on routes of metastatic spread, metastatic cascade, angiogenesis, detachment, invasion, evasion of hose defense, arrest, attachment, extravasation, new growth, and a repetition of the process. The presentation consists of 25 slides.

Angiogenesis

Angiogenesis ⊙ ⊙ ⊙
http://vl.bwh.harvard.edu/angiogenesis.shtml

Part of the World Wide Web Virtual Library of Cell Biology, this site contains links to other sites and articles related to angiogenesis. There are also links to labs studying angiogenesis.

Angiogenesis Factors in Cancer, AIDS, and Diabetes ⊙ ⊙ ⊙
http://zygote.swarthmore.edu/mesend3b.html

Part of Zygote, a virtual library of developmental biology, this site is a tutorial on angiogenesis factors in cancer, AIDS, and diabetes. The detailed information includes diagrams, charts, and illustrations. There is an extensive list of references.

Angiogenesis Facts ⊙ ⊙ ⊙
http://www.angio.org/mainintroangio.htm

Produced by the Angiogenesis Foundation, this site contains well-organized facts about angiogenesis. Information includes scientific facts, the number of cancer patients who might benefit from antiangiogenic therapy, the role of the biotechnology and pharmaceutical industry, antiangiogenic drugs in clinical trials, the community leading antiangiogenic therapy development, and the role of the Angiogenesis Foundation.

Special Project Angiogenesis ⊙ ⊙ ⊙
http://www.med.unibs.it/~airc/links.html

Special Project Angiogenesis contains links to vascular biology societies, biotech companies, angiogenesis companies, and related Web sites. Vascular biology societies include the Australian Vascular Biology Society, the British Microcirculation Society, the Microcirculatory Society, and the North American Vascular Biology Organization.

6.2 Cancer and the Immune System

The Immune System

B Cells and T Cells ⊙ ⊙ ⊙
http://www.epsilon-assoc.com/~jkimball/BiologyPages/B/B_and_Tcells.html

This site offers a tutorial on B lymphocytes and T lymphocytes. There is a hyperlink to a drawing showing the organs of the immune system. There are also hyperlinks to definitions of terms used in the text and detailed discussions of particular topics.

Topics include antigen-presenting cells, helper T cells, and antigen receptor diversity. The site provides illustrative diagrams and pictures.

Characteristics of the Immune System ☼ ☼ ☼
http://www.biology.ualberta.ca/courses.hp/zoo242/belosevic/lecoverheads/sld001.htm

Prepared as a biology tutorial at the University of Alberta in Canada, this comprehensive slide presentation covers the nature of the immune system, including specificity, mobility, replicability, cooperation, compartments, and memory. All of the terms are clearly defined and the mechanisms of immunity are explored in 53 slides.

General Immunology Tutorial ☼ ☼ ☼
http://www.cehs.siu.edu/fix/medmicro/genimm.htm

Providing a clear overview of immune response, the author of this tutorial, Douglas Fix, uses several charts and tables to explain host defense mechanisms, with definitions of terms and identification of the specific cells and tissues involved in the immune response.

Hematopoietic Stem Cells:
An Introduction to Immunology Tutorial ☼
http://www.biology.arizona.edu/immunology/tutorials/immunology/page2.html

Using color graphics, this tutorial provides an introduction to the immune system, beginning with an explanation of hemotopoietic stem cells. This is a basic description for students who wish to begin a study of cancer cell biology.

Immune System and Cancer ☼ ☼ ☼
http://rex.nci.nih.gov/PATIENTS/INFO_TEACHER/bookshelf/NIH_immune/index.html

The National Cancer Institute, a division of the NIH, has produced this excellent tutorial, which clearly explains the nature and operation of the immune system. It covers the Nature of Genes, the Anatomy of the Immune System, Cells and Secretions of the Immune System, Mounting an Immune Response, Immunity, Disorders of the Immune System, Bone Marrow Transplants, Immunity and Cancer, and many other topics, including frontiers in research on immunity.

Immune System Slide Tutorial ☼ ☼ ☼
http://des.sw.cc.va.us/vatnp/courses/Materials/Hematology/sld002.htm

Through 26 slides, this educational presentation explores the components and mechanisms of the immune system. The tutorial covers human leukocyte antigens; the organization of the immune system; antibody-mediated immunity; cell-mediated immunity; inflammation; neutrophils, macrophages, basophils, and eosinphils and phagocytosis; and cell types in cell-mediated immunity, cell types and roles, and cytokines.

Leukocytes, Lymphocytes, and Plasma Cells: A Lecture ◎ ◎
http://www.mpcc.cc.ne.us/steinbeck/hematology/lec013.html

In outline form, this lecture/tutorial provides information on anatomical origin and development of lymphocytes and morphological characteristics of normal lymphocytes. The cell descriptors would be of interest to technically-trained professionals or researchers or medical students.

Normal Lymphocytes ◎ ◎
http://www.tmc.tulane.edu/classware/pathology/krause/blood/lymphocytes.html

With full-color slides, this Tulane University tutorial explores the nature of normal lymphocytes and their role in the immune system. The discussion encompasses both T lymphocytes (helpers, killers, suppressors) and B lymphocytes (antibody production). The viewer can obtain further information about plasma cells and about lymphocyte development by clicking on the underscored terms.

T Cell Classification ◎ ◎ ◎
http://sprojects.mmip.mcgill.ca/immunology/spec_imm_cells.htm

This tutorial describes the classification of T cells, illustrated with a diagram. The site also provides a discussion of T cell development and antigen recognition.

University of Newcastle upon Tyne:
Cancer Immunology and Immunotherapy ◎ ◎ ◎
http://www.ncl.ac.uk/child-health/guides/clinks4i.htm

This British Web site serves as a guide to Internet resources related to cancer immunology and immunotherapy. Links are available to sites specific to immunology, antigens, Prostate Specific Antigen (PSA), and mucin antibody (MUC1). Academic departments, laboratories, research institutes, government resources, news groups, other information sources, and automatic MEDLINE searches are accessible here. The site presents both general links and those appropriate only for health professionals.

Cell-Mediated Immunity

Cell-Mediated Immunity ◎ ◎ ◎
http://ntri.tamuk.edu/immunology/cmediated.html

Norma Laurel of the Natural Toxins Research Initiative at Texas A&M University has prepared an extensive graphic depiction of cell-mediated immune responses. This seven-page technical tutorial illustrates the chain reaction of events during the process of cell differentiation.

Cytotoxic T Cells

Glossary on Cytotoxic T Cells ◎ ◎ ◎

http://www.winabc.org/glossary.html

Provided by the Women's Information Network Against Breast Cancer, this site contains a glossary of terms related to cytotoxic T cells. The terms may be accessed alphabetically.

6.3 Cancer Causes and Risk Factors

Cancer Causes, Screening, and Prevention ◎ ◎ ◎

http://cancer.med.upenn.edu/causeprevent

Part of OncoLink, this site will provide customized cancer screening and early detection reminders via e-mail. The site currently provides links to articles on the following topics: smoking, tobacco, and cancer; screening and prevention of cancer; drugs and cancer; environmental factors and cancer; diet and cancer; genetics and cancer; hormones and cancer; and cancer epidemiology.

Carcinogenic Chemical and Physical Agents ◎ ◎

http://www.uia.org/uiademo/pro/d1239.htm

Focusing on carcinogenic chemical and physical agents, this site offers information on the possible incidence of cancer from environmental causes, including a listing of key causative factors and discussion of chemical and industrial process risks to humans.

Causes of Cancer from OncoLink ◎ ◎ ◎

http://www.oncolink.org/causeprevent

This site index provides articles and links related to different actual and possible causes of cancer, including environmental risks (agent orange, asbestos exposure, second hand smoke, radon risk, pollution, and electromagnetic fields), smoking and tobacco, drugs, diet, genetics, and hormones. It represents a useful survey of these topics with links to studies and government information.

Center for Research on Environmental Disease (CRED) ◎ ◎ ◎

http://sciencepark.mdanderson.org/cred

Funded by the federal government, CRED studies the effect of environmental factors in the cause of human disease, and examines methods of detection, prevention, and control of environmentally-related diseases. Because cancer has been connected with certain environmental conditions, such as site toxicity, this center offers important prospects for establishing links between causes and effects. The site presents the research programs of the Center related to chemical disposition and toxicity, mechanisms of DNA damage and mutagenesis, environmental influences on cell growth and differentiation, and nutrition and disease prevention.

Genetics, Causes, Risk Factors, and Prevention ⊚ ⊚ ⊚

http://cancernet.nci.nih.gov/prevention/risk.shtml

Cancer causes and risk factors are examined at this section of the National Cancer Institute (NCI) site, including food, genetics, hormonal factors, smoking, workplace and environment factors, and other causes and risks. There is information on human papillomaviruses, stress factors, carcinogenicity tests, vasectomy risks, and abnormal moles.

Risk Factors for Cancer ⊚ ⊚ ⊚

http://www.graylab.ac.uk/cancerweb/causes.html

Fifty (50) separate links at this site provide information on environmental exposure, genetic influences, chemical carcinogens, radiation, electromagnetic fields, psychological stress, and numerous other possible risk factors for cancer. This is a substantial resource on the subject for health professionals, medical students, and researchers.

6.4 Screening and Prevention

Alternative Cancer Research Foundation—Prevention ⊚ ⊚

http://www.acrf.ca/acrf.html

Created by the Alternative Cancer Research Foundation, this site offers strategies for cancer prevention. Preventative measures discussed include avoiding pollution, following a beneficial diet, consuming antioxidants, using essential fatty acids, boosting the immune system, avoiding stress, consuming herbs and enzymes, exercising, detoxifying the body, and choosing recommended cancer screening methods.

American Institute for Cancer Research (AICR) ⊚ ⊚ ⊚

http://www.aicr.org

The American Institute for Cancer Research is the country's leading charity in the field of diet, nutrition, and cancer prevention. Their site provides links to articles about soy research and fad diets. There is a link to the Institute's CancerResource, a free information program to answer patient questions. There is an international perspective on food, nutrition, and the prevention of cancer and links to news updates on the topic. There are also links to recent books on the prevention of cancer.

Cancer Prevention and Early Detection ◎ ◎

http://www.narti.com/prevention.html

Provided by the Northwest Arkansas Radiation Therapy Institute, this article provides tips for men and women on the prevention and detection of cancer.

Cancer Screening Tests by Type of Cancer ◎ ◎ ◎

http://cancernet.nci.nih.gov/testing.html

The National Cancer Institute provides detailed information on the screening of many individual types of cancer. Screening information is provided for 13 forms of cancer.

National Cancer Institute Prevention and Control ◎ ◎ ◎

http://www.graylab.ac.uk/cancernet/600045.html

Produced by the National Cancer Institute, this site provides highlights of the Institute's prevention and control programs. These programs include diet and nutrition, smoking cessation, chemoprevention, early detection and screening, and clinical trials for cancer prevention. There is also information about the Cancer Information Service provided by the National Cancer Institute, and there are links to related sites.

Prevention and Early Detection ◎ ◎ ◎

http://www2.cancer.org/prevention/index.cfm

Provided by the American Cancer Association, this site gives information about the prevention and early detection of cancer. There is a lengthy discussion of nutrition and its importance in cancer prevention. There is also general information about cancer screening and specific information about detection of a number of cancers including breast cancer, cervical cancer, anal cancer, child leukemia, liver cancer, and many others. There is also information about environmental cancer risks.

6.5 Symptoms, Side Effects, and Complications

CancerFatigue.org ◎ ◎

http://www.cancerfatigue.org

CancerFatigue.org provides guidance on coping with fatigue from the Oncology Nursing Society. The Web site has a menu of topics that include causes and effects of fatigue and ways of dealing with reduced energy levels. Information is geared to patients and their families.

Clinical Complications Arising from Malignancy ◎ ◎

http://www.merck.com/pubs/mmanual/section11/chapter142/142a.htm

The Merck Manual chapter on General Cancer offers a section that outlines a number of major clinical complications arising from malignancy, including cardiac tamponade, pain, paraneoplastic syndromes, hematologic paraneoplastic syndromes, rental paraneoplastic syndrome, pigmented skin lesions, and other complications. The Manual can be consulted online at this site for further information and references to appropriate chapters.

Coping with Cancer ☼ ☼ ☼

http://cancernet.nci.nih.gov/coping.html

Cancer symptoms and treatment side effects are the subjects of this portion of CancerNet at the National Cancer Institute (NCI). Side effects include fatigue, fever, chills, sweats, nausea, and vomiting. Complications cover hypercalcemia, pain, and sleep disorders. Under emotional concerns, the presentation explores anxiety, depression, loss, grief, and bereavement. Finally, nutrition and eating hints are discussed, along with marijuana use in supportive care. Support group and caregiver resources, along with transitional care are a key part of the site as well.

Living with Cancer ☼ ☼ ☼

http://www2.cancer.org/patientGuides/livingGo.html

Ten major topics and issues are explored at this important site dealing with life issues as a cancer patient. They include disabilities, pain, grief and loss, diet and nutrition, drug and alcohol abuse, hospice care, religion and faith, job rehabilitation, marriage problems, and sexual issues.

Oral Complications of Cancer Treatment ☼ ☼

http://www.aerie.com/nohicweb/campaign

A comprehensive Web site on the subject of oral complications of cancer treatment, this resource covers types of complications; treatment, radiation and chemotherapy and oral effects; the role of dental care; and reference information for patients. Inflammation, infection, dental decay, taste alterations, and other oral effects are explained.

United Ostomy Association (UOA) ☼ ☼

http://www.uoa.org

A volunteer-based organization, the UOA provides education, information, support, and advocacy for people with intestinal or urinary diversions. The Web site provides information on the organization's activities, chapters, membership, and programs. There is a glossary of ostomy terms, supply information, an FAQ section, related sites, and conference and event information.

6.6 **Genetics and Hereditary Cancer**

Cancer Genetics ⚙ ⚙ ⚙

http://www.cancergenetics.org

This site was created to provide primary care physicians, other medical professionals, and the general public with clinical and basic information on cancer, genetics, and the role of genetics in causing cancer. Pages devoted to information for primary care physicians include discussions of the genetics of cancer, basics of molecular genetics, the genetic basis of disease, and genetic counseling. Information for other medical professionals is presented in the form of 11 case studies in inherited cancers and genetic screening. One case study describes the genetic component of breast cancer and genetic counseling for this disease. Visitors to this site can also search the site for specific information, find links to related sites, and access contact information for the organization.

Cancer Genetics Network at the National Cancer Institute ⚙ ⚙

http://www-dccps.ims.nci.nih.gov/CGN

A new initiative of the National Cancer Institute, the Cancer Genetics Network will be a series of centers specializing in the study of inherited predisposition to cancer, in collaboration with other major research institutions. The site discusses the aims and objectives of the new program and provides a listing of the Network Member Facilities.

Cancer Genetics Overview ⚙ ⚙

http://cancernet.nci.nih.gov/clinpdq/cancer_genetics/Cancer_genetics.html

Through this site, the National Cancer Institute (NCI) provides a thorough overview of cancer genetics, including discussion of terms; cancer susceptibility; evaluation of evidence of hereditary factors; the clinical value of genetic testing and family history collection; and genetic counseling, screening, and prevention. There is a bibliography of current reports and documents on the subject of cancer and genetics.

Cancer Risk Assessment and Counseling ⚙ ⚙

http://www.dnai.com/~ptkelly

A medical geneticist, Patricia Kelly, Ph.D. has provided a useful site on cancer risk issues, including discussion of specific areas of genetic risk. The presentation is a balanced view of hereditary vs. nonhereditary factors in the cause of cancer. The focus of the site is on breast and ovarian cancer, although general cancer susceptibility is discussed.

Characteristics of Hereditary Cancer ⦿ ⦿ ⦿

http://www.familycancer.org

This important site deals with family history of breast and ovarian cancer and genetic testing. The site offers a discussion menu on many aspects of the hereditary cancer topic, including the relevance of family history and its impact on diagnosis, risks based upon family history, genetic testing, and genetic counseling. There are a number of beneficial links to other Internet resources for the visitor as well. A section of the site addresses healthcare professionals, and focuses on the same subjects from a professional and clinical point of view.

Hereditary Cancer Prevention Newsletter ⦿ ⦿

http://medicine.creighton.edu/medschool/PrevMed/NewsLet-1.html

The Hereditary Cancer Prevention Clinic at Creighton University in Omaha, Nebraska provides a thorough review of hereditary aspects of cancer, including features of hereditary cancer, evaluation and screening, clinical evaluation, genetic counseling, and other related topics. The Clinic provides a source of additional information on this subject, and maintains a number of sites devoted to hereditary cancer.

National Human Genome Research Institute (NHGRI) ⦿ ⦿ ⦿

http://www.nhgri.nih.gov/Data

An extraordinarily important research initiative, the Institute has gathered together information on genomic and genetic resources on the World Wide Web including genome mapping databases, sequence databases, structure databases, genome centers, chromosome maps, medical genetics, and selected journals.

6.7 Diagnostic Procedures

General Resources

Cancer Tests ⦿ ⦿

http://medweb.bham.ac.uk/Cancerhelp/public/about/tests/index.html

The useful site provides an overview of five major types of cancer tests, including a CT (computed tomography) scan, an MRI (magnetic resonance imaging) scan, ultrasound scan, a bone scan, and a proton emission tomography (PET) scan. Each test is thoroughly explained with text and images.

Cancer Tests for Women Age 65 and Older ◎ ◎

http://www.healthtouch.com/level1/leaflets/nci/nci111.htm

Provided by the National Cancer Institute, this information sets forth questions and answers about cancer tests, including reasons, types, and procedures.

Cancer Tests You Should Know About ◎ ◎

http://wwww.bjcohen.com/annex/library/cic/X0008_cantests.txt.html

A guide for general examination for cancer, the information at this site covers the process of cancer testing and standard types of tests, including mammograms, breast exams, breast self-exams, pelvic exams, rectal exams, and stool tests. Frequency of tests is identified, along with a classification of tests according to cancer types.

Merck Manual of Diagnosis and Therapy ◎ ◎ ◎

http://www.merck.com/pubs/mmanual/section11/sec11.htm

One of the most reliable reference tools for physicians and healthcare professionals is the *Merck Manual of Diagnosis and Therapy*. This site provides online access to sections of this important book related to diagnosis and therapy, covering all types of disorders. The chapters on hematology/oncology are especially relevant, as are portions of many of the other chapters devoted to body systems and disorders. By clicking on "Hematology/Oncology" in this menu of information, the visitor will gain access to focused material on the diagnostic avenues in cancer.

Testing for Cancer ◎ ◎ ◎

http://cancernet.nci.nih.gov/testing.html

Testing information by type of cancer is provided at the NCI site, along with a description of various types of tests, cancer genetics, the role of clinical trials, and statistical sources. Physical examinations and cancer genetic testing are discussed as well.

Types of Cancer Imaging ◎ ◎ ◎

http://www.bristol-myers.com/well/cgda03a.html

This site provides a brief description of the following types of cancer imaging techniques: X-rays, computerized axial tomography, magnetic resonance imaging, ultrasound and sonography, and nuclear scanning.

Biopsy, General

All–important Skin Biopsy ⦿ ⦿
http://www.skincancerinfo.com/sectionb/biopsy.html
Written by Paul J. Weber, M.D., P.A., this site is a tutorial for patients undergoing diagnostic biopsy for suspected skin cancer. The site contains hyperlinks to definitions of terms used in the text. There are pictures and diagrams.

Biopsy Report: A Patient's Guide ⦿ ⦿ ⦿
http://cancerguide.org/pathology.html
These comprehensive report for patients outlines all aspects of biopsies, including types, specimen processing, and pathologic examination. There is also a convenient glossary of important diagnostic terms that would appear in a biopsy report.

Biopsy: Research the Options ⦿ ⦿ ⦿
http://www.breastbiopsy.com/fna1.html
This site provides patient education about biopsy procedures used to diagnose breast cancer. There is information about fine-needle aspiration, advanced breast biopsy instrumentation, core-needle biopsy, open excisional surgical biopsy, and vacuum-assisted biopsy. Each section provides illustrations, diagrams, and hyperlinks to definitions of terms within the text.

Bone-Marrow Aspiration and Biopsy

Bone-Marrow Aspiration and Biopsy ⦿ ⦿ ⦿
http://www.mdadvice.com/library/test/medtest109.html
Part of MDAdvice.com, this site provides a profile of bone-marrow aspiration and biopsy. It includes information about why and where the test is performed, and who performs it. There are sections on risks and precautions and patient preparation. Information about the test itself includes sensory factors, equipment used, and a description of the test. There is information about post-test care, activity after the test, and test results.

Breast Thermography

Breast Thermography ⦿ ⦿ ⦿
http://www.mdadvice.com/library/test/medtest113.html
Part of MDAdvice.com, this site profiles breast thermography. The profile includes information about materials studied, patient time for the test, estimated cost of the

test, and material studied. There is information about why and where the test is performed and who performs it. Information about the test includes sensory factors, equipment, and a description of the test. There is information about post-test care and activity, and test results.

Bronchography

Bronchography ✪ ✪ ✪
http://www.mdadvice.com/library/test/medtest114.html

Part of MDAdvice.com, this site provides a profile of bronchography. It also includes information about why the test is performed, where it is performed, and who performs it. There is a discussion of risks and precautions and patient preparation. There is also information about the test itself, the equipment used, post-test care, and the test results.

Broncoscopy

Broncoscopy ✪ ✪ ✪
http://www.mdadvice.com/library/test/medtest115.html

This site provides a profile of broncoscopy from MDAdvice.com. It also includes information about why the test is performed, where it is performed, and who performs it. There is a discussion of risks and precautions and patient preparation. There is also information about the test itself, the equipment used, post-test care, and the test results.

Colonoscopy

Colonoscopy ✪ ✪ ✪
http://www.mdadvice.com/library/test/medtest134.html

Part of MDAdvice.com, this site provides a profile of colonoscopy. The profile includes information about the category and subcategory of the test, reliability of the results, and estimated cost of the test. The purpose of the test is explained, along with a discussion of risks and precautions. There is information about patient preparation, the test itself, post-testing procedures and instructions, and the test results.

Computerized Axial Tomography

Computed Tomography of the Pancreas ☺ ☺ ☺
http://www.bewell.com/tests/test125.asp

Part of HealthGate, this site provides information about computed tomography of the pancreas. Information includes an estimated cost of the test, patient time for the test, reliability of results, and material studied. There is also information about the purpose for the test, where is is performed, who performs it, risks and precautions, patient preparation, sensory factors, equipment used, the test itself, after the test, and test results.

Computerized Axial Tomography ☺ ☺ ☺
http://www.medicinenet.com

Provided by MedicineNet.com, this site gives a brief overview of computerized axial tomography. Click on "Procedures and Tests" at the top of the home page, and select "CAT Scan." There is also information about the following topics: what a CAT scan is, why and how it is performed, risks involved, and preparation.

Indium Leukocyte Scan

Indium Leukocyte Scan ☺ ☺ ☺
http://www.healthgate.co.uk/dp/dph.0126.shtml

Intended for healthcare professionals, this site is part of HealthGate UK. It provides synonyms and a description for indium leukocyte scan. It includes information on indications, patient preparation, special instructions, causes for rejection, turnaround time, normal findings, limitations, and additional information. There are references included.

Laparoscopy

Laparoscopy ☺ ☺ ☺
http://www.bewell.com/tests/test209.asp

Provided by HealthGate, this site gives a profile of laparoscopy. Information includes the estimated cost of the test, how long it will take, and the reliability of the results. It also provides information about who performs the test, where and why it is performed, and possible risks. There is information about sensory factors of the test itself, and obtaining the results.

Liver Scan

Liver Scan ⚙ ⚙ ⚙
http://www.healthanswers.com/adam/top/view.asp?filename=003825.htm

This site, provided by HealthAnswers.com, contains information about liver scan. There is a list of alternative names and a definition of the procedure. There is information about how the test is performed, preparation required, how it will feel, associated risks, purpose for the test, normal and abnormal results, and cost of the test. There are also links to information about other tests that might be required to confirm the results of the liver scan.

Liver-Spleen Scanning ⚙ ⚙ ⚙
http://www.bewell.com/tests/test216.asp

Part of Healthgate, this site provides a profile of liver-spleen scanning. Included in the profile is the estimated cost of the test, patient time for the test, and the reliability of test results. There is information about where and why it is performed and who performed it. There is also a discussion of risks associated with the procedure. The test itself is discussed, as well as information about the test results.

Lung Biopsy

Lung Biopsy ⚙ ⚙ ⚙
http://www.mdadvice.com/library/test/medtest247.html

Part of MDAdvice.com, this site provides a profile of lung biopsy. It also includes information about why the test is performed, where it is performed, and who performs it. There is a discussion of risks and precautions and patient preparation. There is also information about the test itself, the equipment used, post-test care, and the test results.

Lymph-Node Biopsy

Lymph-Node Biopsy ⚙ ⚙ ⚙
http://www.mdadvice.com/library/test/medtest251.html

Part of MDAdvice.com, this site profiles of lymph-node biopsy. The profile includes material studied, estimated cost of the test, test reliability, and patient time for the test. There is information about the purpose of the test, sensory factors of the test itself, equipment used, and test results.

Lymphangiography

Lymphangiography ⚙ ⚙ ⚙

http://www.mdadvice.com/library/test/medtest252.html

Part of MDAdvice.com, this site provides a profile of lymphangiography. Information about why and where the test is performed is included. Risks and precautions, patient preparation, and the test itself are also discussed. There is information about post-test care and activity, and test results.

Magnetic Resonance Imaging

HealthAnswers MRI Fact Sheet ⚙ ⚙ ⚙

http://www.healthanswers.com/adam/top/view.asp?filename=003335.htm

Part of HealthAnswers.com, this site provides information about magnetic resonance imaging (MRI). It includes pictures, alternative names, and a definition of the procedure. There is information about how the test is performed, preparation required, how it will feel, and risks involved. There are also links to specific types of MRIs including chest MRI, abdominal MRI, heart MRI, cranial MRI, lumbosacral spine MRI, and spine MRI.

Magnetic Resonance Imaging ⚙ ⚙ ⚙

http://www.bewell.com/tests/test227.asp

Provided by HealthGate, this site contains a profile of magnetic resonance imaging. The profile includes information about material studied, cost of the test, patient time for the test, and reliability of the results. There are also discussions of the following topics: purpose of the test, where it is performed, who performs it, risks and precautions, patient preparation, sensory factors of the test itself, equipment used, post-test care, and test results.

Mammography

Certified Mammography Facilities ⚙ ⚙ ⚙

http://www.fda.gov/cdrh/mammography/fda_certified_mammography_faci.html

Providing a search tool to locate mammography facilities in any area of the country, this important Web site links patients to FDA-certified facilities and guidance information.

Digital Mammography Homepage ⊙ ⊙ ⊙

http://www.rose.brandeis.edu/users/mammo/digital.html

Provided by Brandeis University, this page offers a forum for researchers to exchange information. Useful content at this site covers meetings, current Digital Detector Work, institutions providing computer aided diagnosis and image processing, and commercial ventures. This site provides a resource for learning about international imaging centers.

Mammogram ⊙ ⊙ ⊙

http://www.medicinenet.com

This site, part of MedicineNet.com, provides an overview of mammography. Click on "Procedures and Tests" at the top of the home page, and select "Mammography." Topics discussed include what a mammogram is, the risks involved, how it is performed, obtaining results, and implications of an abnormal mammogram. There is also a link to breast cancer information.

Mediastinoscopy

Mediastinoscopy ⊙ ⊙ ⊙

http://www.mdadvice.com/library/test/medtest257.html

Part of MDAdvice.com, this site provides a profile of mediastinoscopy. The profile includes information about the material studied, estimated cost of the test, and patient time for the test. There is information about where and why the test is performed and who performs it. Information about the test itself includes sensory factors, equipment used, and a description of the test. There is information about post-test care and results.

Molecular Diagnostics

Molecular Diagnostic Cell Tracking ⊙ ⊙ ⊙

http://www.heyla.com/health/cancer/molecular.html

The technique of molecular diagnostics for tracking cancer cell development is discussed in this brief descriptive profile of one of the newer cancer diagnostic tools.

Molecular Diagnostics Research ⊙ ⊙ ⊙

http://path.upmc.edu/brochure/diagnostics.html

The Division of Molecular Diagnostics within the Department of Pathology at the University of Pittsburgh provides useful descriptive and research information on this important tool for utilizing molecular-based markers to give added information for determining both prognosis and therapeutic directions. Although the site is under further development, the testing capabilities of the laboratory for oncologic purposes is clearly set forth.

Nucleic Acid Amplification Testing

Nucleic Acid Amplification Testing (NAT) ⚙ ⚙ ⚙

http://www.moffitt.usf.edu/cancjrnl/v6n5/dept5.htm

From *Cancer Control Journal,* this site gives information about nucleic acid amplification testing. Topics discussed include reasons for NAT implementation, NAT technical principles, logistic barriers to NAT implementation, and potential effectiveness of NAT. The site provides references.

Pap Smear

Pap Smear ⚙ ⚙ ⚙

http://www.bewell.com/mdx-books/tests/test246.asp

Part of HealthGate, this site provides information about the pap smear. A profile of the test includes category, subcategory, material studied, cost of the test, patient time for the test, and reliability. There is also information about where and why the test is performed and who performs it. There is information about risks and precautions, patient preparation, sensory factors, equipment used, the test itself, test values, normal values, and drug interactions.

Skin Biopsy

Skin Biopsy ⚙ ⚙ ⚙

http://www.mdadvice.com/library/test/medtest351.html

Part of MDAdvice.com, this site profiles skin biopsy. Information includes where and why the test is performed and who performs it. There is information about risks and precautions and patient preparation. There is also information about sensory factors, equipment used, and the test itself. Test results are discussed.

Small-Bowel Biopsy

Small-Bowel Biopsy ⊙ ⊙ ⊙
http://www.mdadvice.com/library/test/medtest354.html

Created by MDAdvice.com, this site contains a profile of small-bowel biopsy. It also provides an explanation of the procedure, the purpose for the test, and where it is performed. Information about the equipment used, sensory factors, and post-test care is included. There is also information about the test results.

Thyroid Biopsy

Thyroid Biopsy ⊙ ⊙ ⊙
http://www.mdadvice.com/library/test/medtest374.html

Created by MDAdvice.com, this site profiles thyroid biopsy. The profile includes information about the cost, patient time, reliability, and material studied. There is also information about the purpose of the test, who performs it, and where it is performed. There is information about risks and precautions and patient preparation. There is a section on the test itself that includes sensory factors, equipment used, and a description of the test. Post-test care and activity is discussed. There is information about the results.

Tumor Markers

Tumor Markers ⊙ ⊙ ⊙
http://www.medstudents.com.br/onco/onco1.htm

The physicians and students of The Federal University Rio de Janeiro (Brazil) are responsible for this resource on tumor markers, and discusses among other things tumor antigens; carcinoembryonic antigen; alpha-fetoprotein; CA 125; CA19-9; prostate-specific antigen; hormones; human chronic gonadotropin; enzymes; acid photophase; neuron specific enolase; galactosyl reansferase II; and immunoglobulins.

Toward a Proper Use of Tumor Markers ⊙ ⊙ ⊙
http://sos.ist.unige.it/guidelines/english/mmhomee.html

Produced by the Regional Center for the Study of Biological Markers of Malignancy at Regional General Hospital, Venice, this site provides information about serum tumor markers. Topics discussed include general biological and clinical information, clinical use of tumor markers in the most common malignancies, and basic information on individual tumor markers. There is a discussion on methods used to prepare recommendations.

Tumor Markers ◎ ◎ ◎

http://cancernet.nci.nih.gov/clinpdq/detection/Tumor_Markers.html

Provided by the National Cancer Institute, this site provides an overview of tumor markers. There is also information about the following markers: prostate-specific antigen, prostatic acid phosphatase, CA 125, carcinoembryonic antigen, alpha-fetoprotein, human chronic gonadotropin, and several others. The site also provides links to other related Web sites.

Tumor Markers ◎ ◎ ◎

http://nauvoo.byu.edu/Academy/Microbio/Tumor/sld001.htm

Produced by Brigham Young University, this site provides a tutorial on tumor markers. Slides on cancer etiology, cancer phases, approaches for dealing with cancer, detection methods, tumor markers, enzymes, hormones, and immunologic markers are included.

Ultrasound

Thyroid Ultrasonography ◎ ◎ ◎

http://www.bewell.com/tests/test334.asp

Part of HealthGate, this site provides a profile of thyroid ultrasonography. Information includes an estimated cost of the test, patient time for the test, reliability of results, and material studies. There is information about the following topics: purpose of the test, where and why it is performed, sensory factors of the test, the test itself, post-test care and activities, and obtaining the results.

Ultrasound ◎ ◎ ◎

http://www.healthanswers.com/adam/top/view.asp?filename=003336.htm

Part of HealthAnswers.com, this site provides information about ultrasound. It includes an example of ultrasound imaging and a definition of the test. There is a discussion of how the test is performed and links to specific types of ultrasound. Types include duplex/doppler ultrasound, thyroid ultrasound, transvaginal ultrasound, testicle ultrasound, abdominal ultrasound ultrasound of the heart, ultrasound of extremities, and pregnancy ultrasound.

X-ray Imaging

X-ray Imaging ◎ ◎ ◎

http://www.healthanswers.com/adam/top/view.asp?filename=003337.htm

Part of HealthAnswers.com, this site contains information about x-ray imaging. There is an image of the procedure, alternative names, and a definition. There is information about how the test is performed, preparation, and associated risks. There are links to specific types of X-rays including dental X-rays, chest X-rays, gallbladder S-ray, and others.

6.8 Pathology

Case Index by Patient Diagnosis ⊙ ⊙ ⊙
http://path.upmc.edu/cases/dxindex.html

The University of Pittsburgh's School of Medicine's Department of Pathology has formatted many cases for online viewing, organized in an index by patient diagnosis. There is considerable information on cancer pathology.

Clinical Disease Management for Oncology ⊙ ⊙ ⊙
http://www.slis.ua.edu/cdlp/WebDLCore/clinical/oncology/index.htm

This site offers links to chapters in the *Merck Manual* and to other clinical sources for diagnosis and treatment of specific disorders, including libraries of pathology images, clinical practice guidelines, and clinical management resources. Links take the visitor to relevant sections of CHORUS (Collaborative Hypertext of Radiology), WebPath, CliniWeb, the National Institutes of Health, and other Internet information sources.

Digital Database for Screening Mammography ⊙ ⊙ ⊙
http://marathon.csee.usf.edu/Mammography/Database.html

The University o South Florida's Digital Mammography Home Page provides the Digital Database for Screening Mammography (DDSM), a resource for the mammographic image analysis research community. It is organized into "cases" and "volumes." A "case" is a collection of images and information corresponding to one mammography exam of one patient. A "volume" is a collection of cases. The database contains about 2,500 studies. Each study includes two images of each breast along with some patient-associated information. Software for accessing the mammogram and truth images, and for calculating figures for automated image analysis algorithms is also provided.

Guide to Cancer Pathology and Molecular Biology Resources ⊙ ⊙ ⊙
http://www.ncl.ac.uk/child-health/guides/clinks4m.htm

The University of Newcastle has compiled an extensive series of Internet links to cancer pathology and molecular biology topics. There are more than 100 such links to topics including biopsies, molecular biology techniques, molecular genetics, pathology of specific cancers, and numerous other topics of interest to physicians, researchers, and technical healthcare professionals. This is not a site for the general public.

Lung Tumors: A Multidisciplinary Database ⊙ ⊙ ⊙

http://www.vh.org/Providers/Textbooks/LungTumors/TitlePage.html

The Virtual Hospital of the University of Iowa College of Medicine offers this database on lung tumors. Included are interactive diagnostic aids such as a staging tool and nodule tool (predicts the risk of malignancy in solitary pulmonary nodules). Case studies can also be viewed. Information on thoracic neoplasms and pleural-based neoplasms is provided by clicking on the appropriate topics.

Metastases to the Breast ⊙ ⊙ ⊙

http://www.vh.org/Providers/TeachingFiles/Metastases/Metastases.html

The Virtual Hospital provides this useful site on the diagnosis and management of extramammary tumors metastatic to the breast. Seven images concerning the mammography of nonmammary tumors are presented accompanied with explanations. A list of references is provided at the end of the site.

Organ System Pathology Images ⊙ ⊙ ⊙

http://www-medlib.med.utah.edu/WebPath/ORGAN.html

The Internet Pathology Laboratory for Medical Education offers this site on Organ System Pathology Images. The images are available for viewing below by organ system. Each section contains a series of images illustrating gross and microscopic pathologic findings for a number of disease processes. The images are indexed as follows: Bone and Joint Pathology, Breast Pathology, Cardiovascular Pathology, Central Nervous System Pathology, Endocrine Pathology, Female Genital Tract Pathology, Gastrointestinal Pathology, Hematopathology, Hepatic Pathology, Male Genital Tract Pathology, Pulmonary Pathology, and Renal Pathology.

Pathology Manual: Gynecologic Oncology Group ⊙ ⊙ ⊙

http://www.vh.org/Providers/Textbooks/OBGYNOncology/PathologyManualHome.html

The Pathology Manual of the Gynecologic Oncology Group's Table of Contents includes: vulvar neoplasms, vaginal neoplasms, uterine cervix neoplasms, uterine corpus neoplasms, fallopian tube neoplasms (ovary outline and ovarian neoplasms), and trophoblastic diseases. Other topics under the Appendix include uterus-endometrial carcinoma, uterus-cervical carcinoma, ovarian neoplasm, vulvar cancer, and uterus-non-cancer. Sample synoptic reports entitled cervical carcinoma report and endometrial carcinoma report are also given.

Physiological Imaging ⊙ ⊙ ⊙

http://everest.radiology.uiowa.edu

This site is provided by the Department of Radiology at the University of Iowa College of Medicine. This is a huge resource for imaging-related information. The site offers a 3-D gallery of computer movies of a variety of scans, selected papers, project descriptions, course and contact information, and a search engine to search the site for specific information. There are a number of case studies and image collections that deal with tumors and specific cancer conditions.

Radiation Oncology Clinical Articles ◎ ◎ ◎
http://www.rooj.com/index_article_main.htm

The Radiation Oncology Online Journal (RROJ) is a nonprofit service organization responsible for this site, which provides radiation oncology clinical articles. Articles are available by clicking on one of the following areas: breast; central nervous system; gastrointestinal system; genitourinary tumors; gynecologic tumors; head and neck; lymphoma; metastatic tumors; miscellaneous; muskuloskeletal; ophthalmic tumors; pediatric tumors; skin; thorax; physics; and radiation biology.

Tumor Board ◎ ◎ ◎
http://www.tumorboard.com

Tumor Board is a library of digital pathology images. One can browse the library, ask a member to comment on a specific case, add images or view featured cases. Membership criteria is available and there are details regarding Digital Imaging Workshops.

WebPath ◎ ◎ ◎
http://deroh.gsnu.ac.kr/dermpath/webpath.htm

WebPath is provided by the Department of Pathology at the University of Utah. This massive Internet resource provides over 1,800 images, text information, laboratory exercises, and examination items that relate to disease conditions for the education of students and professionals. The user can search the site or pick a destination from the menu. Information concerning faculty and purchase of the WebPath CD-ROM is also provided.

6.9 Cancer Staging

Cancer Staging Information from the National Cancer Institute ◎ ◎ ◎
http://www.nci.nih.gov

Information for health professionals on the stages of each form of cancer is available at this section of the National Cancer Institute. Select the type of cancer, and then click on "health professionals" under the Treatment Section. The database provides full information on the cancer stages for the disorder.

Diagnostic Tools Utilized
in Gauging Stages of Cancer from Merck ◎ ◎
http://www.merck.com/pubs/mmanual/section11/chapter142/142a.htm

The site visitor can scroll to the topic of "Staging" and obtain information on the principal tools and techniques utilized in testing for progressive stages of cancer. The chapter discusses mediastinoscopy, bone marrow biopsy, auxillary lymph node removal, laparotomy, serum chemistries and enzymes, imaging studies, ultrasonography, and the use of liver-spleen scans.

Grading and Staging of Cancers ◎ ◎
http://edcenter.med.cornell.edu/CUMC_PathNotes/Neoplasia/Neoplasia_03.html

Provided by the Weill Medical College of Cornell University, this document explains the basic definition of each stage of cancer, along with the internationally used "TNM System," an acronym for the numerical subscripts that designate the extent of neoplastic disease.

6.10 Therapies

Cancer Therapy Summaries

Cancer Therapy Survey from the NIH ◎ ◎
http://cancernet.nci.nih.gov/clinpdq/therapy.html

The following cancer therapies are surveyed at this site of the National Cancer Institute: Angiogenesis Inhibitors; Biological Therapies; Chemotherapy; Laser Therapy; Antineoplaston Therapy; Hydrazine Sulfate Therapy; Photodynamic Therapy; Mastectomy, Preventive Mastectomy, and Adjutant Therapy for Breast Cancer; Cryosurgery; and Gene Therapy. A question and answer approach is used in some of the discussion links.

Checklist of Cancer Treatments ◎ ◎
http://www.pathfinder.com/time/magazine/1998/dom/980518/box3.html

Time Magazine has compiled an extremely useful overview of all of the principal cancer therapies, including their targets, how they work, and their status in development. The therapies cover anti-angiogenesis factors, anti-metastatic factors, anti-oncologic factors, chemo-prevention therapies, gene therapies, chemotherapy, monoclonal antibodies, radiation therapies, surgical therapies, and vaccines. There is a strong section on Who's Who in Angiogenesis, covering drugs, pharmaceutical developers, working mechanisms, sources, and status in the development cycle.

Conventional and Non-Conventional Treatments ⊙ ⊙ ⊙
http://www.artsci.gmcc.ab.ca/courses/heed110/Cancertreat.htm

As an informational survey, the 1999 article at this site provides useful descriptive information on the following conventional treatments: surgery, radiation therapy, chemotherapy, immunotherapy, and peripheral blood stem therapy. Newer, nonconventional treatments which are discussed are anti-angiogenesis factors, anti-metastatic factors, anti-oncogenic factors, gene therapy, vaccines, complementary/alternative therapies, hormone therapy, combination treatments, and programs seeking other unconventional innovations.

Anti-Angiogenesis

Anti-Angiogenesis Overview ⊙ ⊙ ⊙
http://www.slip.net/~mcdavis/angiogen.html

This site provides an in-depth exploration of anti-angiogenesis therapy in the treatment of cancer, including questions and answers, operating mechanisms, initial drugs, and research strategies.

Cancer Trials on Anti-Angiogenesis ⊙ ⊙ ⊙
http://mednav10.vh.shore.net/NCI_CANCER_TRIALS/zones/PressInfo/Angio

Detailed information on anti-angiogenesis research is provided at this site, including specific trials and research protocols. Endostatin, angiogenesis inhibitor research, anti-angiogenesis archives, and news developments serve as topical sections of the review.

Biological Therapies

BC Cancer Agency: Immunotherapy and Biological Response Modifiers ⊙ ⊙ ⊙
http://www.bccancer.bc.ca/cid/15.html

This detailed article in the British Columbia Cancer Agency Information Database provides an introduction to five major biological therapies and how they operate. Background information, developments, and the results of significant studies are included.

BioOncology On Line ⊙ ⊙ ⊙
http://www.biooncology.com

This site's oncology resource center features colored teaching slides, clinical reviews, a calendar of events, and information resources for patient counseling. Informational sections for lymphoma and breast cancer provide fact sheets, a glossary, news, and meeting details. Discussions of biologic therapies and contract information are also provided.

OncoLink: Biological Response Modifiers (BRM) ☉ ☉ ☉

http://oncolink.upenn.edu/specialty/med_onc/chemo/general/brm_intro.html

A service of the University of Pennsylvania Cancer Center, OncoLink provides an excellent article explaining Biomedical Response Modifiers in detail. The article provides an overview of the immune system, and outlines BRM therapies.

Chemotherapy

Chemotherapy and You:
An In-Depth National Cancer Institute Document ☉ ☉

http://www.meb.uni-bonn.de/cancernet/400064.html

This 30-page booklet, developed at the National Cancer Institute surveys all aspects of chemotherapy from the patient's point of view, including descriptive information, mechanism of operation, side effects, and patient management of the therapy.

Chemotherapy Approaches and Protocols
from University of Pennsylvania ☉ ☉

http://www.oncolink.upenn.edu/specialty/med_onc/chemo/index.html

This 1999 survey of chemotherapy prepared by the University of Pennsylvania provides an excellent summary of research, drugs, patient response, side effects, pain management, technical articles, chemotherapy news, and external links.

Complementary and Alternative Therapies

Center for Alternative Medicine Research in Cancer ☉ ☉

http://www.sph.uth.tmc.edu/utcam

Located at the University of Texas—Houston, the Center's mission is to evaluate the effectiveness of biopharmacologic and herbal therapies in the treatment of cancer. There is a review of therapies, discussion of research in process, resources and links to other information sites on the Internet, and a listing of other alternative medicine centers.

Center for Mind-Body Medicine ☉ ☉

http://www.healthy.net/cmbm

Dedicated to the creation of models of healing that will "transform all parties in the healing process" and to make such models widely available are the principal goals of this Center in Washington, D.C. The application of these alternative medical treatments to cancer patients is the major focus of the organization. The site provides summaries from prior-year conference proceedings on mind-body therapies, outlines of Center programs, a description of mind-body medicine, a library and bookstore, and organization and membership information.

Complementary and Alternative Therapies at CancerNet ⊙ ⊙ ⊙
http://imsdd.meb.uni-bonn.de/cancernet/600914.html

Nonconventional approaches to the treatment of cancer can be an important avenue or adjunct in certain cases. This document explores the nature of complementary and alternative therapies and their possible application for both prevention and treatment. Mind/body control interventions, such as visualization or relaxation, manual healing with acupressure and massage, homeopathy, vitamin and herbal treatments, and acupuncture are among the treatments that are sometimes tried.

Hydrazine Sulfate Treatment ⊙ ⊙
http://cancernet.nci.nih.gov/cam/hydrazine.htm

The use of hydrazine sulfate as a complementary/alternative therapy for cancer has been studied in the U.S. for many years. This site sets forth general information on this MAO inhibitor, its history, laboratory studies, positive and adverse effects, and an extensive bibliography of references.

Medherb.com ⊙ ⊙
http://www.medherb.com

Offering information on the use of herbs as a complementary treatment for cancer and other diseases, Medherb provides links to sites and information regarding positive and adverse effects of herbs, clinical nutrition, herbal journals, research sites on herbs, anatomical and botanical information, and other relevant resources for those interested in exploring this aspect of alternative medicine. The site is sponsored by the journal *Medical Herbalism,* a quarterly publication on clinical herbalism.

National Center for Complementary and Alternative Medicine (NCCAM) ⊙ ⊙ ⊙
http://altmed.od.nih.gov/nccam

A division of the National Institutes of Health (NIH), the NCCAM conducts and supports basic and applied research on complementary and alternative medicine as a therapy option for cancer and other diseases. The organization facilitates and conducts biomedical research as opposed to operating as a referral agency. The site describes the NCCAM, outlines the program areas, provides news, research grant information, and other resources for interested parties. There is a site index along with a search tool as well.

Rosenthal Center for Complementary and Alternative Medicine ◎ ◎

http://cpmcnet.columbia.edu/dept/rosenthal

Created in 1993 as one of the first centers located at a major medical school devoted to research, education, and training in this field, the Rosenthal Center offers courses and events, cancer education initiatives, and complementary and alternative medicine (CAM) research and information sources. It is funded by the National Center for Complementary and Alternative Medicine at the National Institutes of Health.

Cord Blood Transplant

Carolinas Cord Blood Bank (CCBB) ◎ ◎

http://www.canctr.mc.duke.edu/CCBB

The CCBB site provides basic information about cord blood and the donation process. The bank is a National Institutes of Health designated bank and the site is provided by the Duke University Comprehensive Cancer Center. There is an extensive list of articles for professionals and information about the program and its staff.

Cord Blood Applications ◎ ◎

http://www.ahsc.arizona.edu/opa/crnap/dec95cnp.htm

This page is from the Web site provided by the University of Arizona Health Sciences Center and is a report provided for physicians. It details the potential clinical applications and benefits of cord blood banking and transplantation.

Cord Blood Donor Foundation (CBDF) ◎ ◎ ◎

http://www.cordblooddonor.org

The Foundation seeks to provide education and to conduct research into the use of cord blood stem cells. Information concerning the Foundation, donation, cord blood, contacts, and diseases treated is provided. Physician guidelines for initiating a search are given along with an online preliminary search request form and a description of the typical match process.

Cord Blood Registry ◎ ◎

http://www.cordblood.com

The registry provides extensive information for expectant parents, patients, and professionals about the services offered. The organization collects, processes, and stores stem cells for a fee.

UCLA Umbilical Cord Blood Bank ⊙ ⊙ ⊙
http://www.cordblood.med.ucla.edu

Part of the National Institutes of Health cord blood bank system, the UCLA organization banks cord blood from many ethnic backgrounds and conducts research to determine the potentials and limitations of cord blood transplants. The Web site provides contact, donor, staff, and program information along with an FAQ section and a newsletter.

Cryosurgery in Cancer Treatment

Cryosurgery and Hepatocellular Carcinoma ⊙ ⊙
http://www.cryoforum.org/Liver/wongsped.html

The Cryo-Forum offers this comprehensive report on a clinical study involving the application of cryosurgery to the treatment of advanced stage hepatocellular carcinoma. The material is directed at a professional audience, and covers the methodology of the study, detailed information on results, and conclusions. There are discussion sections regarding the procedure and the disease, and evaluation of complications.

Cryosurgery and Prostate Cancer ⊙ ⊙
http://www.coloradohealthnet.org/cancer/prostate/procry.html

Provided in a question and answer format, this report provides a useful overview of cryosurgery, the procedures employed, eligibility and applicability, effects on potency, follow-up testing, anticipated costs, and other information.

Cryosurgery for Malignant Liver Tumors ⊙ ⊙
http://www.cma.ca/cjs/vol-39/issue-5/0401.htm

Focusing on the application of cryosurgery to the treatment of malignant liver tumors, this article offers a broad range of information for both patients equipped to review technical literature and professionals, including the procedures and results of clinical trials, a discussion of the procedure in some depth, and bibliographic references for further study.

Cryosurgery in Cancer Treatment ⊙ ⊙
http://imsdd.meb.uni-bonn.de/cancernet/600734.html

Cryosurgery is the use of extreme cold to destroy cancer cells. This therapy is a subject of active research, and is covered at this site. There is a definition of the treatment, a discussion of the types of cancer that can be treated with cryosurgery, examination of side effects and complications, a review of advantages and disadvantages, and discussion of future possibilities.

Prostate Cancer and Cryosurgery ◎ ◎

http://www.ahcpr.gov/news/press/pr1999/cryopr.htm

As an adjunct to radiation therapy, or as an alternative option when radiation therapy is not effective, cryosurgery for the treatment of prostate cancer is actively being studied as a method of destroying diseased tissue. This procedure is the subject of this site, which focuses on cryosurgery as a second line of therapy.

Gene Therapy

Cancer Gene Therapy ◎ ◎ ◎

http://Web.bham.ac.uk/can4psd4/gt/cancer.html

Gene Therapy approaches are summarized at this site, including immunotherapy, gene directed enzyme pro-drug therapy (GDEPT), and insertion of tumor suppresser genes. Research at the University of Birmingham focuses on nonviral vectors, including polymer vectors.

Gene Therapy Sites ◎ ◎ ◎

http://www.uq.edu.au/vdu/gtlinks.htm

This is an excellent survey, with direct links, covering the gene therapy clinical trials database, technical discussions, types of vectors, laboratories engaged in gene therapy, and numerous other resources.

Medical Research Council Human Genetics Unit ◎ ◎ ◎

http://www.hgu.mrc.ac.uk

A large amount of information concerning genetics and disease is featured at this site. There are research and other sections that provide information concerning cancer genetics, that discuss relevant research and provide links. The site also provides information about seminars and offers downloadable software and data sets.

Tumor Gene Database ◎ ◎ ◎

http://condor.bcm.tmc.edu/oncogene.html

This site is an educational tool for researchers and contains a large amount of information pertaining to tumor suppressor genes, proto-oncogenes and cancer causing mutations. A unified search makes searching the database easy.

Hyperthermia

Hyperthermia in Cancer Treatment ◎ ◎
http://imsdd.meb.uni-bonn.de/cancernet/600073.html

The use of high temperature treatment to attack cancer cells is a new approach under investigation in the cancer-fighting arsenal. This brief but informative report discusses this technique and its possible future application as researchers study ways to deal with metastatic cancer as well as localized cancers.

Laser Therapy/Photodynamic Therapy/Interstitial Thermotherapy

Lasers in Cancer Treatment ◎ ◎ ◎
http://imsdd.meb.uni-bonn.de/cancernet/600078.html

Laser therapy is explored in this document from the National Cancer Institute, a procedure involving the use of high-intensity light to destroy cancer cells. Frequently used to relieve symptoms of cancer, the technique may have applications for shrinking or destroying tumors. The report covers a discussion of laser light, types of lasers, cancer treatment with lasers, laser-induced interstitial thermotherapy, photodynamic therapy, and the outlook for these innovative applications of intense light beams.

MRI-Guided Laser-Induced Interstitial Thermotherapy ◎ ◎
http://splweb.bwh.harvard.edu:8000/pages/current_projects.html

A technical paper chronologically listed among many other projects (look under April 1998), this document offers a summary of the procedure, an explanation of its methodology, the effects of thermotherapy on tissue, MRI monitoring, targeting, conclusions, and references. This information is presented for researchers and professionals seeking a detailed understanding of the use of this procedure for destroying diseased cells. There are extensive references for further inquiry.

Photodynamic Therapy (PDT) ◎ ◎
http://www.chem.ucdavis.edu/groups/smith/PDT_Research/PDT.html

Photodynamic therapy is evolving as a treatment modality for carcinomas and sarcomas as this site sets forth. There is a thorough discussion of this form of treatment, its administration, localization in the tumor, absorbence, photophysics, and other related information.

Photodynamic Therapy (PDT): An Overview ⊙ ⊙

http://www.mps-cpb.com/sijf/photodyn.htm

For healthcare professionals and research-oriented patients, this site offers a clear explanation of Photodynamic Therapy (PDT), including the methodology, the types of cancer it is used to treat, its side effects, and treatment procedures.

Photodynamic Therapy (PDT) in the Treatment of Cancer ⊙ ⊙

http://rpci.med.buffalo.edu/clinic/pdt/pdt.html

This paper outlines the nature and scope of photodynamic therapy as a new two-step cancer treatment utilizing a light-sensitive drug called a photosensitizer and visible red light from a laser to destroy cancer cells. The discussion explores how the therapy works, its side-effects, and its application to particular types of cancer, which are enumerated. References are useful as a source of additional information on this form of treatment.

Monoclonal Antibody Therapy

Herceptin, the First Breast Cancer—Metastatic Breast Cancer ⊙ ⊙

http://pharminfo.com/drugpr/herceptin_pr.html

This pharmaceutical press release discusses the use of Herceptin, a drug under active development as the first monoclonal antibody to slow metastatic breast cancer. Drug mechanisms and clinical trials are the focus of the site information.

Monoclonal Antibody Therapy ⊙ ⊙ ⊙

http://www.lymphomainfo.net/therapy/mab.html

The Lymphoma Information Network provides descriptive information and important links related to the operation and use of monoclonal antibodies. Mechanisms of operation are discussed, combinatorial therapies are explained, specific drugs are cited and examined, and Web resources are provided. Rituxan, Bexxar, and Oncolym are the drugs presently used in recent trials in the U.S. for lymphoma.

Multimodality and Adjuvant Therapy

Multimodality and Adjuvant Therapy ⊙ ⊙

http://www.merck.com/pubs/mmanual/section11/chapter144/144e.htm

The *Merck Manual* provides a clear explanation of multimodality and adjuvant therapy, a treatment technique involving the use of several therapies in combination rather than a single therapy. There are also links to other related chapters, including "Principles of Cancer Therapy" and "Hematology and Oncology."

Radiation Therapies

American Association of Medical Dosimetrists (AAMD) ◎ ◎
http://www.medicaldosimetry.org

The site of the AAMD provides information about membership, credentialing services, educational programs, journal readings, committees, curriculum, and employment. There is also a section detailing news and upcoming events and one that provides a professional FAQ.

Brachytherapy Home Page ◎ ◎
http://www.brachytherapy.com

The resource site is provided by the Cancer Treatment Center of America (CTCA). Details of brachytherapy application to prostate and breast cancer are provided along with information about intensity modulated radiation therapy. There are details of the brachytherapy team at CTCA and contact listings.

BrighamRAD ◎ ◎ ◎
http://brighamrad.harvard.edu

The educational and research site from the Department of Radiology at Brigham and Women's Hospital offers information concerning patient education, professional education, and research. The professional section offers online teaching cases, atlases with normal studies, slide shows and quizzes, lecture tutorials, and an image collection. There are listings of teaching programs and CME programs. Patient materials describe patient care at the hospital, programs, and community services. There is also a listing of patient education documents that describe imaging, procedures, and more. There are comprehensive lists of research areas, laboratories, trials, and projects.

Fermilab Neutron Therapy Facility (NTF) at the Midwest Institute for Neutron Therapy ◎ ◎ ◎
http://adwww.fnal.gov/www/ntf/ntf_home.html

The Fermilab NTF treats malignant tumors via the use of high-energy neutrons. The Web site provides information about neutrons against cancer, clinical information, results of the treatment with prostate patients, a newsletter geared towards physicians, a protocol list, and referral details.

Mallinckrodt Institute of Radiology: Radiation Oncology Center ◎ ◎
http://www.radonc.wustl.edu/radonc.html

Provided by the Washington University School of Medicine, this site offers information about radiation oncology, staff, residency training, news, and publications. Sections of the site are dedicated to cancer biology, information systems, and clinical and physics departments. There are listings of protocols, services and specific programs.

MDAdvice.com: Radiation Therapy and You— Managing Side Effects ◎ ◎ ◎

http://www.mdadvice.com/topics/radiotherapy/info/radside.html

This informative site offers descriptions, encouragement, and suggestions pertaining to common side effects from radiation therapy. Material is presented in the form of answers to common questions related to whether side effects are the same in every patient and whether activity is limited due to treatment. Other topics include fatigue, skin problems, hair loss, immune system problems, eating and digestive problems, and emotional issues. Special issues are discussed related to radiation therapy to the head and neck, breast and chest, stomach and abdomen, and pelvis.

Medical Imaging and Radiation Oncology Data Alliance (MIRODA) ◎

http://www.miroda.org

The goals of MIRODA are to collect, analyze, and present data related to medical imaging and radiation oncology. It serves professional organizations that represent medical imaging and radiation oncology professionals. The site provides a listing of participating organizations with links and information about the organization and its philosophies.

Medical Radiography Home Page ◎ ◎ ◎

http://Web.wn.net/user1/ricter/Web/medradhome.html

This is a massive collection of links to other sites. Sites are organized by topic and are categorized under topics such as radiology resources, professional and continuing education, general anatomy, organizations and societies and more. There are a total of 19 categories.

New York Online Access to Health (NOAH): Tips on Managing Chemotherapy and Radiation Side Effects ◎ ◎

http://www.noah.cuny.edu:8080/cancer/cancercare/patients/briefs/chemo.html

Information at this site focuses on the problem of side effects in patients undergoing chemotherapy and radiation therapy, including fever, infection, nausea, and sickness. Common myths related to these treatments and side effects are also presented.

OncoLink: Symptom Management
for Radiation Therapy Patients ◎ ◎ ◎

http://www.oncolink.upenn.edu/specialty/rad_onc/support

This site provides information for patients concerned with possible side effects of radiation therapy. Links are available to general information about cancer and resources related to symptom management, radiation oncology, cervical stenosis, long-term effects of chemotherapy, post-radiation fertility, heart damage after radiation treatment, radiation-induced hematuria, skin care and radiation therapy, and radiation enteritis. Most resources are available in the form of answers to patients' questions and tips from OncoLink.

Rad EFX: Radiation Health Effects Research Resource ◎ ◎

http://radefx.med.bcm.tmc.edu

This resource site is provided by the Baylor College of Medicine and offers a listing of conferences and meetings, a USA-Canada Chernobyl immigrant Registry, a research software forum, and an extensive listing of online resources. The Ionizing Radiation Health Effects Forum offers extensive details about disaster preparedness, research needs, research projects, population registries, publications and professional organizations.

Radiation and Side Effects ◎ ◎

http://www.bmi.net/mcaron/effects.html

Created by a radiation therapist, this site describes the effects of radiation treatment and the nature of this therapy. Patients will find this site a useful resource for suggestions on self-care during therapy. Unusual symptoms requiring medical attention are described, and patients can access the site for a short description of what to expect during radiation treatment.

Radiation in Cancer Treatment ◎ ◎ ◎

http://www.thedailyapple.com/public/content/healthLibrary

The use of radiation, a standard treatment for cancer, is examined at this site, including operational mechanism, benefits and goals, risks, application, treatment provision, and insurance factors.

Radiation Oncology Study Session ◎ ◎

http://www.RadOnc.Duke.EDU/~carter

A personal physician's page provided by the Duke University Medical Center offers some relevant abstract, links and other information. The feature of the page is a study session that provides 33 sessions of 243 questions and answers. The list of topics covered is comprehensive and has sections for nearly every disorder. There is also a link to a breast cancer tutorial.

Radiation Therapy for Soft-Tissue Sarcoma ⊙ ⊙ ⊙

http://www.mskcc.org/document/wicsar3b.htm

This Memorial Sloan-Kettering article examines various forms of radiation therapy, including brachytherapy for soft-tissue sarcoma. Two forms of brachytherapy are described—the use of radiotherapeutic seeds and high-dose-rate intraoperative radiation therapy.

Vaccine Therapies

Cancer Vaccines and Gene Therapy
Current Clinical Status ⊙ ⊙ ⊙

http://westbyserver.westby.mwt.net/~ctustis/dal.htm

This article by a professor in London provides a short introduction and history of cancer vaccines as well as the current status of their clinical effects.

Cancer Vaccines: Market and Technology Report ⊙ ⊙ ⊙

http://www.newmedinc.com/reports/401.html

A report on the state of cancer vaccines, this site provides the clinical aspects of vaccines, indications and epidemiology, as well as an analysis of markets and development environment. Company and product profiles are offered as well.

DNA Vaccine Web ⊙ ⊙ ⊙

http://www.genweb.com/Dnavax/dnavax.html

Boasting a massive collection of scientifically oriented material concerning vaccine research and development, this comprehensive site provides information from all areas of study including the study of oncogenes. Information pertaining to meetings, clinical news, patents, articles, reviews, research, FDA guidelines, plasmids, protocols, and more is provided, as well as contact information, job center information, and links to other resources. A contact address is provided to request a collection of DNA vaccine references.

iafrica.com: Cancer Vaccine Therapies ⊙ ⊙

http://health.iafrica.com/doconline/cancer/index.htm

A brief explanation of cancer vaccines is provided at this iafrica.com site under the health and fitness category. This article provides information in a patient-oriented format about how cancer vaccines operate.

Sloan Kettering Cancer Vaccine Research ○ ○ ○
http://www.mskcc.org/document/cn970205.htm

The Memorial Sloan Kettering Cancer Center is engaged in extensive research on new cancer vaccines. This site provides an overview of the different vaccine therapies that are under study. Profiles of the principal research investigators are included with direct links that provide further background information for this research-oriented Web site.

6.11 Pain Management

American Alliance of Cancer Pain Initiatives (AACPI) ○ ○ ○
http://www.aacpi.org

The AACPI establishes standards and provides leadership for nationwide cancer pain initiatives. Its Web site offers links and contact information for all U.S. Cancer Pain Initiatives, and an information resource center. The resource center is a comprehensive information bank that offers links, meeting listings, videos, archives, and patient and professional education documents.

American Pain Society (APS) ○ ○ ○
http://www.ampainsoc.org

The APS is a multidisciplinary, scientific organization. This Web site provides annual meeting, publication, advocacy, news, opportunity, and events information. A pain facility database allows the user to search for facilities by classifications. Resources for patients and professionals provides contact information for organizations that are related to pain management. The APS site also provides an abstract search engine for their database of internal documentation on pain-related topics. A resources section offers links that are organized for patients or professionals.

Cancer Pain Management: Pain Lecture Slide Show ○ ○ ○
http://pain.roxane.com/SlideShow/TOC.html

This site allows the user to navigate through a slide show on cancer pain management. There are 74 titled slides, with most accompanied by diagrams, charts, or other illustrations. The menu provides the titles of the slides, which allows the user to select and view those slides of interest.

CancerFatigue.org ○ ○ ○
http://www.cancerfatique.org

Those suffering from cancer fatigue can find a great deal of helpful information from this particular site. The site provides tips, a service that allows the user to ask a nurse a specific question, and a locator service that searches for local educational events.

Chronic Pain Support ⚙ ⚙ ⚙

http://www.chronicpain.net

This online patient support and information resource provides a bookstore, chat rooms, discussion lists, links, and resources. There is extensive information about the site and how to use its services.

International Association for the Study of Pain (IASP) ⚙ ⚙

http://www.halcyon.com/iasp

This international, multidisciplinary, and professional organization site promotes pain research to improve patient care. The IASP Web site offers information on continuing education, local chapters, awards, programs, working groups, publications, employment information, and meetings. For the public, medical newsletters and a listing of resources by country are supplied.

M. D. Anderson Cancer Center (MDACC) Cancer Pain Page ⚙ ⚙ ⚙

http://prg.mdanderson.org/index.htm

This is a site from MDACC for patients, researchers, and clinicians and provides information about books, cancer pain conferences, news, articles, a newsletter, and MD Anderson services. The Articles Section is extensive as is the list of links.

Management of Cancer Pain ⚙ ⚙ ⚙

http://text.nlm.nih.gov/ftrs/pick?ftrsK=0&collect=ahcpr&dbName=capc&t=946661740

This clinical guideline was published by the Agency for Health Care Policy and Research. It provides information on the following topics: assessment of pain in the patient with cancer, pharmacologic management, nonpharmacologic management, nonpharmacologic interventions, procedure-related pain in adults and children, pain in special populations, and monitoring the quality of pain management. There is an overview, reference list, glossary, and list of acronyms. There are also tables, figures, and a list of contributors.

National Guideline Clearinghouse (NGC): Pain Management ⚙ ⚙ ⚙

http://www.ngc.gov

The National Guideline Clearinghouse provides clinical guidelines in all medical areas, covering all diseases and disorders. This site provides clinical guideline information concerning management of cancer pain, including assessment, pharmacologic management, invasive therapies, and quality control. The pain management guidelines are located under the American Society of Anesthesiologists. This is a useful reference for practitioners, and not a site for the general public.

New Hampshire Cancer Pain Initiative ◎ ◎ ◎

http://www.nhcpi.org

The organization's site offers consumer information, informational documents, links for professionals, abstracts of research studies, links to research institutions, and contact information. There are discussions of the physical, mental, sociocultural, and spiritual aspects of pain and of nondrug pain relief.

Symptom Management ◎ ◎ ◎

http://oncolink.upenn.edu/support

Part of OncoLink, this site provides links to articles within OncoLink on the following topics: helping people cope, frequently asked questions about symptom management, symptom management for radiation therapy patients, and psychological issues. It also provides information about end of life issues, bone marrow suppression, fatigue and cancer, lymphedema, oral complications, and pain management.

Talaria: The Hypermedia Assistant for Cancer Pain Management ◎ ◎ ◎

http://www.statsci.com/talaria/talaria.html

This thorough and informative resource for professionals concerns pain management for patients. It offers an online form of the *Clinical Practice Guideline on the Management of Cancer Pain* publication. Also featured is a drug dosage calculator, dermatome map, a library of technical references and documents, and a variety of interactive educational tools. An assortment of multimedia instructional tools includes video clips of patients and professionals addressing pain management issues and animated tutorials of pain-related neurological processes.

Washington–Alaska Cancer Pain Initiative (WACPI) ◎ ◎

http://www.fhcrc.org/cipr/wacpi

Information about local symposia, news, and other sites is provided here. There are fact sheets, National Cancer Institute patient materials, a Q/A section, links, audio files on pain management, videos and a resource library of PDF files.

West Virginia Cancer Pain Initiative (WVCPI) ◎ ◎

http://ruralnet.marshall.edu/pain

This informative WVCPI site is provided by Marshall University School of Medicine. It offers a large collection of articles, hospice details, guidelines for severe cancer pain, links, legislative information, and special announcements.

6.12 Supportive Care and Behavioral Oncology

American Society for Psychosocial and Behavioral Oncology/ AIDS (ASPBOA) and International Psycho-Oncology Society ◎ ◎ ◎
http://www.ipos-aspboa.org

These two organizations dedicated to supportive care for cancer and AIDS patients share this Web site. A description is provided for each organization and its activities, with links to further information by organization. Directed to healthcare professionals, the organizations offer conference, event, policy, and program information, as well as fellowship offerings.

Cancer Supportive Care ◎ ◎ ◎
http://www.cancersupportivecare.com

The site describes Cancer Supportive Care Programs (CSCP), providing multidisciplinary information and services for patients, their families, and friends. This program employs the Fifth Dimension Programs to complement surgery, radiation therapy, chemotherapy, and immunotherapy, and is currently a component of the Stanford Complementary Medicine Clinic (UCSF Stanford Health Care). Details are provided about individual programs within this system, including Psychosocial Support, Nutrition, Exercise, Fatigue, Anemia, Pain Control, Sleep Disorders and Management, Sexuality, Intimacy and Communications, Lymphedema, Diversions, Creativity and Coping, Spirituality and Chaplaincy Program, Planning for the "End Of Life," Pharmacy Program, and the Second Opinions Program.

Guide to Internet Resources for Oncology: Supportive Care ◎ ◎ ◎
http://www.ncl.ac.uk/child-health/guides/clinks4s.htm

This address contains links to sites providing resources on oncology supportive care issues. Visitors can find sites with information and product sources related to hair loss (alopecia), psychosocial issues, hypercalcemia, lymphedema, nausea and vomiting, cancer pain and palliative care, late effects treatment, rehabilitation after cancer, and other supportive care issues. Sources are available for patients, caregivers, and health professionals, including links to MEDLINE searches.

H. Lee Moffitt Cancer Center and Research Institute: Behavioral Oncology and Supportive Care ◎ ◎
http://www.moffitt.usf.edu/research_programs/Programs/ccontrol/behavioral/index.htm

This component of the Institute's Cancer Control Research Programs conducts activities in an effort to develop psychosocial and educational programs for patients and primary caregivers, determines how interactions between patients and physicians impact treatment decisions, improves supportive care in an effort to reduce the burden of cancer, and gains an improved understanding of normal aging and its relationship to cancer. This site presents the goals and future plans of the Institute, and profiles the group leaders and investigators in the program. Press releases, contact information, a site search engine, links to other clinical programs within the Institute, employment listings, and other resources are also available at this site.

Supportive Care Information for Emotional & Physical Manifestations ◎ ◎ ◎

http://cancernet.nci.nih.gov/clinpdq/supportive.html

Anxiety, depression, pain, sleep disorders, and 16 other emotional and physical manifestations of cancer are profiled in detail at this site of the National Cancer Institute. Summary descriptions and detailed management approaches are included for each manifestation.

6.13 Clinical Guidelines and Consensus Statements

Agency for Health Care Policy and Research ◎ ◎ ◎

http://text.nlm.nih.gov/ftrs/pick?collect=ahcpr&ftrsK=0&t=947080215

This site provides links to clinical practice guidelines on 19 different topics. In addition to clinical practice guidelines, there is a quick reference guide and a consumer guide for each topic. Spanish and English versions of the consumer guides are available.

American Society of Clinical Oncology (ASCO) ◎ ◎ (fee-based)

http://www.asco.org

This comprehensive, interactive resource provides educational and informational resources to patients and oncology professionals. The site offers news and information regarding ASCO current events, abstracts, guidelines, and links to oncology training programs. There is an ASCO member section that requires registration and a non-member section that does not. There is also a link to the *Journal of Clinical Oncology*.

Cancer Consensus Statements ◎ ◎ ◎

http://text.nlm.nih.gov/nih/cdc/www/cdc.html

This site provides links to full-text consensus statements published by the National Institute of Health Office of Medical Applications of Research. Cancer-related documents include breast cancer screening for women, cervical cancer, ovarian cancer, diagnosis and treatment of early melanoma, adjuvant therapy for patients with colon and rectum cancer, oral complications of cancer therapies, and others.

Cancer Economics for Oncology Group Practices

http://www.moffitt.usf.edu/cancjrnl/v2n6/economics.html

This is a clinical information document providing a discussion of cancer care approaches, insurance coverage, specialty insurance contracts in cancer, cost of case management, development of group practices, and reference information. It was developed by the Radiation Oncology Service of the H. Lee Moffitt Cancer Center & Research Institute.

Journal of Clinical Oncology: Topical Reports

http://www.jco.org/collected/index.dtl

Original reports are provided for clinical practitioners on thirty-five (35) subjects, ranging from AIDS-related cancers and Bone Marrow Transplantation to Supportive Care and Surgical Oncology. This is an excellent resource for healthcare professionals, and is not intended for the general public.

Neoplasm Guidelines

http://www.guideline.gov/FRAMESETS/search_fs.asp?view=disease

Part of the National Guideline Clearinghouse, this site provides links to 86 guidelines related to neoplasms. The site also provides links to related subconcepts including neoplastic processes, paraneoplastic syndrome, neoplasms by histologic type, neoplasms by site, and precancerous conditions.

Oncology Practice Guidelines

http://www.cancernetwork.com/indexes/nccn.htm

This professional resource provides practice guidelines related to all forms of cancer. Many screening, testing, and therapeutic practices are discussed, and individual disease guidelines are very technical. Twenty-eight (28) types of cancer and the accompanying guidelines are provided.

7. OTHER TOPICAL RESOURCES FOR ONCOLOGY AND HEMATOLOGY

7.1 **Advocacy, Legislation, and Public Policy**

Advocates: Cancer Research Foundation of America (CRFA) ⊙ ⊙ ⊙
http://www.preventcancer.org/advocates.htm

Seeking to prevent cancer, the CRFA offers valuable information on public advocacy, including how to be an advocate, Congressional issues, legislative alerts, legislative correspondence, events, and commemorative months. This organization explains its position regarding the support of bills that advance cancer research and prevention activities.

Health Care Policy and Advocacy from Cancer Care, Inc. ⊙ ⊙ ⊙
http://congress.nw.dc.us/cci

A Legislative Action Center at Cancer Care, Inc. provides information on bills concerning patient rights, cancer research, and cancer prevention. The site provides directions on writing to Congressional members, a Search Guide to Congress, and a section on Issues and Legislation, including recent bills and votes.

Take Action ⊙ ⊙ ⊙
http://www2.cancer.org/advocacy/new_advo/index.cfm

Important legislative issues and opportunities for individual advocacy are explored at this site of the American Cancer Society (ACS). Specific current bills in Congress are examined, instructions are given on how to take action and send a message to a member of Congress, and information is provided on the ACS Campaign Against Cancer. Each year, more than 10,000 cancer-related proposals are introduced before Congress, according to the home page of this site.

7.2 **Epidemiology and Cancer Registries**

AIDS Oncology Handbook: National Cancer Institute Intramural AIDS/AIDS Malignancy Activities in the Division of Cancer Epidemiology and Genetics (DCEG) ⊙ ⊙
http://ctep.info.nih.gov/aidsoncoresources/aidshandbooktext/IntramuralDCEG.htm

Studies in the DCEG Viral Epidemiology Branch (VEB) determining the nature and magnitude of HIV-1-associated malignancies are presented here. Major findings relate to Kaposi's Sarcoma, non-Hodgkin's lymphoma, anogenital cancer, and other malignancies. Contact information, a publications bibliography, objectives of the project, and a description of methods employed are all available at the site.

Cancer Epidemiology ◎ ◎ ◎

http://www.leukaemia.demon.co.uk/epidppt

This tutorial on cancer epidemiology was written by Ken Campbell. It contains information on the following topics: epidemiology, descriptive and analytical epidemiology, and prevalence, incidence, and mortality rates. It also provides population statistics, cumulative incidence rates, age standardization tables, and information about types of study.

H. Lee Moffitt Cancer Center and Research Institute: The Epidemiology of Cancer in Florida ◎ ◎

http://www.moffitt.usf.edu/cancjrnl/v5n3s/article5.html

Epidemiological data of cancer rates in Florida are presented at this site, including a description of trends, cancer by race and malignancy site, cancer mortality, race and gender comparisons, cancer among Hispanics, and variations within Florida. A bibliography of selected references and accompanying data tables are available at the site.

International Association of Cancer Registries (IACR) ◎ ◎ ◎

http://www-dep.iarc.fr/iacr.htm

The IACR provides a worldwide directory of cancer registries at this site. By selecting a region of the world, such as the United States, one can access a scroll-down menu of state by state registry listings, each with its own Web site link. There is also a list of names and addresses of registries without Web locations.

National Cancer Registrars Association (NCRA) ◎ ◎ ◎

http://www.ncra-usa.org

Providing extensive information and links related to cancer registration in the United States, the NCRA offers a central focal point for data about the purpose and importance of cancer registries. The site provides detailed information about the Association and its membership; educational resources; the *Journal of Registry Management;* and the process of cancer data collection, storage, use, and dissemination.

National Program of Cancer Registries ◎ ◎ ◎

http://www.cdc.gov/cancer/npcr/index.htm

Detailed information on the Cancer Registries Amendment Act and the National Program are provided at this Web site of the Centers of Disease Control and Prevention. There is information on national and state data, legislation, programs and events, contact specifics, and resource links.

OncoLink: Cancer Epidemiology ◎ ◎ ◎
http://www.oncolink.upenn.edu/causeprevent/epidemiology

This online resource for physicians offers news articles and links to useful statistical and epidemiology sources on the Internet. Resources are presented from the *Journal of the American Medical Association* and other journal articles, the National Cancer Institute and other government programs, state agencies, and consumer information sources.

SEER: Cancer Surveillance, Epidemiology, and End Results ◎ ◎ ◎
http://www-seer.ims.nci.nih.gov

The SEER (Surveillance, Epidemiology, and End Results) Program at the National Cancer Institute focuses on the collection of information on cancer incidence and survival in the United States. Information on more than 2.5 million cancer cases is included in the database. This site provides information on the program, regional registries of data, systems and methodologies, and links to other Internet resources related to the subject.

University of California (UC), Davis: Cancer Epidemiology ◎ ◎
http://wellness.ucdavis.edu/cancer/epidemiology/cancer_epidemiology.html

Epidemiological studies at the University of California, Davis related to cancer rates in different populations are discussed at this site. The highlighted projects, all involving California populations, are monitoring rates of lung cancer, liver cancer in Asian populations, veterinary cancers, tobacco smoke exposure, cervical cancer in Hispanic women, breast cancer recurrence and plant-based diets, childhood cancers, and cancers associated with pesticide exposure. Investigators are profiled, and visitors can access statistics related to cancer rates in California.

7.3 Hospice Care

(See also "Patient Education and Planning" in Part 2: General Medical Web Resources.)

Hospice Education Institute ◎ ◎ ◎
http://www.hospiceworld.org

Information and education about hospice care is provided by the Hospice Education Institute at this Web site, including an extremely valuable linked database, called Hospicelink, which provides information on all hospice and palliative care programs in the U.S.

HospiceWeb ⊙ ⊙ ⊙

http://www.hospiceweb.com

A discussion of hospice care and a directory of hospice facilities, organized state by state, can be found at this very useful site for severely-ill cancer patients. There are numerous links to sites offering general and specific information on the nature and value of hospice care, including many relevant organizations, all in addition to the links to hospice programs.

7.4 Informatics and Research Databases

Bioinformatics ⊙ ⊙ ⊙

http://biotech.icmb.utexas.edu/pages/bioinform/BIintro.html

This site provides introductory information about bioinformatics, a field related to the organization and indexing of sequence information in biology. There is also information about the process of computational biology. The site includes diagrams and pictures.

Cancer Genetics Informatics Centers ⊙ ⊙

http://unisci.com/stories/0727983.htm

The National Cancer Institute's focus on the field of informatics is the subject of this report dealing with the designation of the University of California/Irvine (UCI) as a key center for the dissemination of information on the genetic basis of cancer. UCI will develop and manage two of the most comprehensive human cancer genetics research databases ever assembled. The site describes this new initiative and outlines the goals of the project and its anticipated benefits for researchers, clinical practitioners, patients, and the public.

Carcinogenic Potency Project ⊙ ⊙ ⊙

http://potency.berkeley.edu/cpdb.html

The Carcinogenic Potency Database (CPDB) is a useful resource on the results of chronic, long-term animal cancer tests. Qualitative and quantitative information on positive and negative experiments are given, including all bioassays from the National Cancer Institute/National Toxicology Program (NCI/NTP). Results from the general literature that meet a set of inclusion criteria are also given. Links to the International Agency for Research on Cancer, The National Toxicology Program, Environmental Health Perspectives, and The National Library of Medicine are provided.

Clinical Trials and Informatics

http://www.nih.gov/news/pr/oct98/nci-06b.htm

The new initiative in this field, called the Cancer Informatics Infrastructure (CII), is described at this site, focusing on the collection, management, and dissemination of clinical trials data to improve the efficiency of the research "pipeline" for new cancer drug results.

Informatics and Information Flow

http://2001.cancer.gov/challenge4.htm

Knowledge Management, the field that is often called "Informatics," represents the discipline engaged in the study of ways to collect, handle, use, and share raw data that is generated from researchers and other sources around the globe. In the complex cancer arena, informatics is extremely important, for it calls for developing systems and frameworks for assimilating information and making it available in a fast and efficient manner to those who can use it to best advantage. This site explains how the National Cancer Institute is utilizing the field of informatics to assist in making new discovers and vital data available instantaneously, such as clinical trial results, toxicity information, physician experience with developing drugs, and research laboratory progress.

Yale Center for Medical Informatics

http://ycmi.med.yale.edu

Focused on the use of computers in clinical medicine, molecular biology, biomedical research, and medical education, the Yale Center offers information on its staff, laboratories, the childhood immunization informatics initiative, other informatics initiatives, and descriptions of projects utilizing informatics. Because of the applicability of this field to cancer, this site offers a useful resource for researchers and clinical practitioners interested in the efficient use and handling of vital data from clinical trials, medical management environments, and primary research studies.

7.5 International Resources

Cancer Care Ontario

http://www.cancercare.on.ca

Information provided at this government site is directed to Canadian medical professionals. However, much of the information applies to all medical professionals. Included in this site are informational documents referring to screening, referral, treatment plans, and funding.

CancerEurope ⚙ ⚙

http://www.cancereurope.net

CancerEurope provides access to the European School of Oncology (EOS), the European Association for Cancer Research (EACR), the European Oncology Nursing Society (EONS), the European Society of Mastology (EUSOMA) and the Europa-Donna site. The EOS is an educational institution for health professionals that enables them to better their skills in the area of cancer prevention. EACR is an institution of cancer research and its Web site provides information regarding the organization's philosophy, publications, and institutional fellowship. EONS is a society that supports cancer nursing and its Web site details the society's nursing program and meetings it holds. EuropaDonna is a coalition of organizations devoted to breast cancer. Its site provides information about chapters worldwide, upcoming events, support, and the society's newsletter.

Clinical Trials Service Unit (CTSU) Cancer Overviews ⚙

http://www.ctsu.ox.ac.uk/cancer/cancov.htm

The Clinical Trials Service Unit (CTSU) is a UK medical research unit that studies chronic diseases, including cancer. This page from the CTSU site provides overviews of each of the eight cancer collaborative groups, each of which studies a different form. A listing of CTSU and relevant publications is provided.

Health Canada Online ⚙ ⚙ ⚙

http://www.hc-sc.gc.ca/english/cancer.htm

The cancer section of the Canadian online health information site contains information for cancer prevention, statistics, epidemiological information and treatment, and risk information. There is specific information categorized by cancer type, and there are a number of research reports and news releases. News releases detail initiatives, practice guidelines, and funding information.

International Union Against Cancer: International Directory of Cancer Institutes and Organizations ⚙ ⚙ ⚙

http://www.globalink.org/directory

This alphabetized international directory lists a number of entries for cancer institutes and organizations for 65 countries. Clicking on a country will provide the links to these entries. Information on organizations and institutes includes addresses, telephone and fax numbers, e-mail addresses, descriptions of the various departments, and the names and contact information of the directors.

State of the Art Oncology in Europe ⊙ ⊙ ⊙
http://www.cancereurope.org

Launched by the European School of Oncology, this site and the project it represents involves 170 leading European oncologists, and offers a database on current treatment of human malignant tumors. There are separate chapters devoted to each type of tumor, as well as many other oncology topics and practices, including pain therapy, nutritional support, pharmacology, and screening. Click on the icon for the project to access the database and search engine.

Telescan: Telemantic Services in Cancer ⊙ ⊙ ⊙
http://telescan.nki.nl

A European service for researchers, physicians, and patients, Telescan provides information and links to a variety of organizations that provide treatment, education, and research information about cancer. The home page allows the user to locate specific information via keyword search. European sources are primarily provided.

University of Newcastle upon Tyne: International Resources ⊙ ⊙ ⊙
http://www.ncl.ac.uk/child-health/guides/clinks5.htm

International Internet resources related to cancer are available through links at this site, including home pages of key organizations, disease-specific organizations, specialty-specific organizations, and miscellaneous sites. Users can choose from more than 100 countries for resources specific to a particular nation or region. Most site links are presented with a short description of resources found at the address.

World Oncology Network (WON) ⊙ ⊙ ⊙
http://www.worldoncology.net

WON is a worldwide directory of oncologists, hematologists, and related specialists, assembled to promote effective communication among healthcare providers. Registration with the service is free for professionals, and all members receive printed information about all participants. The WON site provides an application, a bookstore, job information, and an international doctor's exchange.

7.6 Minority and Women's Health

American Association of Gynecologic Laparoscopists (AAGL) ⊙ ⊙ ⊙
http://www.aagl.com

The AAGL site offers a calendar of events, membership information, a newsletter, news, and publications information. There are links to the AAGL official journal, the Accreditation Council of Gynecological Endoscopy (ACGE), and the International

Federation of Gynecologic Endoscopists (IFGE). The ACGE page provides information concerning procedure, operative case lists, advanced operative hysterectomy case lists, and more. The association funds the development of technology in the field of gynecological laparoscopy.

American College of Obstetricians and Gynecologists (ACOG) ⚙ ⚙ (free registration)

http://www.acog.com

Both physicians and patients can locate useful information at the site of this professional association. Information is provided on all aspects of women's health including gynecologic cancers. Also included are a physician directory, news, and meeting information. The health professionals section provides information about postgraduate courses, ACOG membership, coding/nomenclature, residency, practice management, and case list software. Access to this section is restricted to ACOG members and online registration is required.

Cancer and Women ⚙ ⚙ ⚙

http://www.amwa-doc.org/publications/WCHealthbook/canceramwa-ch37.html

The American Medical Women's Association (AMWA) provides clinical information for physicians and consumers. Information includes methods of early detection, risk factors, gynecologic cancers, the future of research and care, warning signs, and what to do after cancer is provided. Information about AMWA publications is also offered.

Gillette Women's Cancer Connection ⚙ ⚙ ⚙

http://www.gillettecancerconnect.org

Sponsored by an organization for women and their families, this site offers extensive psychological and support information. Information regarding breast and gynecological cancers is provided in the form of brochures, surveys, and documents. The site also provides telephone numbers for information about regional support groups, online registration for "Connecting to Wellness" seminars, and a link to iVillage.com which provides information for women who wish to create their own Web pages and who want access to an instant messaging service.

Intercultural Cancer Council (ICC) ⚙ ⚙ ⚙

http://icc.bcm.tmc.edu/home.htm

This comprehensive site explores all aspects of cancer and intercultural issues, with extensive resources and links, a calendar of events, search features for information from the National Caner Institute, the Centers for Disease Control, and the Department of Health and Human Services, policy information and advocacy, news stories and public interest topics, and press releases of the ICC.

National Asian Women's Health Organization (NAWHO) ☉ ☉ ☉
http://www.nawho.org/homepageN.html

In the Partnership Initiatives Section of the Web site of the NAWHO, information and statistics are provided for cancer and Asian women in the Breast and Cervical Cancer Program. Information on cancer incidence, early detection, screening, prevention, and public awareness are provided.

National Women's Health Information Center (NWHIC) ☉ ☉ ☉
http://www.4women.gov

The National Women's Health Information Center is a project of the Office on Women's Health in the Department of Health and Human Services. This Web site offers extensive information on the subject of women's health issues, including resources on cancer for women. This information is accessed by typing the word "cancer" in the site search engine at the top of the page. Twenty important topics are explored regarding breast cancer and other forms of cancer, nutrition, imaging techniques, AIDS, coping with cancer, therapies, and support resources.

OBGYN.net ☉ ☉
http://www.obgyn.net

This resource site for patients, professionals, and others in the medical industry is presented in English and Spanish. It provides information concerning all aspects of women's health, including cancer. For patients, there are lay term descriptions of individual disorders and their respective treatments, patient events calendars, and listings of discussion and support groups. Professionals will find articles, news sections, medical videos, an image library, and professionally-oriented, moderated chat rooms.

Office of Minority Health Resource Center ☉ ☉ ☉
http://www.omhrc.gov

By clicking on the "no frames" choice on the home page, the site provides a menu of topics and issues related to minority health, including issues related to the provision and availability of cancer cancer for minorities. There is also information on AIDS, breast cancer, drugs, and other health concerns. Federal initiatives are also examined as they relate to minority health.

Women's Cancer Center ☉ ☉ ☉
http://www.womenscancercenter.com

Current information about the treatment of gynecological cancers is provided here. Areas of the site deal with treatments and tests, clinical trial information, minimally invasive laproscopic surgery, and a guide to other Internet resources. Patient information exists regarding surgery, emergencies, insurance procedures, and prescriptions.

General information, phone numbers, physician profiles, contact, and other information about the Center is also provided.

Women's Cancer Information Project   ◉ ◉

http://www.eurohealth.ie/cancom

This European site offers information and statistics to patients concerning most if not all cancers. The site offers a question/answer feature. Information about rare cancers such as uterine sarcoma, vaginal cancer, fallopian tube cancer, gestational trophoblastic tumor, and cancer of the vulva is available at this site. It offers professional and patient information regarding breast cancer, cancers specific to women, and statistics.

Women's Cancer Network (WCN)   ◉ ◉ ◉

http://www.wcn.org

WCN provides information for physicians concerning the prevention, detection, and treatment of cancer in women. It provides links to relevant articles, reviews, announcements, treatment and research information, and to news. In addition, there are links to sources of general information, information for survivors, support information, and a referral service that helps one locate a gynecologic cancer specialist.

7.7   Neuro-Oncology

M. D. Anderson Cancer Center: Neurosurgery Specialists   ◉ ◉

http://www.mdanderson.org/centers/neuro/treatment/specialists/neurosurg.htm

The Department of Neurosurgery uses this site to describe treatment at the Center for patients with tumors of the nervous system, including tumors of the spinal column, sacrum, and pituitary gland. Specific technologies are described, including monitoring of neurological functioning and cortical mapping. The site also offers a general overview of the Department of Neurosurgery, research activities, and specialties and recent publications bibliographies of faculty members.

Neuro-Oncology Foundation   ◉ ◉

http://www.networx.on.ca/~neuro

Research accomplishments, fellowships provided by the Foundation, publications, clinical opportunities open to patients, and information about the Foundation's advisory board are covered here. Other resources include news, patient services, education materials, links, and contact information.

OncoLink: About Brain and
Central Nervous System Tumors ⊙ ⊙ ⊙

http://oncolink.org/disease/brain/general/about_brain_tumors.html

This address offers a detailed discussion of brain and spinal cord tumors. Topics include the anatomy of the central nervous system, cancer of the brain and spinal cord, signs and symptoms of brain tumors, and a chart outlining different types of tumors, cell of origin, and normal function of that cell type.

San Diego Gamma Knife Center ⊙ ⊙

http://www.sdgkc.com

This site provides point-by-point explanations of the gamma knife in a surgery slide show with text explanations. There are also listings of upcoming events, an FAQ page, patient testimonials, and information about the Center.

UCLA Neuro-Oncology Program ⊙ ⊙

http://www.neurooncology.ucla.edu/neuro_web/index.asp

The UCLA Neuro-Oncology Program provides clinical care, scientific and clinical research, and psychosocial support in a multidisciplinary approach. The well-organized Web site provides detailed information about the aforementioned aspects of the program as well as information about facilities, staff, and research partners. Current research involves the molecular and physiological mechanistic approaches to understand oncogenesis. Educational information about brain tumors, statistics, and symptoms is also provided.

University of Chicago Hospitals: Department of
Neurology: Brain Tumors/ Neuro-Oncology ⊙ ⊙ ⊙

http://ucneurology.uchicago.edu

Treatment of brain tumors and tumors of the spinal cord at the University of Chicago are described at this site, located under Neurological Disorders/Brain Tumors. The site discusses malignant and benign brain tumors, symptoms, diagnosis, surgery, radiation therapy, interstitial brachytherapy, medication, specific clinical trials for brain tumors, and brain tumors in children. Links are also offered to related Web sites.

7.8 Nutrition

American Institute For Cancer Research (AICR) ⊙ ⊙

http://www.aicr.org

The American Institute for Cancer Research provides information about cancer prevention, particularly through diet and nutrition. Its site is oriented to information that will help reduce cancer risk. Topics covered include: pesticides, diet and nutrition, and AICR press releases on recent findings. They offer a toll-free nutrition hotline, pen pal support network, funding of research grants, and brochures and health aids for professionals and the general consumer about diet and nutrition. AICR CancerResource is the Institute's information and resource program for cancer patients.

Cancer Nutrition Center ◎ ◎
http://www.cancernutrition.com

A certified nutrition specialist offers information about lectures, a nutrition handbook, the connection between cancer and nutrition, relevant books, and links at this helpful site.

Memorial Sloan Kettering Cancer Center: Dietary Guidelines for Preventing Cancer ◎ ◎
http://www.mskcc.org/document/peddiet.htm

This site provides information for the general public on the role nutrition plays in the prevention of cancer. Fats, fiber, caloric intake, alcohol consumption, and the specific benefits of fruits and vegetables are discussed. The site also offers information on risks posed by barbecued, smoked, salt-cured, and pickled foods, and provides links to additional nutritional information and research findings.

National Cancer Institute (NCI): Nutrition ◎ ◎ ◎
http://cancernet.nci.nih.gov/clinpdq/supportive/Nutrition_Physician.html

Nutritional issues related to cancer patients are discussed at this site meant for health professionals. The site offers an overview of nutritional problems associated with loss of appetite, obstructive tumors, and metabolism changes. Specific effects of the tumor, effects of cancer therapies, and psychosocial effects are presented, as well as information on nutritional assessment, general management guidelines, and support. All information is supported with a reference bibliography.

7.9 Patient Education and Support

Anderson Information Network ◎ ◎ ◎
http://www.mdanderson.org/centers/pathway/andnet

Provided by the University of Texas M.D. Anderson Cancer Center, this information site is useful for patients and professionals. Information about support groups, support conferences, online support services, a newsletter, medical facts and the center can be accessed from this site. In addition, there is information about research at the center, contacts, referrals and news.

Association of Cancer Online Resources (ACOR) ◉ ◉

http://www.acor.org/index.html?Poe_Session=d405998b4ff8fb3158d26f3a02f1e14a

ACOR provides a wide range of Internet-based cancer resources to patients, families, and professionals. Within the CancerNet section of the site there is an extensive list of types of cancer, with detailed descriptions of typical treatments. The site offers archives of support and electronic information groups, links to other Web sites, an external search service, and links to journals.

Association of Community Cancer Centers (ACCC) ◉ ◉

http://www.assoc-cancer-ctrs.org

An interdisciplinary organization for the improvement of patient care, the ACCC also seeks to define standards of care. Information available includes lists of cancer centers and member profiles, the ACCC vision and mission, meeting schedules, news, professional job opportunities, program standards and contacts. There is an ACCC member newsgroup that has restricted access. The user is also given access to *Oncology Issues,* the official journal of the ACCC.

Cancer 411 ◉ ◉

http://www.cancer411.com

Cancer 411 is part of the Rory Foundation, a patient and public awareness, information and support organization. The site offers extensive patient information, a calendar of events, a newsletter, message board, publication news, and links. The site features a chat room that provides oncologists, other health practitioners, acupuncturists, authors, and researchers to answer questions from anyone.

Cancer Care, Inc. ◉ ◉ ◉

http://www.cancercare.org

Focusing on the care of cancer patients, this Web site offers support and coping information, treatment information, details of educational seminars and conferences held by Cancer Care, Inc., and information about professional consultations and educational programs. The easily navigated site library contains a search engine specific to the site and areas devoted to individual types of cancer, professional papers and briefs, and clinical trial information. Information regarding cost management and physician communication is available for patients.

Cancer Chat Room Web Page ◉ ◉

http://members.aol.com/Sunny9652/index.html

This page lists many support and information chat rooms and message boards for a variety of people. There are chat rooms on pain relief, alternative healing, and more for women, family members, and other groups. There are also many links to cancer related information pages and Web sites.

Cancer Education from The Arkansas Cancer Research Center

http://www.acrc.uams.edu

Patient information and education, professional education, and multimedia resources are provided at this university research site. Multimedia resources consist of text and image modules that concern a variety of disorders, and offer information about cancer biology, pathology, prevention principles, diagnosis, and treatment. Professional educational resources include conferences, curriculum information, and a primary care physician's resource center. Patient resources include informational booklets, general information, and information about the Center.

Cancer Hope Network

http://www.cancerhopenetwork.org

This unique New Jersey-based not-for-profit provides support and hope to cancer patients and their families throughout the United States by matching patients and/or family members one-on-one with trained volunteers who have themselves undergone and recovered from a similar cancer experience. There is no charge for the organization's services and patient confidentiality is observed. Cancer Hope's Web site covers frequently asked questions about the organization's matching process, the training their volunteers receive, and how to schedule a visit. The patient and/or family member seeking support can fill out the site's Web page form or call its toll-free number. The "More Help" option on the site menu provides links to many other sites for general cancer information and help, cancer-specific organizations, and treatment-specific organizations/corporations.

Cancer Information and Support International ○ ○ ○

http://www.cancer-info.com

This is the site of an international support organization with a mailing list, domestic and international phone numbers, and information. Links to information pages and documents are listed under alternative therapies, books, news group, disorders, support, research, conventional therapies, and general categories.

Cancer Support Center of Saint Louis ○ ○

http://recluse.mvp.net/cancersc

This St. Louis-based center for adult cancer patients and families provides a variety of comprehensive support and information services. A great deal of information about the program and its mission is provided along with general support information for the public. A number of informative documents, contact listings, and an FAQ are provided.

Cancerdirectory ⊙ ⊙ ⊙
http://www.cancerdirectory.com

Included at this site is a products, information, discussion, and support source for patients and their families. There are lists of hospitals and centers, symposia, alternative therapies, directories, and other links.

Community Support
Organizations for Breast Cancer ⊙ ⊙ ⊙
http://www.nabco.org/support

Clearly indexed by states and cities, this extraordinarily useful resource for breast cancer support organizations provides resources in every state and hundreds of cities and towns across America. Names and telephone numbers are provided for each support group.

Corporate Angel Network ⊙ ⊙
http://www.corpangelnetwork.org

Providing free air transportation for cancer patients traveling to and from recognized treatment centers in the U.S., the Corporate Angel Network draws upon the generosity of companies with private aircraft who donate seat space without regard to the financial resources of the patient. Information and guidelines for patients are outlined at this supportive Web site.

Financial Assistance for Cancer Care ⊙ ⊙
http://imsdd.meb.uni-bonn.de/cancernet/600083.html

Exploring 15 different avenues to secure financial assistance for cancer care, this report is an important document for cancer patients who are faced with insufficient medical insurance coverage. There is information on social security, supplemental security income (SSI), Medicaid, federal government general assistance programs, veterans benefits, American Cancer Society resources for patient consultation, foundation sources, and national associations in different areas of cancer.

Gilda's Club ⊙ ⊙
http://www.gildasclub.org

Serving the support needs of individuals and families dealing with cancer, Gilda's Club provides social and emotional support through a community of concerned persons. The club offers support and networking groups, lectures, workshops, and social events. The organization was founded by Gilda Radner.

Keepin' the Faith:
Cancer Support for the Heart and Soul ⊙ ⊙ ⊙

http://ktf.org

This is a Web site that provides support information for patients, relatives, and friends. There are more than 200 pages of advice, stories, education materials, poetry, humor, news, and more. In addition, there is a staff of 80 volunteers who provide one-to-one e-mail support. The home page is easy to navigate and provides direct links to specific sections of the site.

National Coalition For Cancer Survivorship (NCCS) ⊙ ⊙ ⊙

http://www.cansearch.org

The National Coalition for Cancer Survivorship is a grassroots, nationwide network of independent organizations and individuals working in the area of cancer support and information for all types of cancer. Their Web site carries an index to the organization's current newsletter, *NCCS Networker,* as well as back issues. The newsletter contains information on regional and local support groups, new clinical trials and research, recent legislative activity, and reviews of the latest publications by and for cancer survivors. A yearly membership fee is required to receive the newsletter. Free on the site is the "Cancer Survival Toolbox." This is a tutorial in audio and transcript form that coaches the patient on developing skills needed during treatment. Topics include communicating, finding information, solving problems, making decisions, and negotiating and standing up for your rights. Another useful, free tutorial unique in the field of cancer education is the "Cancer: Keys to Survivorship" program. It addresses skills and strategies for self-employment, communicating with healthcare providers and loved ones, understanding workplace concerns and employment rights, and under-standing health insurance issues. The site's "CanSearch Websites" provides excellent step-by-step directions for researching cancer on the Internet, with sites to visit first to gather basic information, and secondary sites for information of a specific nature. The NCCS site and a selection of their publications are available in Spanish.

National Support Organizations ⊙ ⊙ ⊙

http://cis.nci.nih.gov/fact/8_1.htm

Dozens of major national organizations that provide support services to people with cancer and their families can be found at this useful site, including organization name, address, toll-free number, Web address, and e-mail.

Oncochat ⊙ ⊙

http://www.oncochat.org

Oncochat is a peer support group that features Internet Relay Chat (IRC) and allows users to chat online 24 hours a day. Information about IRC is provided at the site along with other support information and links.

Patient Advocacy Phone Numbers ◎ ◎ ◎
http://infonet.welch.jhu.edu/advocacy.html

Provided by the Johns Hopkins Medical Institutions' InfoNet, this site includes patient advocacy telephone numbers for most if not all disorders, including specific telephone numbers for specific cancers. Links to each advocacy organization are provided.

Patient Advocate Foundation ◎ ◎ ◎
http://www.patientadvocate.org

A national organization serving as a liaison between patients and insurers, employers, and creditors, the Patient Advocate Foundation seeks to resolve patient problems arising from illness through mediation, in order to assure access to care, employment, and financial stability. The site provides a menu of subjects, including current issues, cancer news, patient resources, children's resources, debt crisis intervention, job discrimination assistance, insurance support, and contact methods.

R.A. Bloch Cancer Foundation, Inc. ◎ ◎ ◎
http://www.blochcancer.org

This site is a thorough patient resource and support site for cancer in general. There are many informational documents and articles that refer to topics such as multidisciplinary second opinions, patient checklists, treatment information, and more.

Wellness Community ◎ ◎ ◎
http://www.wellness-community.org

Directed to cancer patients fighting for recovery, The Wellness Community offers a program as well as resources for emotional support, education, and hope for patients and families. There are a series of links related to issues of support and care, as well as programs, events, and information about the organization. Support groups, networking, workshops, and educational programs are all a part of the Wellness Community.

7.10 Pediatric Oncology

A Starting Point: To Connect with
Resources Related to Pediatric Oncology ◎ ◎
http://www.med.miami.edu/neurosurgery/start_intro.htm

Supplied by the University of Miami School of Medicine, this resource provides a large number of links and information pages regarding second opinions, types of cancer, treatments, university hospitals, research, organizations, contacts, projects, and terms. Much of the information is provided for patients; some is provided for professionals.

American Academy of Pediatrics (AAP) Section on Hematology/Oncology ◎ ◎

http://www.aap.org/sections/shem-onc.htm

This section of the AAP professional society's Web site provides information related to care and serves as an educational forum for discussion of neoplastic and hematological disease in infants. Membership information and information about training programs, section annual meetings, CME courses, contacts, and research is provided. Access to the rest of the AAP site is also provided. There, one can find more informative documents and patient resources relating to pediatric hematology/oncology. Some areas of the site are restricted to AAP members.

American Society of Pediatric Hematology/Oncology (ASPH/O) ◎ ◎

http://www.aspho.org

The official Web site of the professional society offers information about the ASPH/O, membership criteria, announcements, symposia, and news. A resource section groups links to related sites and to information pages by suitability for patients, professionals, or both. There is also a link to the *Journal of Pediatric Hematology/Oncology,* the organization's official journal.

Cancer Books for Children ◎ ◎ ◎

http://mel.merit.edu/health/cancerbooks

Provided by the Michigan Electronic Library, this site is a resource for online and offline informational sources for children. There are sections that list books for children with cancer, grieving children, or children whose parents/relatives have cancer. The listings are quite extensive and, in most cases, there exist direct links for each book to retailers.

Cancer Kids ◎ ◎

http://www.cancerkids.org

This site for children with cancer provides a forum to share stories and find information. A discussion forum, contact information, and organization information are provided. The Resource section provides links to sites that offer summer camp, support, wish fulfillment, and e-mail list information.

Candlelighters Childhood Cancer Foundation (CCCF) ◎ ◎

http://www.candlelighters.org

The CCCF provides education, information, support and advocate services for professionals, patients, and families. Its Web site provides announcements about raising awareness, CCCF news, events, and research studies. There is also information on the many CCCF services, addresses, and contacts.

Children's Cancer Center ◎ ◎

http://www.childrenscancercenter.org

The site of this nonprofit organization provides educational and support information to children and their families. There is news about the Center, upcoming events, and available services.

Children's Cancer Research Fund ◎ ◎

http://www.ccrf.org

This organization is sponsored by New York Medical College and is devoted to raising funds for and fostering research, providing support, and bettering clinical services available to patients. One can find information at the site regarding social support services, research programs, events sponsored, contacts, and the organization's newsletter.

Children's Cancer Web ◎ ◎ ◎

http://www.ncl.ac.uk/child-health/guides/guide2.htm

This comprehensive site functions as a guide to Internet resources on all aspects of children's cancer. Information and links to sources of information for patients, parents, and health professionals are provided. The 500+ links in this easy-to-navigate site are separated by category or disorder type.

Institute for Neurology and Neurosurgery at the Beth Israel Medical Center: Pediatric Neurosurgery: Childhood Brain Tumors ◎ ◎ ◎

http://www.nyneurosurgery.org/tumor/child/brain/present.html

Definitions of brain tumors affecting children, including gliomas, midline tumors, pituitary tumors, and meningioma are presented at this informative site. Brain tumor symptoms and treatments are also discussed in detail, and users can also access a glossary of terms and links to support services and other sites of interest.

National Childhood Cancer Foundation (NCCF) ◎ ◎ ◎

http://www.nccf.org

The NCCF is a nonprofit organization that provides support for pediatric cancer treatment and research in the U.S., Canada, and Australia. Its Web site provides information about the Childhood Cancer Group, the network of over 2,800 pediatric cancer specialists that work in partnership with the NCCF. From the site, one can search through CCG clinical trial protocols, find CCG institutions, learn about the NCCF and pediatric cancers, and find information on current events. There is a section of CCG information that is restricted to members.

National Children's Cancer Society ⊚ ⊚ ⊚

http://www.children-cancer.com

The goal of this nonprofit organization is to provide support, advocacy, education, and financial assistance to children with cancer and their families. Some specific programs offered promote education and wellness, pediatric oncology camps, and communication assistance with hospitals and insurance companies. Detailed information about all programs, contacts, and news is offered at the site.

Never Ending Squirrel Tale ⊚ ⊚ ⊚

http://www.squirreltales.com

A support site for parents of children with cancer, the site claims to be a "practical Web site" and provides encouragement, practical tips, feature articles, information, and news. Some "practical tips" concern children's appetite, taste alterations, recipes, shopping items, hydration tips, and warnings. There is also an extensive links directory for other informative sites.

Pediatric Database ⊚ ⊚ ⊚

http://www.icondata.com/health/pedbase/index.htm

This massive database provides professional information on most if not all pediatric disorders including extensive information about various pediatric cancers and anemias. The site also provides a long list of links to pages that offer epidemiology, pathogenesis, clinical feature, investigation, prognosis, and management data.

Pediatric Oncology Resource Center ⊚ ⊚

http://www.acor.org/diseases/ped-onc/index.html

An information resource for childhood cancers, this site has many information pages, links, and references to medical literature. Topics covered in information pages include treatment, family issues, activism, and support.

Pediatric Oncology Web Resources (POWR) ⊚ ⊚

http://www.hmc.psu.edu/depts/pedsonco/index.html

This site provides links to sites and information pages associated with many aspects of pediatric oncology. The site is divided into three sections: patient resources, professional resources, and "cool sites." Patient resources provide education and general information about therapy, diagnosis, and home care. Professional resources consist of links to some professional organizations.

Pediatric Pain ⊚ ⊚ ⊚

http://is.dal.ca/~pedpain/pedpain.html

Pediatric Pain is a site for patients, family members and professionals providing resources related to cancer and other disorders. Sections of the site detail professional resources, research into pediatric pain, and self-help assistance. Information about mailing lists, newsletters, forums, handbooks, and publications is also provided.

SpecialLove for Children with Cancer ◎ ◎
http://www.speciallove.org

This Virginia based organization provides children and their families with the opportunity to develop a network of support, to participate in activities, and to find information. The organization sponsors a number of activities including day trips, camps, weekend outings, and support meetings. Information about all services, contacts, and news is available at the site.

Tomorrow Fund ◎ ◎ ◎
http://www.tomorrowfund.org

A support organization for children with cancer and their families, Tomorrow Fund details the organization's programs for family financial support, emotional support, education and outreach, and research. The Web site can be used by all but is especially child-friendly. An information library, games, live Web cameras, inspiration, news, and discussion sections are some of the attractions of this site.

William Guy Forbeck Research Foundation ◎ ◎
http://www.wgfrf.org

This Foundation promotes research in the field of pediatric oncology, and provides a forum for the exchange of scientific ideas. The site features information regarding the organization's annual meeting, and other forums for scientific exchange. Proceedings from past meetings can be accessed along with information about the organization's scientific advisory board. Grant and award information is also provided.

7.11 Radiation Oncology

American College of Radiation Oncology (ACRO) ◎ ◎
http://www.acro.org

The ACRO provides a comprehensive source of information on radiation oncology, including organization details and useful links to Internet resources in the field. There are links to general oncology sites, associations, radiation oncology departments, and sites focusing on different aspects of radiation oncology, including support for patients, radiography, journals, and centers.

American Society for Therapeutic Radiology and Oncology (ASTRO) ✪ ✪ (some features fee-based)

http://www.astro.org

ASTRO is a society for physicians and scientists that serves to advance the practice of competent radiation oncology via excellence in care, and the use of research through professional development. The site provides information about the society's meetings, educational opportunities and abstracts. Member portions are secure.

Association of Residents in Radiation Oncology ✪ ✪ ✪

http://www.arro.org

This site is focused on residents, but has extensive resources for physicians and healthcare professionals as well. For residents, there are fellowship sources, residency programs, article bibliographies, and certification details. For a larger audience, there are many useful links to online journals and journal clubs, search engines, clinical trials, screening and treatment sites, associations, and directories.

European Society for Therapeutic Radiology and Oncology (ESTRO) ✪ ✪

http://www.estro.be

The ESTRO Web site provides information regarding the society, membership, fellowships, past awards winners, events, publications, and research news. An educational section provides a number of informative documents.

Radiation—Oncology Newsgroup Archive ✪ ✪ ✪

http://www.bio.net:80/hypermail/RADIATION-ONCOLOGY

This site boasts a large collection of articles that range from 1996 to the present. Articles are located by month and year or by keyword search. One can also post new articles.

Radiation Oncology Online Journal (ROOJ) ✪ ✪

http://www.rooj.com

Physicians and technicians will find this to be a comprehensive source of information on radiation oncology, providing both professional and patient resources, clinical articles, a search engine, political action information, and a larger number of Internet links to other important sites. The professional section provides radiation calculators, therapy treatment records, and patient information forms. The patient section offers valuation information on radiation treatments, side effects, restrictions, consultation, and post-procedure care. Articles offer information on each different type of cancer, and are an additional resource for a wide audience of readers.

Radiological Society of North America (RSNA) ◎ ◎ ◎

http://www.rsna.org

Details about the society, its affiliations, and members are available at this site. There are links to a number of journals, conference registration materials, and events listings. Learning and practice tools available include a CME database, practice guidelines, case studies, and medical images. There are a large number of organized links to other image and information resource sites.

Society for Radiation Oncology Administrators (SROA) ◎

http://www.sroa.org

SORA serves medical management professionals and seeks to improve administration and nonmedical management and to provide information. Information about career opportunities, membership, annual meetings, legislation and the SROA member network is provided. News briefs, links, and discussion forum pages are also available.

Stanford University School of Medicine
Department of Radiation Oncology ◎ ◎

http://www-radonc.stanford.edu

This Stanford site provides details of academic programs, clinical trials, training programs, treatment modalities, research programs, grants, faculty, and patient support. There are more than 50 useful links and a newsletter for patients.

7.12 Survivorship

National Cancer Institute (NCI): Office of Cancer Survivorship ◎ ◎ ◎

http://dccps.nci.nih.gov/ocs

Designed for researchers, health professionals, advocates, and survivors and their families, this Web site focuses on what is new in cancer survivorship, including ongoing research. There is information on cancer prevalence and survivorship issues, incidence and survival among children and adolescents in the U.S., and research links in the Researchers' Toolbox.

Survivorship Programs of the
National Coalition for Cancer Survivorship (NCCS) ◎ ◎ ◎

http://www.cansearch.org/programs/index.html

Programs directed at communities, groups, and individuals focused on survivorship are profiled at this section of the National Coalition for Cancer Survivorship. Programs include "Rays of Hope," "NCCS Ribbon of Hope," "The Cancer Survival Toolbox," and "NCCS Town Halls." There is also information on the Spirituality Committee, the NCCS Speakers Bureau, and Minority Cancer Survivorship Programs.

8. ORGANIZATIONS AND INSTITUTIONS

8.1 **Associations and Societies**

Introduction
Below are profiles of more than 80 associations and societies in the fields of oncology and hematology. Those organizations that have a specific focus appear a second time in this volume under the "Diseases" section or under an appropriate topical heading.

American Academy of Dermatology (AAD) ☺ ☺ ☺
http://www.aad.org

The AAD site includes patient information, a referral service, and a link to the society's official journal. There is a link to a special physician and patient education section that provides information that concerns melanoma. A professional section details, news, AAD information, a virtual exhibit hall, meetings information, residents news, a marketplace, and more.

American Academy of Ophthalmology (AAO) ☺ ☺ ☺
http://www.aao.org

The site of the professional organization provides a large number of resources for patients and professionals that concern all eye disorders. The professional area offers an academy overview, clinical education information, listings of meetings, member services details, practice services, and a products and publications listing. The patient area provides information about the AAO, ophthalmology, eye health, anatomy, conditions and diseases, low vision resources, support groups, surgery, and news.

American Academy of Orthopedic Surgeons (AAOS) ☺ ☺ ☺
http://www.aaos.org

The site for this professional organization provides information about most orthopedic issues for professionals and the public. Public information about the AAOS, disorders, and prevention is offered. For professionals, there are details on the AAOS Annual Meeting, links to other sites, and discussions of current legislative issues. A restricted section for AAOS members provides information about specialty societies, research, member directories, AAOS services, outcomes assessment, educational resources, discussion groups, and AAOS archives. Membership information is provided. An Orthopedic Yellow pages section provides listings of clinical product suppliers, firms, office suppliers, and more.

American Academy of Pediatrics (AAP)
Section on Hematology/Oncology ⊙ ⊙

http://www.aap.org/sections/shem-onc.htm

This section of the AAP professional society's Web site provides information related to care and serves as an educational forum for discussion of neoplastic and hematological disease in infants. Membership information and information about training programs, section annual meetings, CME courses, contacts, and research is provided. Access to the rest of the AAP site is also provided. There, one can find more informative documents and patient resources relating to pediatric hematology/oncology. Some areas of the site are restricted to AAP members.

American Association for Cancer Research (AACR) ⊙ ⊙ ⊙

http://www.aacr.org

The scientific society's easy to navigate site provides a tremendous number of resources and links for professionals and patients. The site includes information about the society, patient education, grants and funding, research awards and fellowships, symposia schedules, educational workshops, abstracts and publications, the Association Newsletter and links to Scientific Journals. The site also has live and archived audio programs and provides a public forum.

American Association of Blood Banks (AABB) ⊙ ⊙ ⊙

http://www.aabb.org

The AABB is an international association of blood banks that seeks to implement high standards for patients and donors in all aspects of the process. The AABB Web site provides facts about blood, donation, receiving, subscription services, and news. Percentage testing reports, practice guidelines, statements on transfusion practices, reviews, and ISO reports are provided for medical professionals. Educational materials available include information on workshops, meetings, and certification information.

American Association of
Clinical Endocrinologists (AACE) ⊙ ⊙

http://www.aace.com

The AACE site offers organization, publication, clinical, education, research, events, and membership information. Clinical information is about all endocrine disorders including cancer. There are listings of regional meetings, clinical abstracts, and includes calendars and directories. A restricted access members area provides information about CPT coding, legislative and socioeconomic issues, and a professional chat room.

American Association of Gynecologic Laparoscopists (AAGL) ◎ ◎ ◎

http://www.aagl.com

The AAGL site offers a calendar of events, membership information, a newsletter, news, and publications information. There are links to the AAGL official journal, the AAGL foundation, the Accreditation Council of Gynecological Endoscopy (ACGE) and the International Federation of Gynecologic Endoscopists (IFGE). The ACGE page provides information concerning procedure, operative case lists, advanced operative hysterectomy case lists, and more. The foundation funds the development of technology in the field of gynecological laparoscopy.

American Association of Oral and Maxillofacial Surgeons (AAOMS) ◎ ◎

http://www.aaoms.org

The society consists of professionals who care for patients with disorders of the areas of mouth, teeth, jaw, and face including those with tumors and cysts. The site provides information about the AAOMS, news, continuing education programs, and conferences, residency, and contacts. A patient information section supplies details about the specialty and procedures.

American Brain Tumor Association ◎ ◎

http://www.abta.org

The American Brain Tumor Association provides information to patients and healthcare professionals and funds and encourages research. Featured are links for professionals to pages describing funding and current research. Resources at the site for patients include links to brain tumor information, patient support resources, and patient education tools.

American Cancer Society (ACS) ◎ ◎ ◎

http://www.cancer.org

The ACS is one of the most important supersites for information on all aspects of cancer, primarily directed to the public. The site home page includes headlines and brief stories on new cancer developments and treatments, as well as links to types of cancer, pediatric cancer, prevention, treatment options, therapies, research, statistics, and media resources. Details about the ACS itself are provided, including Annual Report, financial statements, employment, meetings, and e-mail. There is a state by state scroll menu to link to state organizations, services, and support, an online directory of medical resources, including a hospital locator, information on legislative and public action issues, and extensive sublinks focusing on more than 50 different forms of cancer. Each cancer description is quite thorough, and is augmented by additional links to other resources on the same topic, such as specialized glossaries, imaging, drugs, and alternative therapies.

American College of Radiation Oncology (ACRO) ◉ ◉
http://www.acro.org

This informative site is geared towards radiologists and other professionals. News, links and information about ACRO, membership, its programs, publications and meetings are available at this site. A section for residents details awards and resident membership criteria. Programs offered deal with practice accreditation, captivation, and charge capture.

American College of Surgeons Oncology Group (ACOS–OG) ◉ ◉
http://www.acosog.org

The ACOS-OG has been established by The American College of Surgeons as a surgical clinical trial group. Its site details clinical site technical requirements, society membership and application, meeting information, study titles, contact information for ACOS-OG staff, and news about the organization.

American Gastrointestinal Association (AGA) ◉ ◉
http://www.gastro.org

The site of the AGA primarily serves gastroenterologists and related professionals. There are details about sections, committees, documents, and courses that concern gastrointestinal oncology.

American Institute For Cancer Research (AICR) ◉ ◉
http://www.aicr.org

The American Institute for Cancer Research provides information about cancer prevention, particularly through diet and nutrition. Its site is oriented to information that will help reduce cancer risk. Topics covered include: pesticides, diet and nutrition, and AICR press releases on recent findings. They offer a toll-free nutrition hotline, pen pal support network, funding of research grants, and brochures and health aids for professionals and the general consumer about diet and nutrition. AICR CancerResource is the Institute's information and resource program for cancer patients.

American Lung Association ◉ ◉
http://www.aarc.org

Association-related information concerning news, medical releases, all lung diseases, local chapters, research, publications, programs and events, support and data, and statistics is located at this site.

American Neurological Association (ANA) ⊙ ⊙ ⊙

http://www.aneuroa.org

ANA is a professional organization that serves those who deal with all disorders of the brain. Information available at the ANA Web site concerns brain tumors as well as other neurological disorders. Extensive ANA information is provided along with abstract information and listings, ANA archives, meeting information, member databases, links, and a newsletter.

American Pain Society (APS) ⊙ ⊙ ⊙

http://www.ampainsoc.org

The APS is a multidisciplinary, scientific organization. This Web site provides annual meeting, publication, advocacy, news, opportunity, and events information. A pain facility database allows the user to search for facilities by classifications. Resources for patients and professionals provides contact information for organizations that are related to pain management. The APS site also provides an abstract search engine for their database of internal documentation on pain-related topics. A resources section offers links that are organized for patients or professionals.

American Prostate Society ⊙ ⊙ ⊙

http://www.ameripros.org

This society provides patient and professional information for all diseases of the prostate including enlarged prostate, prostatitis, and cancer. There are informational sections regarding these disorders as well as conferences, the society mission, professional abstracts, and membership. An online newsletter is also available.

American Society for
Blood and Marrow Transplantation (ASMBT) ⊙ ⊙ ⊙

http://www.asbmt.org

The ASMBT is a professional association for researchers and clinicians that seeks to foster research, represent physicians, establish clinical standards, promote communications, provide accreditation programs, and provide recommendations for insurance reimbursement. Information about the society's meetings, directors, membership, policy, and contacts is provided. Reviews and informative documents are also provided. There is a link to *Biology of Blood and Marrow Transplantation;* this journal publishes research, reviews, commentaries, news of the ASMBT, and more.

American Society for Colposcopy and Cervical Pathology ◉ ◉

http://www.asccp.org

The society's Web site provides information about symposia, disorders, educational materials, and a forum for discussion of educational topics. Membership and contact information is supplied. Forum registration is free.

American Society for Dermatologic Surgery (ASDS) ◉ ◉

http://www.asds-net.org

The ASDS provides information regarding all skin disorders including cancer. It includes information about ASDS, patient education materials, news, and continuing education.

American Society for Gastrointestinal Endoscopy ◉ ◉ ◉

http://www.asge.org

The professional society for gastroenterologists, surgeons, and other health professionals provides information about GI disease and the use of endoscopy. Information about endoscopy related to all GI disease, including cancer, is provided. Patient information comes in the form of educational documents that discuss upper endoscopy, flexible sigmoidoscopy, colonoscopy, and more. One can view an online database of clinical updates, policy and position statements, and patient care guidelines. There is a member section that has restricted access by password.

American Society for Histocompatibility and Immunogenetics (ASHI) ◉ ◉

http://www.swmed.edu/home_pages/ASHI/ashi.htm

The society seeks to provide a forum for discussion of recent advances, to aid professionals, to maintain histocompatibility testing laboratory quality and fidelity and to provide a voice for its members in governmental regulatory agencies. Its site provides detailed information about the society, ASHI services, discussion, directories, employment updates, H&I archives, ASHI products and news, information and meetings updates. There is also a restricted section for members that requires a password, and includes information about its members, committees, bylaws, and council.

American Society for Therapeutic Radiology and Oncology (ASTRO) ◉ ◉ (some features fee-based)

http://www.astro.org

ASTRO is a society for physicians and scientists that serves to advance the practice of competent radiation oncology via excellence in care, and the use of research through professional development. The site provides information about the society's meetings, educational opportunities and abstracts. Member portions of the sight are currently under construction and will be secure to the society's members in the future.

American Society of Clinical Oncology (ASCO) ◎ ◎ (fee-based)

http://www.asco.org

This comprehensive, interactive resource provides educational and informational resources to patients and oncology professionals. The site offers news and information regarding ASCO current events, abstracts, guidelines, and links to oncology training programs. There is an ASCO member section that requires registration and a non-member section that does not. There is also a link to *The Journal of Clinical Oncology.*

American Society of Colon and Rectal Surgeons (ASCRS) ◎ ◎ ◎

http://www.fascrs.org

The ASCRS provides information about many colon and rectal disorders and their relation to surgery. Information available at the site concerns the ASCRS council, committees, research, residency programs, core subjects, a practice registry, and regional societies. One can locate a colorectal surgeon and find general patient information via the site. The Practice Parameters section features documents devoted to the treatment of rectal carcinoma and detection of colorectal neoplasms. The documents are quite detailed and come with extensive information concerning supporting documentation.

American Society of Hematology (ASH) ◎ ◎

http://www.hematology.org

The ASH Web site provides information about the professional society, ASH awards, the annual meeting, training programs, news, membership, and educational materials. There is an extensive list of educational documents that are organized by topic. There is also a link to *Blood,* the journal of the American Society of Hematology.

American Society of Ophthalmic Plastic & Reconstructive Surgery ◎ ◎

http://www.asoprs.org

This Web site provides information about reconstructive surgery involving the eyelids, orbits, and lacrimal system. There is information about membership, fellowships, scientific meetings, journals, and contacts. A patient information section provides information about the field, procedures, eyelid skin cancers, tumors, and other conditions. There is a restricted section for members that provides professional information.

American Society of Pediatric Hematology/Oncology (ASPH/O) ◎ ◎

http://www.aspho.org

The official Web site of the professional society offers information about ASPH/O, membership criteria, announcements, symposia, and news. A resource section groups links to related sites and to information pages by suitability for patients, professionals, or both. There is also a link to the *Journal of Pediatric Hematology/Oncology,* the organization's official journal.

American Society of Transplant Surgeons (ASTS) ◎ ◎ (fee-based)

http://www.asts.org

The ASTS Web site offers information about its committees, bylaws, membership, meetings, fellowship accreditation, awards, and an ethics section to aid in clinical decision making. A substantial portion of the site has restricted access for members, and these sections offer a journal, a member directory, conference rooms for discussion, and organization reports. An online membership application is required.

American Society of Transplantation (AST) ◎ ◎

http://www.a-s-t.org

The professional society serves physicians and scientists and promotes research, patient care, advocacy, and education. Information concerning bylaws, CME, meetings, ethics, officers, membership, job postings, publications, and certification is provided. A restricted section for members provides committee reports, slide lectures, a newsletter, CME transcripts, and a member directory. Preregistration for meetings is also possible via the site.

American Thyroid Association (ATA) ◎ ◎

http://www.thyroid.org

The official Web site of the ATA provides information about thyroid disease and thyroid cancer. The Site Menu provides links to information for patients, research, the ATA journal, announcements, the ATA newsletter, physician guidelines, and contacts.

American Urological Association (AUA) ◎ ◎

http://www.auanet.org

This site of the AUA details information about the AUA, publications, coding and reimbursement, guidelines, events, managed care issues, education, member services, and the AUA Annual Meeting. The education section offers a residency program database and details of home study and other CME programs. A Web Forum has restricted access for members. A section for the public offers disorder, general urology, and member information.

Aplastic Anemia (AA) Association of Canada ◉ ◉

http://www.aplastic.ualberta.ca

This site provides patient education and support information. Details of AA and myelodysplasia, their causes, and treatments are provided along with a newsletter. Contact information for support, an FAQ section, and further details are provided.

Association for Research in Vision and Ophthalmology (ARVO) ◉ ◉

http://www.faseb.org/arvo

Information about ARVO, membership, abstracts, scientific programs, awards, and ARVO forms is supplied. There are links to Investigative Ophthalmology and Visual Science and to the *Guide to Finding Sources in Eye and Vision Research*.

Association of Cancer Online Resources (ACOR) ◉ ◉

http://www.acor.org/index.html?Poe_Session=d405998b4ff8fb3158d26f3a02f1e14a

ACOR provides a wide range of Internet based cancer resources to patients, families, and professionals. Within the CancerNet section of the site there is an extensive list of types of cancer, with detailed descriptions of typical treatments. The site offers archives of support and electronic information groups, links to other Web sites, an external search service, and links to journals.

Association of Community Cancer Centers (ACCC) ◉ ◉

http://www.assoc-cancer-ctrs.org

An interdisciplinary organization for the improvement of patient care, the ACCC also seeks to define standards of care. Information available includes lists of cancer centers and member profiles, the ACCC vision and mission, meeting schedules, news, professional job opportunities, program standards, and contacts. There is an ACCC member newsgroup that has restricted access. The user is also given access to *Oncology Issues,* the official journal of the ACCC.

Association of Residents in Radiation Oncology ◉ ◉ ◉

http://www.arro.org

This site is focused on residents, but has extensive resources for physicians and healthcare professionals as well. For residents, there are fellowship sources, residency programs, article bibliographies, and certification details. For a larger audience, there are many useful links to online journals and journal clubs, search engines, clinical trials, screening and treatment sites, associations, and directories.

Breast Cancer Society of Canada ⊗ ⊗

http://www.bcsc.ca

This society funds breast cancer research and provides information concerning detection, prevention, and treatment of breast cancer. Included are questions patients should ask their doctor, details about the society, information about research the society funds, FAQs, recent news, and contacts and location information.

British Society for Histocompatibility and Immunogenetics (BSHI) ⊗ ⊗

http://www.umds.ac.uk/tissue/bshi1.html

A nonprofit society that provides a forum for the sharing of scientific information, new technology and education, this site provides information about the BSHI annual scientific meeting, the Histocompatibility and Immunogenetics Group (HIG) and other internal groups, membership, a newsletter, relevant sites, and more. A listing of useful software, such as CD antigen files and sound files, can be downloaded directly from the site.

Canadian Oncology Society (COS) ⊗ ⊗ ⊗ (fee-based)

http://www.cos.ca

The COS Web site contains information for patients and physicians. Open to all are links to the COS newsletter, information about the organization, membership application materials, and numerous links to affiliated societies. A section of the Web site is restricted to members, and provides access to search engines, information about clinical trials, an events calendar, professional and educational opportunities, and a membership directory.

Cancer Research Institute (CRI) ⊗ ⊗

http://www.cancerresearch.org

CRI focuses on the science of cancer immunology. The Institute's Web site provides extensive information regarding the Institute's goals, grants and fellowships, the science of cancer immunology, current prostate cancer and melanoma initiatives, and the CRI international symposia series. One can access articles from *The Researcher,* the official newsletter of the CRI, and download forms regarding grant and fellowship information. The CRI's research funding decisions are made by a 64-member Scientific Advisory Council; information about the council's members and other contact information is provided.

Coalition of National Cancer Cooperative Groups, Inc. ◎ ◎

http://www.ca-coalition.org

This organization serves to enhance the translation of research into clinical treatments, to provide patient access to clinical trials, to manage health outcomes data, and to promote the exchange of scientific information internationally via its leadership of cooperative groups. Information about the society and its members, membership, current studies, meetings, and activities is available.

Colorectal Cancer Association of Canada (CCAC) ◎ ◎ ◎

http://www.ccac-accc.ca

The CCAC organizes educational and support activities for patients, and this information is provided with membership information, links, and news. The information program supplies updates about the disorder, treatment risks or benefits, and research and clinical trials news.

European Organization for Research and Treatment of Cancer (EORTC) ◎ ◎

http://www.eortc.be

The EORTC site provides information about the organization, its meetings, services, directories, protocols, and informational documents. There is a restricted section that provides access to recognized IP addresses. The Documents section includes anticancer therapy economic data and a Telemantics for Clinical Research video.

European Society for Medical Oncology (ESMO) ◎

http://www.esmo.org

Information about the organization, its structure, activities, its journal and news is offered at this site for professionals. There is an extensive listing of ESMO organized courses and fellowships.

European Society for Therapeutic Radiology and Oncology (ESTRO) ◎ ◎

http://www.estro.be

The ESTRO Web site provides information regarding the Society, membership, fellowships, past awards winners, events, publications, and research news. An educational section provides a number of informative documents.

Histiocytosis Association of America ⊙ ⊙

http://www.histio.org

The organization funds research and provides information to patients and professionals. The site offers conference and funding details and a number of discussion lounges. An information library provides news, research information, and links.

International Association for the Study of Lung Cancer (IASLC) ⊙ ⊙ ⊙

http://www.iaslc.org

Goals of the IASLC are to study etiology, epidemiology, prevention, treatment, and other aspects of the disorder, and to present information to the public and professionals. Its site offers organization, past meetings, committees, upcoming events, IASLC publications, and news information. There is a link to the *Lung Cancer* journal and details of membership.

International Association for the Study of Pain (IASP) ⊙ ⊙

http://www.halcyon.com/iasp

This international, multidisciplinary and professional organization site promotes pain research to improve patient care. The IASP Web site offers information on continuing education, local chapters, awards, programs, working groups, publications, employment information, and meetings. For the public, medical newsletters and a listing of resources by country are supplied.

International Association of Laryngectomies (IAL) ⊙ ⊙

http://www.larynxlink.com/ial/ial.htm

This nonprofit organization is made up of member clubs and seeks to provide patient information, support, and other services. The IAL Web site provides information concerning its Voice Institute, various clubs, speech instructors, events and products, and their distributors. An online information library offers health and laryngectomy articles. There is a newsletter and a section of links to other information sources.

International Ostomy Association (IOA) ⊙ ⊙

http://www.ostomyinternational.org

This Web site provides information and a forum for patients. There is information about meetings, membership, regional events, local support and information organizations, and about care. A feature of the site is the global discussion forum where participants can post new questions or reply to those of others. There is an active forum as well as archives.

International Paraneoplastic Association ⊙ ⊙ ⊙

http://paraneoplastic.hypermart.net¨

Those suffering from Neurological Paraneoplastic Syndromes can learn more about their condition and gain support here. Comprehensive information including notices, news, information about Paraneoplastic Cerebellar Degeneration (PCD), medical contact information, coping and rehabilitation information, and journal access is easily accessible. A large number of links are provided for research information.

International Society for Hematotherapy and Graft Engineering (ISHAGE) ⊙ ⊙

http://www.ishage.org

This professional organization for researchers and physicians serves as a forum for communication, education, training, research and standardized technology, and as a representation vehicle. Symposia schedules, abstracts, news, FAQs, organization and director information, guidelines, and an information library are provided at the site. Discussion lounges are available for members that are password protected. There is also a link to the new official ISHAGE journal, *Cytotherapy*.

International Society for Prevention Oncology (ISPO) ⊙ ⊙

http://www.cancerprev.org/ISPO

ISPO is an organization that serves to study etiologic factors in the development of cancer for its primary and secondary prevention. The ISPO Web site offers information about its journal, *Cancer Detection and Prevention,* its international meetings and workshops, awards, membership, and news. The user can search abstracts and view the organization of past meetings. One can download a membership application and the membership fee includes a yearly subscription to the ISPO journal.

International Union Against Cancer (UICC) ⊙ (fee-based)

http://www.uicc.org

UICC is an international, independent organization based in Geneva, Switzerland and consists of medical, scientific, and other members who are devoted to the fight against cancer. The organization promotes the advancement of scientific research and prevention and treatment of cancer. Also emphasized are professional and public education. The site provides information regarding membership, fellowships available, and educational opportunities and materials provided by the UICC. There is a member section of the site that has restricted access to UICC members.

Kidney Cancer Association (KCA) ⊙ ⊙ ⊙

http://www.nkca.org

The KCA is composed of and provides information for physicians, patients, family members, and researchers. The site details membership, drug trials, research, public policy, disorders, patient meetings, and annual convention information. The site has online chat sessions and a mailing list. There is also information about current financial grants and past recipients. For patients, disease facts, diagnosis, surgery, therapy, and other details are available.

Leukemia Society of America   ⚙ ⚙
http://www.leukemia.org

The Society seeks to provide information, education, patient services, community services, and fund research dealing with leukemia, lymphoma, Hodgkin's disease, and myeloma. The society's site provides information about educational materials, publications, services offered, news, and events. The Research link provides workshop information and applications, a professional education calendar, and grant information.

Lymphoedema Association of Australia   ⚙ ⚙
http://www.lymphoedema.org.au

Information on treatment, therapy, treatment results, a newsletter, and membership information are available at this association's comprehensive site. Reviews of complex physical therapy and of compression instruments are supplied, as well as information about reference material.

Multiple Myeloma Association   ⚙ ⚙ ⚙
http://www.webspawner.com/users/myelomaexchange

Information for professionals and patients is provided. There is also an e-mail discussion group and information archives. Links are to transplant information sites, chat rooms, informative sites, PDQ statements, articles, programs, physicians, research centers, and more.

National Cervical Cancer Coalition (NCCC)   ⚙ ⚙
http://www.nccc-online.org

The official Web site of the NCCC is geared mostly towards patients, and provides comprehensive information concerning their Pap test, DES, support, dealing with one's HMO, treatment options, books available, and clinical trials. For professionals, news, clinical trial information and the Clinical Laboratory Improvement Act guidelines are provided. There are also links to articles and to related sites.

National Children's Cancer Society   ⚙ ⚙ ⚙
http://www.children-cancer.com

The goal of this nonprofit organization is to provide support, advocacy, education, and financial assistance to children with cancer and their families. Some specific programs offered promote education and wellness, pediatric oncology camps, and communication assistance with hospitals and insurance companies. Detailed information about all programs, contacts, and news is offered at the site.

National Coalition For Cancer Survivorship (NCCS)   ⊙ ⊙ ⊙

http://www.cansearch.org

The National Coalition for Cancer Survivorship is a grassroots, nationwide network of independent organizations and individuals working in the area of cancer support and information for all types of cancer. Their Web site carries an index to the organization's current newsletter (_NCCS Networker_) as well as back issues. The newsletter contains information on regional and local support groups, new clinical trials and research, recent legislative activity, and reviews of the latest publications by and for cancer survivors. A yearly membership fee is required to receive the newsletter. Free on the site is the "Cancer Survival Toolbox." This is a tutorial in audio and transcript form that coaches the patient on developing skills needed during treatment. Topics include communicating, finding information, solving problems, making decisions, and negotiating and standing up for your rights. Another useful, free tutorial unique in the field of cancer education is the "Cancer: Keys to Survivorship" program. It addresses skills and strategies for self-employment, communicating with healthcare providers and loved ones, understanding workplace concerns and employment rights, and understanding health insurance issues. The site's "CanSearch Websites" provides excellent step-by-step directions for researching cancer on the Internet, with sites to visit first to gather basic information, and secondary sites for information of a specific nature. The NCCS site and a selection of their publications are available in Spanish.

National Ovarian Cancer Coalition (NOCC)   ⊙ ⊙

http://www.ovarian.org

A large collection of ovarian cancer information is available here. The site offers facts, opportunity for discussion, chapter locations, contact information, and news. The Resources section provides an opportunity to ask questions of experts in the field, supplies information about state resources, and allows for the search of a database, by state, that contains names of more than 600 gynecologic oncologists.

Neuroblastoma Children's Cancer Society (NCCS)   ⊙ ⊙

http://www.graniteWebworks.com/nccs.htm

The NCCS provides advocacy, support, information, and research funding. Its site provides professionals and patients with PDQ information, a list of accomplishments, projects, and a list of resources. There is also a page for information exchange and contact data.

Oncology Nursing Society (ONS) Online ⊙ (fee-based)
http://www.ons.org

The Web site of the ONS has sections for members, healthcare providers, and for patients/consumers. Access to each section requires a registration that can be completed online. Members receive access to journals, educational opportunities, employment information, and more. Details of membership and registration are provided.

Orthopedic Research Society (ORS) ⊙ ⊙ ⊙
http://www.ors.org

Goals of the ORS are to support and promote research in the areas of orthopedic surgery and muskuloskeletal diseases and injuries. The site offers details of seminars, announcements, news, membership, abstracts, directors, and W.H.O. initiatives. There is an online discussion group, a newsletter, and a link to the *Journal of Orthopedic Research*. There are links to relevant sites and to specific resources for researchers.

Pituitary Tumor Network Association ⊙ ⊙
http://www.pituitary.com

This nonprofit organization supports, encourages, and funds research. Information about many pituitary disorders is provided along with patient resources. There are links to the Association's magazine that provide information about medical advances and other in-depth articles. The physician's section provides information dealing with publication opportunities, an Internet referral program, and resource guide listings.

Radiological Society of North America (RSNA) ⊙ ⊙ ⊙
http://www.rsna.org

Details about the Society, its affiliations, and members are available at this site. There are links to a number of journals, conference registration materials and events listings. Learning and practice tools available include a CME database, practice guidelines, case studies, and medical images. There are a large number of organized links to other image and information resource sites.

Second Wind: A National Lung Transplant Patients Association ⊙ ⊙
http://www.2ndwind.org

This organization is for lung transplant recipients, lung surgery candidates, and the concerned public. It provides support, education, and advocacy. Information about the organization, transplantation, membership, activities, news, meetings, and disorders is listed.

Society for Endocrinology ✪ ✪ ✪

http://www.endocrinology.org

Information for all aspects of endocrinology including cancer is available here. There are details of the Society, membership, its journals, conferences, events, grants, books, education, topical briefings, and training courses. In addition, *Endocrine-Related Cancer,* one of the Society's journals, details subscription criteria and includes some online articles.

Society for Neuro-Oncology ✪

http://www.soc-neuro-onc.org

The site of the multidisciplinary professional society offers a calendar of events, listings of employment and research opportunities, links, annual meeting information, a discussion forum, announcements, and a newsletter. There is a link to the *Neuro-Oncology Journal.*

Society for Radiation Oncology Administrators (SROA) ✪

http://www.sroa.org

SROA serves medical management professionals and seeks to improve administration and nonmedical management and to provide information. Information about career opportunities, membership, annual meetings, legislation, and the SROA member network is provided. News briefs, links, and discussion forum pages are also available.

Society for Surgery of the Alimentary Tract (SSAT) ✪ ✪ ✪

http://www.ssat.com

The SSAT seeks to promote and offer leadership, teach and research diseases, provide a forum for discussion, and to promote training, funding, and publications related to the functions of the alimentary tract. The SSAT Web site provides membership information, a directory, news, and a link to its official journal. Information concerning cancer and other diseases is offered. There are patient guidelines written in English, Spanish ,and Japanese for the treatment of cancer of the colon or rectum, the surgical treatment of pancreatic cancer, and the management of colonic polyps and adenomas. An electronic abstract submission program is also offered.

Society of Gynecologic Oncologists (SGO) ✪

http://www.sgo.org

The SGO site offers a tremendous amount of information to practitioners of Gynecologic Oncology. Consistent with the Society's philosophy of encouraging research and raising the standards of practice, the site offers up-to-date news from the SGO, upcoming symposia schedules, coding references, and abstracts.

Southern Association for Oncology   ○

http://www.sma.org/sao

This Association sponsors a quarterly newsletter and annual meeting. Its Web site offers information concerning the annual meeting, the Association, and membership. The Oncology Online section offers select abstracts and articles from recent journals.

United Ostomy Association (UOA)   ○ ○ ○

http://www.uoa.org

UOA is a nonprofit information and support organization for patients. The UOA Web site offers information about ostomy, local chapters, conferences, and links to related sites and distributors of ostomy equipment. There is also information about the local chapter visitor and support service where certified visitors are made available to patients in need. An FAQ and documents concerning insurance issues and rights are available along with links to special committees for parents of ostomy children, and for gay and lesbian ostomates.

World Marrow Donor Association (WMDA)   ○ ○

http://www.bmdw.org/WMDA

WMDA is a professional organization whose mission is to promote information exchange and to develop standards for the exchange of hematopoietic stem cells, internationally. The WMDA Web site provides extensive membership information, house rules, numerous reports of the Association's guidelines, and online access to minutes from past meetings.

Y-Me National Breast Cancer Organization   ○ ○ ○

http://www.y-me.org

The Y-Me National Breast Cancer Organization was founded in 1978 by two breast cancer patients to provide information and support to patients, their families, and friends. Its site provides information in both English and Spanish about the organization, its chapters, general facts for patients, FAQs (frequently asked questions), access to the organization's newsletter, and information about offline resources such as a current calendar of its monthly open door education and support groups held throughout the country, early detection workshops, peer support programs, wig and prothesis bank, and teen program. There is a section devoted to males with the disorder. The site also lists the 800 numbers for their 24-hour toll free hotlines and links to other resources.

8.2 **Research Organizations**

American Association for Cancer Research (AACR) ⊚ ⊚ ⊚
http://www.aacr.org

The scientific society's easy-to-navigate site provides a tremendous number of resources and links for professionals and patients. The site includes information about the society, patient education, grants and funding, research awards and fellowships, symposia schedules, educational workshops, abstracts and publications, the Association newsletter and links to scientific journals. The site also has live and archived audio programs and provides a public forum.

Cancer Research And Biostatistics (CRAB) ⊚ ⊚ ⊚
http://www.crab.org

This nonprofit organization seeks to apply a biostatistical approach to the study of cancer. The Web site provides information about the organization, publication details, lists of biostatistical programs, reports, biostatistical calculators, and current project information.

Cancer Research Foundation of America (CRFA) ⊚ ⊚
http://www.preventcancer.org

Research at over 100 U.S. academic institutions and public education is facilitated by this organization's funding. Information about men's, women's and children's health, programs, research, and news is supplied. Some available programs cover breast health, issues concerning Spanish speaking women, mammography awareness and Congressional action. Researchers browsing this site will find information regarding future grants, applications, past recipients, and current protocols.

Cancer Research Institute (CRI) ⊚ ⊚
http://www.cancerresearch.org

CRI focuses on the science of cancer immunology. The Institute's Web site provides extensive information regarding the Institute's goals, grants and fellowships, the science of cancer immunology, current prostate cancer and melanoma initiatives, and the CRI international symposia series. One can access articles from *The Researcher,* the official newsletter of the CRI, and download forms regarding grant and fellowship information. The CRI's research funding decisions are made by a 64-member Scientific Advisory Council; information about the council's members and other contact information is provided.

Cancer Treatment Research Foundation (CTRF) ○ ○

http://www.ctrf.org

The CTRF is a nonprofit organization that seeks to make research findings clinically available to cancer patients by funding research, offering treatment protocols, and promoting education. The organization supports The Society for Nutritional Oncology Adjutant Therapy (NOAT), an organization that promotes the collaboration between scientists and clinicians to better oncologic treatment via the inclusion of nutritional oncology. The CTRF Web site provides information about NOAT, nutritional oncology, grant support, other CTRF resources such as publications, and CTRF contacts.

Carcinogenic Potency Project ○ ○ ○

http://potency.berkeley.edu

This database of the results from long-term cancer tests on animals is provided by the University of California at Berkeley. Qualitative and quantitative information is displayed for 5152 experiments and 1298 chemicals. Information regarding species, strain, and sex of test animals is provided for each experiment, along with extensive details of the experiment protocol. A database of experiments can be searched in a variety of ways.

Centerwatch: Profiles of Centers Conducting Clinical Research ○ ○ ○

http://www.centerwatch.com/procat12.htm

This site is organized geographically by state. It provides an in-depth profile of hundreds of clinical institutions and research centers engaged in cancer research. The contact information of each Center is provided along with an overview, research experience description, information on facilities, staff expertise, and patient demographics.

Centerwatch: Profiles of Industry Providers ○ ○ ○

http://www.centerwatch.com/provider/provlist.htm

Centerwatch has cataloged an extensive listing of preclinical and clinical research, laboratory, monitoring, project management, trial design, patient recruitment, post-marketing services, and regulatory services providers in the U.S., organized topically and geographically. For each industry provider, Centerwatch has prepared an in-depth profile listing services, facilities, and contact information.

Coalition of National Cancer
Cooperative Groups, Inc. ◉ ◉

http://www.ca-coalition.org

This organization serves to enhance the translation of research into clinical treatments, to provide patient access to clinical trials, to manage health outcomes data and to promote the exchange of scientific information internationally via its leadership of cooperative groups. Information about the society and its members, membership, current studies, meetings, and activities is available.

European Organization for Research
and Treatment of Cancer (EORTC) ◉ ◉

http://www.eortc.be

The EORTC site provides information about the organization, its meetings, services, directories, protocols, and informational documents. There is a restricted section that provides access to recognized Web addresses. The Documents section includes anticancer therapy, economic data, and a Telemantics for Clinical Research video.

International Agency for
Research on Cancer (IARC) ◉ ◉ ◉

http://www.iarc.fr

The IARC is part of the World Health Organization and its goals are to conduct research and to develop methods of cancer control. Information available at the IARC site relates to its meetings, research units, press releases, fellowships, publications, training courses, and databases. Databases and other resources available are monographs, cancer epidemiology and p53 databases, the WHO program on cancer control and information on occupational exposure to carcinogens.

International Cancer Alliance for
Research and Education (ICARE) ◉ ◉

http://www.icare.org

The alliance seeks to bring together patients, doctors, and researchers to provide accurate, up-to-date information on a personal basis. Through the collection and analysis of information, patients are brought into contact with physicians. The site offers information about all of ICARE's programs, cancer therapy reviews, and updates about clinical and pharmaceutical research.

Ludwig Institute for Cancer Research,
New York Branch: Cancer Immunology ◉ ◉

http://www.mskcc.org/rande/immunology/103.html

This site lists the head of research, laboratory supervisor, associate members, assistant members, visiting investigators, research associates, and research fellows of the cancer

Immunology Unit within this research Institute. A description of research in the Unit focuses on the development of cancer vaccines and antibody-based therapies. The highly technical nature of the information makes this site suitable only for fellow investigators and health professionals.

Protein Reviews on the Web: CD Molecules ◎ ◎ ◎
http://www.ncbi.nlm.nih.gov/prow/cd/index_molecule.htm

This is a U.S. government site that provides a listing of cell surface molecules that are recognized by the International Workshops of Human Leukocyte Differentiation Antigens. Links are provided to CD guides and molecules are listed by primary name.

Sustaining Oncology Studies (SOS) Server ◎ ◎ ◎
http://sos.unige.it

This Web site is an international information resource for researchers, clinicians, and other related professionals. Variations of the site are offered in English and Italian. Information provided concerns grants, online training, international conferences, publications, and more. There is an extensive links section with links to databases, institutes, associations, cancer registries, and search engines.

8.3 Selected Hospital Oncology Departments

Albert Einstein Comprehensive Cancer Center ◎ ◎ ◎
http://www.ca.aecom.yu.edu

The center is provided by the Albert Einstein College of Medicine and ranks among the top 10 in National Cancer Institute funding. The site for the academic cancer center offers an overview of the center and details of programs, research, clinical services, protocols, lab facilities, the administration, directions, and events.

Research	There are research programs for immunology, viral oncology, receptor mediated growth and differentiation, growth control in malignant cells, molecular membrane biology, drug design and development, hematological malignancies and general oncology, cancer control, and epidemiology and colon cancer.
Patient Resources	There are descriptions of services and clinical trials protocols. There is also a newsletter.
Location	Bronx, New York, NCI-designated

Allegheny University Hospitals (AUH) ⊙ ⊙ ⊙

http://www.allhealth.edu

This Web site provides access to all University Hospital facilities. Professional educational materials are provided in a Health Sciences Library covering topics such as document delivery services, literature searches, professional development, information consulting, and current awareness. The main page offers information about AUH services, various health topics, news, and a physician directory.

Research	The Department of Radiation Oncology conducts research in the areas of prostate seed implantation, intraoperative brachytherapy for nonsmall cell lung and esophageal cancer, interstitial breast implantation, high-dose-rate brachytherapy, external beam radiation for macular degeneration, intensity modulated radiation therapy, and external beam radiation for temporal mandibular joint syndrome. The department has also recently added a medical physics research component.
Patient Resources	There is a wealth of patient resources available at the Health Sciences Library along with news, treatment information, clinical research updates, informational videos, and a toll-free information hotline. One can also pose questions directly to a staff physician online.
Location	Pittsburgh, Pennsylvania

Arizona Cancer Center ⊙ ⊙ ⊙

http://www.azcc.arizona.edu

The Cancer Center is at the University of Arizona Health Sciences Center and its Web site offers information regarding patient care, cancer prevention, research, public education, professional education, conferences, the Cancer Biology Graduate Program, and related pages. There are details of fellowship training in hematology and oncology, cancer prevention research, and of individual disorders.

Research	Basic science research is conducted in the areas of new drug development, cancer biology, gene therapy, melanoma, and breast cancer. The site also provides descriptions of prior research contributions, clinical research, and cancer prevention and control research.
Patient Resources	The patient education section offers lay descriptions of medical terms as well as information on coping and support groups. There are details of detection, treatment, risks, other facts, and prevention of individual cancers.
Location	Tucson, Arizona, NCI-designated

Arthur G. James Cancer Hospital ⊙ ⊙ ⊙

http://www.jamesline.com

This center ranks among the NCI designated Comprehensive Cancer Centers. The site offers information about the center, cancer in general, specific cancers, departments, prevention, detection, research, education, and about treatment at the center. The home page offers news, hot topics in cancer, and tips of the week. There are also links to departments of the hospital partner, The Ohio Sate University Comprehensive Cancer Center.

Research	Programs of research are in the areas of cancer prevention and control, experimental therapeutics, hormones and cancer, immunology, molecular biology and cancer genetics, molecular and cellular carcinogenesis, and RNA oncogenic virus. Detailed information concerning notable research accomplishments, clinical trials, and the James Cancer Hospital and Solove Research Institute's Cancer Genetics Program is available.
Patient Resources	Hospital service and facility information is offered along with detailed information about types of cancer, directions, hospice services, events, special programs, screening schedules, stories of hope, support groups, links, and a physician directory.
Location	Columbus, Ohio, NCI-designated

Barbara Ann Kamanos Cancer Institute ⊙ ⊙ ⊙

http://www.karmanos.org

From the home page, one is provided with news and articles and can access information concerning the Institute, treatment, staff, programs, contacts, clinical trials, and research. For physicians, details of continuing education seminars, core facilities, and initiatives are provided.

Research	Basic research, clinical research, clinical care, community research and education are incorporated into five programs: Breast Cancer; Cancer Control; Epidemiology & Environmental Carcinogenesis; Experimental & Clinical Therapeutics; Genitourinary Cancer; and Tumor Progression and Metastasis. One can search for and view clinical trials protocols by anatomical location.
Patient Resources	Information about patient breast care, home care, hospice, counseling, pain control, screening, guest housing, and educational services is provided. Other details of treatment and cancer in general can be found.
Location	Detroit, Michigan, NCI-designated

Barnes-Jewish Hospital ⊙ ⊙ ⊙

http://www.bjc.org

This Web site is for the BJC Health System and includes links to associated hospitals including Barnes-Jewish Hospital. The main menu offers information about the hospital's extensive services and departments. There is useful information concerning events, lodging, spiritual care, services, phone numbers, support groups, employment, and the cancer committee report. This report discusses the cancer center, community outreach, staff achievements, the staff oncology data service, research, and more. The hospital has programs that deal with many individual cancers, and diagnosis, treatment, and procedure information is available.

Research — Research is conducted in the areas of Cancer and Developmental Biology, Cancer Genetics, Cellular Proliferation, Oncologic Imaging, Prevention and Control, Stem Cell Biology and Gene Therapy, and Tumor Immunology. There is an extensive listing of the various clinical investigations and research information resources and data services.

Patient Resources — Extensive patient resources are provided such as support groups, spiritual services, detailed treatment and disorder information for individual cancers, clinical trials participation, and listing information and links.

Location — St. Louis, Missouri

Baylor University Medical Center ⊙ ⊙ ⊙

http://baylorhealth.com

This Web site offers access to all sections of the Baylor Health Care System. There are directories, search services, and listings of health information for a variety of disorders along with an online physician referral service, insurance information, and a list of medical services. The page for the Division of Oncology offers information regarding oncology facilities, education and support groups, coping with cancer, resource books, and individual disorders.

Research — Notable research areas and clinical trials are conducted in the areas of breast cancer prevention, prostate cancer prevention, and adjuvant chemotherapy with breast and colon cancer. There are six oncology facilities and contact information for further research details is provided.

Patient Resources — Patient resources at this site are extensive with information about individual disorders, educational programs, support groups, offline resources, prevention, awareness and screening, clinical trials, and lymphedema.

Location — Dallas, Texas

Beckman Research Institute, City of Hope ○ ○ ○

http://www.cityofhope.org

From the Site Map, one can find information concerning location and positions available at the center, patient referral, CME—accredited Educational Symposia, publications, consulting services, a reference library, medical services, individual disorders, professional education, research, BMT, the graduate school, and technology development.

Research	Research divisions are: Biology; Cell and Tumor Biology; Immunology; Molecular Medicine; Molecular Biology and Neurosciences. From the home page for each division, one can find details of publications, researchers and individual programs. There is access to details of Molecular Tools and Databases, the DNA Sequencing Lab, the DNA Chemistry Lab, and a reference library.
Patient Resources	There are details of medical services offered and of detection, treatment, investigational treatments, and other research for individual disorders.
Location	Duarte, California, NCI-designated

Brigham and Women's Hospital (BWH) ○ ○ ○

http://www.partners.org/bwh

The main page of the Web site provides hospital information concerning visitors, healthcare, primary care practices, women's health, BWH doctors, research, and news. The page devoted to the Dana-Farber/BWH Cancer Center provides information about its gynecologic oncology, hematology, oncology, radiation oncology, and surgical oncology divisions. For each division, there is general, patient, and physician education information. Physician education resources concern training programs and other educational opportunities available at BWH.

Research	Investigative groups at BWH study the areas of Autologous Transplantation and Interleukin-2 for Lymphoma, Prevention of Acute GVHD with IL-1RA, Radioimmunotherapy Studies for Low Grade Lymphomas, Solid Tumor Transplant, Mammography, Dermatopathology, Cell and Developmental Biology, Functional Genomics, Immunogenetics and Transplantation, Molecular and Cellular Physiology, Signal Transduction, Molecular Genetics of Disease, and Molecular Transport Physiology.
Patient Resources	There is extensive information about gynecologic cancers and their treatment, prevention, and management. There is also information about the BWH Familial Ovarian Cancer Center, its New England Trophoblastic Disease Center, and its Pap Smear Evaluation Center.
Location	Boston, Massachusetts

Chao Family Comprehensive Cancer Center ☺ ☺ ☺
http://www.ucihs.uci.edu/cancer

This family center is located on the University of California, Irvine campus and is associated with the College of Medicine. Its site provides information about clinical trials, research, staff, education, maps, and organizational resources. There are CME programs, newsletters, and descriptions of its Lifestyle Medicine Clinic.

Research — Research is conducted in the areas of BMT, epidemiology, basic science, and prevention. There are listings of open protocols by specific disorder.

Patient Resources — There are patient and parent support groups and listings of community education and outreach programs. Basic information about cancer and individual disorders is supplied.

Location — Orange, California, NCI-designated

Clarian Health Partners ☺ ☺ ☺
http://www.clarian.com

Patient and professional information available at this site and related to its oncology program includes information about the hospital's mission, employment opportunities, community services, healthcare services, and news. A section for healthcare professionals provides information about libraries and graduate medical education, CME, and programs information.

Research — Research programs exist in the areas of Adult Oncology, Pediatric Oncology, Hematopoiesis, Regulation of Cell Growth, and Experimental Therapeutics. Extensive lists of clinical trial protocols and of associated investigators are displayed. Research is conducted at the Indiana University Cancer Center.

Patient Resources — Patient resources include details of cancer, specific disorders, and the hospital's pediatric and radiology oncology departments.

Location — Indianapolis, Indiana

Cleveland Clinic ☺ ☺ ☺
http://www.clevelandclinic.org

This Cleveland, Ohio-based clinic provides care in a number of areas including oncology. The Taussig Cancer Center site offers patient, cancer, professional information ,and a listing of questions and answers. The professional information section offers information about related centers, allied health, the Cleveland Clinic *Journal of Medicine,* CME offerings, graduate medical education, and medical student education. Contact information is available.

Research — The Taussig Cancer Center includes these departments: Brain Tumor and Neuro-Oncology Center; The Breast Center; Experimental

Therapeutics; Hematology and Medical Oncology; Medical Genetics; Radiation Oncology; and Pediatric Neurosurgery. Each department has its own Web page and there are extensive lists of research protocols on each page.

Patient Resources   Information about individual cancers, written especially for patients, is provided. Also, there are mailing lists, support groups, and risk assessment sections. A patient education page offers a health information library, multiple publications, and information about classes, seminars, and events.

Location   Cleveland, Ohio

Dana-Farber Cancer Institute ◎ ◎ ◎

http://www.dfci.harvard.edu

Details about the Institute, staff, adult oncology programs and facilities, pediatric oncology programs and facilities, patient services, research, news, events, and employment opportunities are available. There are descriptions of individual disorders, statistics, and links.

Research   Departments of research are: Adult Oncology; Pediatric Oncology; Biostatistical Science; Cancer Biology; and Cancer Immunology and AIDS. Descriptions of core facilities, details of research news, and clinical trials listings are included. A Web page for each research department offers specific research information.

Patient Resources   Patient resources include information about cancer, specific disorders, prevention, and detection. Patient services include support groups, events, and scheduling. Listings of clinical services offered are displayed.

Location   Boston, Massachusetts, NCI-designated

Duke University Medical Center (DUMC) ◎ ◎ ◎

http://www.mc.duke.edu

This center is a major agent of cancer related information. The main menu offers links to sections for patients, professionals, faculty, education, research, and news. For professionals, there is information about DUMC, library services, continuing education, managed care, clinical trials, clinical services, a referral directory, and a referral center. The Duke Comprehensive Cancer Center Web site offers patient, medical, clinical trials, and general information. There are listings of upcoming events, programs, and departments as well.

Research   Established research programs exist in the areas of Breast and Ovarian Oncology, Cancer Immunobiology, Cancer Prevention, Detection and Control, Cell Regulation and Transmembrane Signaling, Cellular and Structural Biology, Experimental Therapeutics, Molecular Oncology and Cancer Genetics, Neuro-Oncology, Nucleic Acid Biology and Chemistry, and Radiation Oncology and Hyperthermia. Also listed is information on development, clinical programs, shared resources, and medical center departments, divisions, and research centers.

Patient Resources   A hyperlinked list of patient resources includes a patient support program, education program, oncology social work, pediatric neuro-oncology newsletters, managed care and academic medical centers, news, and links information.

Location   Durham, North Carolina, NCI-designated

Emory University Hospital ⊙ ⊙ ⊙
http://www2.cc.emory.edu/WHSC/EUH/euh.html

Primarily for the university healthcare system, this site also provides general information with links to more specific areas. The hospital is part of the Robert W. Woodruff Health Sciences Center that also includes the Emory University School of Medicine, Nell Hodgson Woodruff School of Nursing, Rollins School of Public Health, Yerkes Regional Primate Research Center, The Emory Clinic, Emory Children's Center, and other healthcare components. This single site has access to each of the aforementioned institutions, and the Emory University Hospital Site provides driving directions, basic departmental information, and appointment instructions. A search service allows the user to search the system for specific information. The site is vast and many sections are still under construction.

Research   Research efforts at the Emory University School of Medicine are focused within the departments of Biochemistry, Cell Biology, Genetics, Microbiology and Immunology, Pharmacology, and Physiology. Research also takes place in all clinical departments and in the many Emory Centers.

Patient Resources   This hospital site offers a directory, news releases with full-text stories, and a search service for specific information at the Robert W. Woodruff Health Sciences Center.

Location   Atlanta, Georgia

Evanston Hospital ⊙ ⊙ ⊙
http://www.enh.org/about.asp#EvanstonHospital

Introductory information about the hospital and its specialized areas is displayed. Special sections are the Kellogg Cancer Care Center, the Breast Health and Mammography Section, and the Neurosciences section. Special services are in cardiac care, rehabilitation, high risk obstetrics, and women's health. Telephone numbers and basic information is offered. Access to other areas of the Evanston Northwestern Healthcare system is provided.

Research   The Kellogg Cancer Care Center is part of the National Institutes of Health Community Clinical Oncology Program and offers diagnostic, treatment, and research services. Telephone numbers are provided. There is information about The Research Institute, the Evanston Northwestern Healthcare system's research vehicle. Cancer is among its priority areas.

Patient Resources   Basic hospital divisions are described along with ample contact information. One can search the system for directions, physician directories, news, and support groups.

Location   Evanston, Illinois

F.G. McGaw Hospital at Loyola University ◎ ◎ ◎

http://www.luhs.org

The Loyola University Health System offers information about system wide services, programs, and staff. Information is provided for the major departments and the bone marrow transplantation unit. Bone Marrow Transplant (BMT) unit statistics, contact information, and a staff directory are provided. Oncology services and information are provided at the page for The Oncology Institute. The center offers comprehensive cancer-related services in conjunction with the Cardinal Bernadin Cancer Center, and its page offers general, patient, education, research, media, and departmental information. Links to major CME and other teaching institutions are provided. Major subsections within the center are devoted to breast, gastrointestinal, gynecologic, urologic, and lung cancer.

Research   Programs of research are in cancer immunology, prevention and control, hematology, and skin cancer. Specific programs of research study the Human Papilloma Virus, breast cancer, prostate cancer, brain cancer, lymphoma, ovarian cancer, skin cancer, lung cancer, and cancers of the head and neck.

Patient Resources   In-depth information about clinical departments, specialty programs and services, physician selection, and about a series of free health lectures is available. News and basic cancer information can also be found.

Location   Maywood, Illinois

Fox Chase Cancer Center ◎ ◎ ◎

http://www.fccc.edu

This Web site offers patient, cancer, hospital, professional, research, referral, technology transfer, contact, news, and employment information. The facility offers multidisciplinary cancer treatment programs, clinical support services, and a protocol management system. A calendar of social and educational events, a listing of affiliations, and a comprehensive directory of telephone and fax numbers can be found at its site.

Research Research programs are in the areas of gene expression, molecular aspects of oncogenesis, viral molecular biology and pathogenesis, molecular structure and function analysis, pharmacology and therapeutics, regulation and development of the immune system, cell cycle control, and human genetics. The center participates in the Human Genome Project. The Protocol Management System provides access to current research protocols.

Patient Resources There is extensive information about prevention, clinical services, telephone directories, and staff members. The Cancer Information section offers information about individual cancers, lists cancer treatment programs, and provides a list of reference publications and materials.

Location Philadelphia, Pennsylvania, NCI-designated

Fred Hutchinson Cancer Research Center ⊙ ⊙ ⊙
http://www.fhcrc.org

There is information about the Center, research, professional and graduate education programs, shared resources, and the administration. Details of the online Arnold Library are provided along with facts about clinical trials, funding, interdisciplinary training, past research, events, and technology transfer.

Research Research is conducted in four divisions: the Division of Basic Sciences; the Division of Human Biology; the Division of Clinical Research, and the Division of Public Health Sciences. Web pages for each division offer faculty and scientific program training opportunities. There is a collection of links to known international and domestic research projects.

Patient Resources Informational documents cover topics such as accessing medical care, the treatment process, support groups, social work and psychiatric services, and long-term follow-up. For cancer and individual disorder information, the patient is supplied with select links.

Location Seattle, Washington, NCI-designated

Greater Baltimore Medical Center (GBMC) ⊙ ⊙ ⊙
http://www.gbmc.org

The cancer center is among the various departments that comprise the Medical Center. The page for the cancer center provides information about news, services offered, screening programs, psychosocial support, educational opportunities, clinical trials, and directions.

Research The GBMC Cancer Center participates in clinical trials for treatment, control, and prevention via a number of national cooperative groups.

Patient Resources | There is information available regarding a number of disorders and related subjects such as transplantation, radiology, and hospice care. Information about psychosocial support services and organizations is offered along with information about cancer screening programs and community lecture schedules.

Location | Baltimore, Maryland

H. Lee Moffitt Cancer Center and Research Institute ⊘ ⊘ ⊘

http://www.moffitt.usf.edu

The Center is located at The University of South Florida and its Web site provides a comprehensive information resource for patients and professionals. Press releases, events calendars, center details, links, Moffitt publications, patient guidelines, and library services are available at the site. In addition, information about research, clinical programs, shared resources, cancer screening, and support is available.

Research | Programs of basic research are in molecular oncology, immunology, early detection and prevention, behavioral oncology, and diagnostic imaging. Clinical investigations are in experimental therapeutics, the metastatic process, treatment-related toxicities and means of reducing them, and the pathogenesis of hemotopoietic malignancies. Detailed descriptions of research departments and investigators is provided and there is a list of open protocols.

Patient Resources | Patient resources include support information and information about the center's treatment and screening services. A question and answer forum and a number of informative patient publications add to the scope of patient information.

Location | Tampa, Florida

Hospital of the University of Pennsylvania ⊘ ⊘ ⊘

http://www.med.upenn.edu/health/vi_files/vi_hup/vi_hup.html

The hospital is part of the University of Pennsylvania Health System, and its Web site offers information about the hospital, visitor requirements, health topics, events, medical services, news, and staff. There are lists of services available by location or by specialty and links are to the various components of the health system. The hospital's Hematology-Oncology Division Web page provides information about individual disorders and related treatment facilities and their staff. Many treatment facilities are located within the University of Pennsylvania Cancer Center. Some services available at the University of Pennsylvania Cancer Center include multidisciplinary evaluation centers, treatment programs, research, and support services. Center-related and other educational information is available on the University of Pennsylvania's OncoLink Web site.

Research   Research is conducted at various facilities within the University of Pennsylvania Health System, within many departments of basic and clinical science. Lists of research facilities and their respective departments may be accessed via OncoLink.

Patient Resources   A myriad of patient resources is available via the OncoLink Web service. Information about individual cancers, treatments, diagnosis, therapy, clinical trials, pain management, patient links, surgery, and much more can be accessed via this comprehensive and detailed Web resource.

Location   Philadelphia, Pennsylvania, NCI-designated

Johns Hopkins Hospital   ◎ ◎ ◎
http://hopkins.med.jhu.edu

The hospital is an integral part of the Johns Hopkins Health System and the Johns Hopkins School of Medicine. A large number of treatment centers and clinics are included in the system. Cancer information available throughout the system concerns treatments, screening, prevention, diagnosis, surgery, rehabilitation, Bone Marrow Transplant (BMT), news, pain services, hospice care, clinical trials, and support. One can search for information by cancer type. Professional information concerning referrals, CME, publications, speakers, and postgraduate training programs is supplied.

Research   Research is conducted in the basic sciences for a variety of cancer types. Specific research protocols may be found at the Web site for the Johns Hopkins Oncology Center.

Patient Resources   There are thorough descriptions of individual cancers, diagnosis, screening, support services, treatment information, clinical trials, care, and surgery.

Location   Baltimore, Maryland, NCI-designated

Kettering Medical Center (KMC)   ◎ ◎ ◎
http://www.kmcnetwork.org

The Kettering Medical Center is part of a comprehensive system of healthcare centers within the local area. The site provides information about hospital services, location, staff, programs, medical education, and employment opportunities. There are also links to other members of the healthcare system. The oncology services page offers information about cancer, diagnosis, treatments, surgery, and radiation therapy. KMC is a member of the Dayton Clinical Oncology Program (DCOP), a system of local hospitals that works with the NCI to organize clinical trials.

Research   A link to DCOP, a research arm of KMC, details clinical trials available through the Kettering Medical Center. In addition, research details may be obtained from the Web site for Wright State University, a member of the Kettering comprehensive healthcare system.

Patient Resources   There is an on-site library for patients that offers detailed information about cancer and individual disorders. The Web site provides screenings, patient stories, and KMC departmental information. In addition, there is an online newsletter and descriptions of support, diagnosis, and treatment services that are offered.

Location   Dayton, Ohio

Loma Linda University Medical Center (LLUMC) ⊙ ⊙ ⊙
http://www.llu.edu/llumc

The Web site provides information regarding all LLUMC services, departments, programs, facilities, residency programs, and visitor guidelines. The home page for the LLU Cancer Institute provides information about its Proton Treatment Center, research, goals, contacts, news, lectures, and education resources for professionals.

Research   The LLU Cancer Institute undertakes basic science research in the areas of the immune system and cell transformation and cancer therapy, protons for treatment, radiation molecular biology, radiolabeled monoclonal antibody studies, electromagnetic fields and gene transcription, development of cancer and medical therapy, bone metabolism markers, growth factors, and proto-oncogenes. Information about clinical trials participation is offered along with information about translational research programs.

Patient Resources   There is an information resource center for patients to locate detailed information about cancer and individual disorders. Also, the Web site provides patient news, a lecture calendar, support group information, and links. There are special LLU Cancer Center services for breast cancer patients, referrals, and for caregivers.

Location   Loma Linda, California

Lombardi Cancer Research Center at
Georgetown University Medical Center ⊙ ⊙ ⊙
http://lombardi.georgetown.edu

This informative site provides details about the center, research, professional education opportunities, treatments, new therapies, the graduate program, prevention and control, events, employment opportunities, and other resources. There is a Specialized Program of Research Excellence (SPORE) that allows for access to resources among SPORES and the National Cancer Insitute. There are also details of the Tumor Biology Training Program.

Research   There is a breast cancer research initiative and programs for the study of cancer growth, invasion and metastasis, new therapy development, neuro-oncology, radiation oncology, cancer prevention and control, psycho-oncology, AIDS-related cancers, BMT, and viral connection in gynecological oncology. There is also information about Lombardi collaboration in national Hematology/Lymphoma trials. Information about specific projects and faculty are available.

Patient Resources There are listings of patient events and activities and there are educational materials about prevention. Details of patient care services, facilities, counseling services, diagnosis, imaging, surgery, and clinical trials are available.

Location Washington, DC, NCI-designated

Lutheran General Health System ⊙ ⊙ ⊙

http://www.advocatehealth.com/sites/hospitals/luth/index.html

Lutheran General Hospital is a teaching, research, and referral hospital. Its Web site offers information relevant to staff, residency, articles, affiliate hospital, services, directions, and more. The page for the Lutheran General Cancer Care Center details its approaches to prevention, evaluation, treatment, and follow-up care. It boasts a multidisciplinary Breast Clinic, Head and Neck Tumor Clinic, a Pigmented Lesion Clinic, and extensive imaging resources.

Research Clinical trials are available in the areas of bone and soft tissue tumors, breast cancer, colorectal cancer, lung cancer, small-cell lung cancer, non-small cell lung cancer, prostate cancer, BMT studies, colon cancer, stomach cancer, lymphoma, melanoma, prevention studies, and rectal cancer. Listings of specific studies are available at the Cancer Care Center Web page.

Patient Resources The Advocate Health Care Cancer Care Information Service provides the user with detailed information regarding early warning signs, patient guides, screening, links, and articles. There are also educational classes, support groups, and discussion forum details.

Location Park Ridge, Illinois

M. D. Anderson Cancer Center, University of Texas ⊙ ⊙ ⊙

http://www.mdanderson.org

This is a comprehensive resource that provides extensive patient and professional information. There are individual sites for a number of specific cancers, news releases, programs lists and descriptions, practice guidelines, research updates, listings of educational events and meetings, and information documents for cancer, individual disorders, secondary disorders, and related diseases.

Research The research report (accessible from the site menu) provides comprehensive information about the Center's research programs and news. Research programs are in Behavioral Science, Biochemistry, Molecular Biology, Biomathematics, BMT, Cancer Bioimmunotherapy, Cancer Biology, Cancer Supportive Care, Carcinogenesis, Clinical Cancer

Prevention, Diagnostic, Drug Development, and Pharmacology, Epidemiology, Gene Therapy and Molecular Therapeutics, Immunology, Molecular Genetics, Pediatrics, Radiation Oncology and Biology, and Sarcoma. There are also research programs for a variety of individual cancers.

Patient Resources   There is a cancer prevention quiz, information about becoming a patient, a newsletter, and information about diagnosis, treatment, prevention, and more for individual cancers and associated disorders.

Location   Houston, Texas, NCI-designated

Massachusetts General Hospital (MGH) ◉ ◉ ◉

http://www.mgh.harvard.edu

The site menu contains information about MGH and affiliate institutions, clinical services, research, education, directions, news, MGH publications, and various department and staff directories. The Web site for the MGH Cancer Center serves as a comprehensive information resource. A link for the Cancer Center is provided from the main page. Associated links lead to substantial trials, services, education, and disease center information. All sections of this Web site are clearly organized.

Research   The MGH Cancer Research Center has laboratory divisions for cancer risk analysis, developmental biology, immunopathology, molecular genetics, molecular oncology, signal transduction, and tumor biology. There are complete listings of publications from 1994 and details about model organisms such as C. elegans, Xenopus, and Drosophila. Substantial information about research in all departments of the hospital is supplied.

Patient Resources   The Cancer Resource Room has detailed information documents for patients that cover living with cancer, diagnosis, locations, support programs, and treatment fact sheets. Clinical trials information and links are accessible.

Location   Boston, Massachusetts

Mayo Clinic ◉ ◉ ◉

http://www.mayo.edu

The Web site for the Mayo Clinic provides access to all related facilities and institutions. General health information and information about medical services, patient care, research, education, programs, journalists, news, and employment is offered. The Web site of the Mayo Clinic Cancer Center details information about the center, patient information, research, and education. Information about Mayo Clinic educational programs concerns Hematology-Oncology Training, other training programs, the medical school, the Mayo Graduate School of Medicine, the Mayo School of Health-Related Sciences, and the Mayo School of Continuing Medical Education.

Research | Research in the basic sciences focuses on Developmental Therapeutics, Immunology, and Cancer Genetics. Clinical Research programs are in Clinical and Translational Research, Imaging, and Prostate Cancer. Population science research programs are in the areas of Genetic Epidemiology, Prevention, and Control. Shared resources for all research programs of the Cancer Center are in pharmacology, tissue acquisition and Cellular/Molecular Analysis, Cytogenetics, Gene Discovery, Pharmacy, Statistics, Molecular Biology Core, Protein Core, and Flow Cytometry/Optical Morphology. Detailed information is provided for each area of research.

Patient Resources | Substantial travel, appointment, clinical trials, clinical care, and other resource information is available in addition to extensive lists of online resources, printed resources, support groups, and national associations.

Location | Rochester, Minnesota, NCI-designated

Memorial Sloan-Kettering Cancer Center (MSKCC) ○ ○ ○

http://www.mskcc.org

This is a comprehensive resource site providing extensive patient, educational, and research information that is easily accessed through the Site Menu, which covers Access, Treatment Information, Laboratory Research, Prevention and Early Detection, Resources for Medical Professionals, and the MSKCC Network of Facilities.

Research | Detailed information is provided on the areas of research being conducted at MSKCC. Research is organized into seven programs: Molecular Biology, Cell Biology, Cellular Biochemistry and Biophysics, Immunology, Molecular Pharmacology and Therapeutics, Clinical Research, and Cancer Prevention and Control. Major specific research thrusts include signals and pathways involved in the control of cell proliferation; regulatory pathways involved in developmental biology and the control of cell differentiation; cell-cell interactions, adhesion, and protein targeting; tumor immunology, immunotherapy and transplantation biology; human cancer genetics and molecular pathology; drug development, drug resistance and clinical therapeutics, and clinical research and clinical trials.

Patient Resources | Detailed descriptions of different forms of cancer, treatment side effects, pain management, rare cancers, and clinical trials are provided.

Location | New York, New York, NCI-designated

MeritCare Health System ⊙ ⊙ ⊙

http://www.meritcare.com

This Web site offers news and information about employment, practice opportunities, listings of affiliated clinics and healthcare centers, patient guides, referral guides, health information for a variety of conditions, and events schedules. The main page has a link to the Roger Maris Cancer Center (RMCC). The page for the RMCC offers a wealth of information about cancer, treatment, workshops, events, clinical services, education, and support.

Research	The center offers clinical research programs for the study of new treatments, management, and prevention.
Patient Resources	An online booklet thoroughly explains clinical trials and news. Also, patient information is available concerning prevention, detection, pain management, support, coping, treatment, and clinical services.
Location	Fargo, North Dakota

Nebraska Health System ⊙ ⊙ ⊙

http://www.nhsnet.org

The Nebraska Health System is made up of more than 20 outreach programs, two hospitals, University Medical Associates, and private practice physicians. The Web site provides extensive Health System information and a link to the University of Nebraska Medical Center Eppley Cancer Center. Its Web page offers information about the center, research, education and outreach, patient services, and links.

Research	Research is conducted in the areas of experimental therapeutics; hematologic malignancies and transplantation; molecular and bio-chemical etiology; molecular, cellular, and structural biology. There is a listing of clinical trials and a facilities description.
Patient Resources	Information about clinical trials, support groups, and physicians is offered. The Cancer HelpLink service offers a toll-free telephone information service for anyone.
Location	Omaha, Nebraska

New York Presbyterian Hospital (NYP) ⊙ ⊙ ⊙

http://www.nyp.org

New York Presbyterian is the university hospital of Columbia and Cornell and is made up of Columbia Presbyterian and New York Weill Cornell Hospitals. Its main page supplies information about the hospital, news and events, health services, departments, centers of excellence, and the NYP Healthcare Network. A link to the Herbert Irving Comprehensive Cancer Center (HICCC) provides access to information about cancer outreach, education and control, clinical and laboratory research, referrals, and facilities.

Research   The Division of Laboratory research has programs in Molecular Oncology and Virology; Developmental Biology and Genetics; Radiation Physics and Biology; and Immunology. The Division of Clinical Research has programs in breast cancer, urologic malignancies, neuro-oncology, BMT, allogenic stemcell, sarcoma and mesothelioma, and experimental therapeutics. Its Web page has a full listing of protocols.

Patient Resources   There are a large number of cancer outreach programs, support groups, and education programs. In addition, information concerning cancer causation, prevention, and control is available.

Location   New York, New York, NCI-designated

New York University School of Medicine
Kaplan Comprehensive Cancer Center (KCCC) ⊙ ⊙ ⊙

http://kccc-www.med.nyu.edu

This site of the KCCC offers information concerning clinical trials, research programs, community services, training and education, publications, and other resources. A link to the Comprehensive Breast Cancer Center provides access to information about clinical care, education, social support, and about the disorder.

Research   Research programs are conducted in the areas of epidemiology, cell interactions, environmental carcinogenesis, growth regulation, molecular oncology, and tumor immunology. Details of each program with lists of focus areas are provided. A separate Breast Cancer Research Program (BCRP) covers tumor biology, epidemiology, immunology and prevention, and therapy. A page for the Genitourinary Cancer Program for prostate and bladder cancer offers lists of basic and clinical research activities.

Patient Resources   Information concerning clinical trials is available along with details of community education lectures, the Outreach & Community Services program, and of the Cooperative Education Center at the Tisch Hospital.

Location   New York, New York, NCI-designated

Norris Cotton Cancer Center (NCCC) ⊙ ⊙ ⊙

http://nccc.hitchcock.org

The NCCC takes a multidisciplinary approach to research, education, and service and is part of the Dartmouth-Hitchcock Medical Center. The Web site offers information about NCCC services, treatment, clinical trials, referral services, research, news, events, education, its SunSafe Project, and other resources. Educational materials are provided via a link to Dartmouth Medical School, as well as lists of symposia and lectures.

Research   Programs of research are conducted in the areas of: Cancer Control; Cancer Epidemiology and Chemoprevention; Call Signaling, Growth & Differentiation; Immunology & Cancer Immunotherapy; Molecular Therapeutics and Radiobiology; and Bioengineering. Lists of specific projects are offered.

Patient Resources   There are details of clinical trials, treatment options, support groups, and obtaining second opinions. A patient resource guide provides a summary of NCCC healthcare providers, libraries, resource centers, and more. The SunSafe project provides information for the public about prevention of skin cancers.

Location   Lebanon, New Hampshire, NCI-designated

North Carolina Baptist Hospital ⊙ ⊙ ⊙

http://www.bgsm.edu

The Web site of the Wake Forest University Baptist Medical Center serves as the healthcare system site. It offers news and information about the center, departments, employment, clinical trials, education, patient care, and research. The page for the Department of Hematology and Oncology is provided by the Comprehensive Cancer Center of Wake Forest University. This site offers information about news, prevention, control, clinical trials, clinics, treatment programs, research, publications, radiation oncology, referrals, cancer biology, and continuing education.

Research   Information for research may be obtained from the Department of Cancer Biology at Wake Forest University. Links are provided. The Comprehensive Cancer Center offers specific information about a large number of protocols.

Patient Resources   For patients, there are a large number of informative articles and there is specific information about treatment programs, clinical trials, support programs, and outreach clinics.

Location   Winston-Salem, North Carolina, NCI-designated

Robert H. Lurie Cancer Center
of Northwestern University ⊙ ⊙ ⊙

http://www.nums.nwu.edu/lurie/index.html

The Center serves as the coordinator of cancer-related activity at the university and related hospitals. Information concerning research, clinical trials, educational programs, shared resources, faculty, and patient events is available.

Research   There are four programs in the Division of Basic Sciences: Adhesion, Motility and Angiogenesis; Molecular Oncogenesis; Differentiation and Development; and Hormone Action and Signal Transduction. Specific clinical sciences information is also available.

Patient Resources   There are descriptions of services offered and details of patient activities.

Location   Chicago, Illinois, NCI-designated

Roswell Park Cancer Institute ⊙ ⊙ ⊙

http://rpci.med.buffalo.edu/external.html

The Institute is a division of The New York State Department of Health and is an NCI-Designated Comprehensive Cancer Care Center. The Web site offers information about the facility, directions, news, diagnosis and treatment, research, trials, clinical divisions, conferences, and continuing medical and professional education programs.

Research   Basic science research is conducted in the areas of biophysics, diagnostic immunology, experimental therapeutics, human genetics, molecular and cellular biology, molecular immunology, and molecular medicine. Specific projects, faculty, and relevant organisms are discussed in detail for each research area. Research facilities are described in detail and there is a posted scientific report.

Patient Resources   Information for each clinical department is provided with associated diagnosis, treatment, and facility information. In addition there are support groups, newsletters, and links.

Location   Buffalo, New York, NCI-designated

Rush Presbyterian—St. Lukes Medical Center ⊙ ⊙ ⊙

http://www.rpslmc.edu

The Web site's main page offers information regarding news, patient services, patient education, the center, and professionals. The page for the Rush Cancer Institute (RCI) supplies fellowship, news, affiliates, physician, and treatment information. Areas of focus are Medical Oncology, Hematology, BMT, and comprehensive cancer care for specific disorders.

Research   Clinical trials research is conducted in the areas of breast, lung, pancreatic, head and neck, renal, bladder and prostatic cancers, sarcomas, and melanomas.

Patient Resources   Physician profiles, RCI news and descriptions of disorders, FAQ sections, virtual tours of facilities, insurance details, and other various online learning aids compose the site's collection of patient resources.

Location   Chicago, Illinois

San Antonio Cancer Institute (SACI) ⊙ ⊙ ⊙

http://www.ccc.saci.org

The SACI is the result of a collaboration between the Cancer Therapy Research Center and the University of Texas Health Science Center at San Antonio. Its Web site provides information about the Institute, facilities, locations, research programs, shared resources, clinical research, SACI membership, funding, publications, news, events, referral, clinics, and clinical and research conferences. A publications database allows the user to browse or search for publications of interest and there is a list of patient registration data submission requirements.

Research	There are established research programs in the areas of Breast Cancer, Cancer Prevention and Health Promotion, DNA Repair and Tumor Suppressor Genes, Experimental Therapeutics, and Growth Factor and Molecular Genetics. Details of program characteristics and Selected Phase I/II Studies are available.
Patient Resources	Details of facilities, clinical trials, and of services are offered. For disorder information a number of organized links are supplied. Support group information is available.
Location	San Antonio, Texas, NCI-designated

Scott and White Memorial Hospital ⊙ ⊙ ⊙

http://www.sw.org

The hospital's main page offers access to clinical centers and programs, directories and articles, and information about clinical education programs, institutional resources, conditions, referrals, locations, associated clinics, residency, employment, and patient resources. The Scott and White Center for Cancer Prevention and Care Web page offers access to staff, and information related to facilities, patient care, and links to other sites.

Research	The Center conducts clinical research in the areas of developmental therapeutics, prevention, BMT, and peripheral blood stem-cell transplant.
Patient Resources	The facility features a Cancer Resource Center, an Educational Resource Center, support groups, a quarterly publication, and information about American Cancer Society programs. The Educational Resource Center offers health information, education, and training through special programs.
Location	Temple, Texas

Shands Hospital at the University of Florida ⊙ ⊙ ⊙

http://www.hsc.ufl.edu

General facility, appointment, and department information is provided at the site's main page. The Pediatric Oncology Group offers news, publications, statistics, and meeting information at http://www.pog.ufl.edu.

Research	Information regarding Shands publications, notable achievements, and University of Florida Centers is offered. Links to University of Florida research departments are offered. The University of Florida—Shands has specialized research programs in pediatric oncology.
Patient Resources	Department, physician, events, and services information, is available along with links, as well as answers to commonly asked questions.
Location	Gainesville, Florida

Stanford University Hospital ⊙ ⊙ ⊙

http://www-med.stanford.edu/shs

Stanford University Hospital is part of the University of California San Francisco Stanford Health Care system that is comprised of numerous hospitals, clinics, Stanford University, and other facilities. The site menu offers information about visiting hours, contacts, directories, staff, medical services, medical groups, news, and medical units. The page for the Division of Oncology provides information about clinical services, care centers and facilities, fellowship, research, faculty, staff, and referrals.

Research	The Division of Oncology Home Page provides information about Stanford University faculty members and their respective basic science research projects. The same page also lists individual clinical trials for the study of specific cancers.
Patient Resources	Online access to a health library is supplied. This resource offers online videos, audio, links, and numerous text resources that provide information about the facility, cancer, and individual disorders. There is also a list of recommended books for patients.
Location	Stanford, California

Thomas Jefferson University Hospital ⊙ ⊙ ⊙

http://www.jeffersonhealth.org/tjuh

The main page provides links to departments, centers and programs, community programs, directories, and the Kimmel Cancer Center (KCC). The Web page for the KCC serves as an information resource for patients and professionals. It offers information regarding programs within the health network, research news, KCC news, clinical trials, clinical programs, medical science programs, and seminars.

Research	Basic science research programs are in the areas of cell biology, signal transduction, molecular biology/genetics, structural biology and bio-

informatics, immunology, and sequence analysis. There are listings of individual protocols and there is a news page that provides detailed information about findings, affiliations, and more. There are also listings of clinical trials at the KCC.

Patient Resources There is extensive diagnostic, treatment, prevention, and other information about cancer and specific disorders. There is research and other news for patients, information about the Center and its facilities, and listings of patient support programs.

Location Philadelphia, Pennsylvania, NCI-designated

UCLA Medical Center ☼ ☼ ☼

http://www.healthcare.ucla.edu

This site offers information for the entire University of California Los Angeles healthcare system and for the university. The Web page for the Department of Cancer Services lists the clinical divisions within the department and provides basic treatment information. Information about research, patient care, professional education, community cancer control, and clinical trials is provided.

Research Research information for the UCLA Medical Center may be obtained from the listed toll-free physician helpline. In addition, Web pages for individual divisions within the Department of Cancer Services provide research information.

Patient Resources Information concerning different forms of cancer is available, along with descriptions of treatment, diagnosis, research, and clinical trials.

Location Los Angeles, California, NCI-designated

University Hospital ☼ ☼ ☼

http://www.ohsu.edu/hospitals

The site is for the hospitals and clinics of Oregon Health Sciences University (OHSU). Information about care facilities and services, patient resources, provider resources, locations, and medical services and departments is offered.

Research There are research programs in many OHSU schools and institutes and these sites may be searched for basic science or other research programs.

Patient Resources The Consumer Health Resources Center at OHSU offers health information via mail and the Internet through links, brochures, and other documents. Patients are also given access to Consumer Health Materials in the OHSU Library Collection. Other features include an interpreter program and facilities information.

Location Portland, Oregon

University Hospitals and Clinics ◎ ◎ ◎

http://www.muhealth.org

The Web site is sponsored by the University of Missouri Health Sciences Center and provides information for a variety of disorders. Cancer information is provided by tumor type and comes in the form of descriptions of hospital programs, treatments, research, and staff. The page for the Ellis Fischel Cancer Center provides cancer questions and answers and information about clinical trials, screening, services offered, employment opportunities, and reviews.

Research   Information about basic science research programs is available at the site for the School of Medicine. There is an extensive directory of clinical trials research by modality at the page for the Ellis Fischel Cancer Center.

Patient Resources   There is a section of cancer questions and answers related to individual disorders and cancer in general. Also, there are detailed descriptions of clinical trials, counseling services, and clinical departments.

Location   Columbia, Missouri

University Hospitals of Cleveland ◎ ◎ ◎

http://www.uhhs.com

This site serves the University Hospitals Health System and the University Hospitals of Cleveland. Information about the academic arm, Case Western Reserve University, is provided along with a link. The Ireland Cancer Center is an NCI-Designated Comprehensive Cancer Center and its site has information about clinical trials, BMT, core research, cancer information, and the medical staff.

Research   Research at the Ireland Cancer Center occurs in seven programs: Molecular Biology of Oncogenesis; Molecular Virology; Cancer Genetics; Radiation Biology; Hematopoietic and Immune Cell Biology; Developmental Therapeutics; and Cancer Prevention and Control. Details are provided for each program with investigator listings.

Patient Resources   The Cancer Information Service provides information about clinical trials, free education materials, and community resources. There are also detailed documents about family and cancer, colorectal cancer, prostate disease, and breast cancer.

Location   Cleveland, Ohio, NCI-designated

University of Alabama at Birmingham Comprehensive Cancer Center ◎ ◎ ◎

http://www.ccc.uab.edu

This particular Web site provides details about the Center, research, patient services, news, the Cancer Center Seminar Series, clinical trials, appointments, treatments, prevention and control, cancer, and publications. There is also information about its multidisciplinary prostate cancer clinic.

Research	Programs of research are in the areas of immunology, structural biology, virology, molecular genetics, experimental therapeutics, neuro-oncology, cancer control and population science, women's cancer, and developmental chemoprevention. For each program, details of specific projects and participating faculty are provided. There are also grant announcements and postings of cancer data.
Patient Resources	Information about cancer, clinical trials, treatments, support services available, patient education programs, and making an appointment can be found here, as well as a glossary of terms and a links section.
Location	Birmingham, Alabama, NCI-designated

University of California (UC), Davis Medical Center   ○ ○ ○

http://www.ucdmc.ucdavis.edu/medical_center/index.html

UC Davis Medical Center is an academic medical center that offers education, research, patient care, and public service programs. Its site offers information about the center, referrals, clinical programs, research, and community service. The site for the UC Davis Cancer Center offers program, services, clinical trials, referral, clinics, and physician information.

Research	There are programs for individual disorders and listings of specific clinical trial protocols.
Patient Resources	There is an on-site resource center that offers video, audio, and print materials about many aspects of cancer and individual disorders. There are also online guides that cover prevention, risk, breast cancer, general cancer, and prostate cancer. A set of organized links is also offered.
Location	Sacramento, California

University of Chicago Hospitals   ○ ○ ○

http://www.uchospitals.edu

The Web site offers overview information about the University of Chicago Hospitals and Health System. There is information about the facility, locations, directions, news, events, community outreach, aeromedical transport, departments, and contacts. A variety of multimedia videos are offered. Oncology departments are spread throughout various hospitals in the system and there are individual departments for specific disorders.

Research	Research information may be obtained at the Web site concerning The Cancer Research Center at the University of Chicago. Research programs: Include Molecular Biology of Cell Growth and Differen-

tiation; Cancer Molecular Genetics; Immunology and Cancer; Clinical and Experimental Therapeutics; Advanced Imaging; Breast Cancer; Prostate Cancer; and Cancer Prevention and Control.

Patient Resources   The Cancer Research Center offers support services and a patient events calendar. There are a number of links and clinical trials, as well as appointment and staff information. Newsletters and an online discussion forum are also available.

Location   Chicago, Illinois, NCI-designated

University of Colorado Cancer Center ⊙ ⊙ ⊙
http://www.uchsc.edu/chancllr/UCCC/UCCCwelcome.html

This Web site provides information about the Center and its programs of basic research, clinical research, patient care, education and prevention, and early detection.

Research   Clinical research information is available from the Clinical Investigations Core (CIC) and comes in the form of a Clinical Trials Priority List. Listings of individual protocols are available.

Patient Resources   Basic information about the Center and its services is offered.

Location   Denver, Colorado, NCI-designated

University of Iowa (UI) Hospitals and Clinics ⊙ ⊙ ⊙
http://www.vh.org/Welcome/UIHC/UIHCMedDepts/CancerCenter/

The site is a comprehensive information resource and offers information for all UI health affiliates and departments via its Virtual Hospital Service. The Web site for the UI Cancer Center (UICC) offers details of cancer center organization, grant opportunities, core facilities, clinical trials, training and education, positions available, meetings, protocols, clinical programs, links, and UICC facts. Clinical programs and treatment information specifics are discussed at the page for the John and Mary Pappajohn Clinical Cancer Center.

Research   Descriptions of UICC programs of Cancer Epidemiology, Cellular Activation in Cancer, Experimental Therapeutics, Free Radicals and Membranes, Molecular and Tumor Virology, and Molecular Mechanisms of Metastasis are available.

Patient Resources   Descriptions of the Clinical Cancer Center's multidisciplinary treatment, support care programs, online support groups, and patient events are available. The Cancer Information Service offers educational materials for individual cancers, general facts, diagnostic tests, pain control, prevention, chemotherapy/radiation, clinical trials, coping, nutrition/diet, statistics, and helpful organizations.

Location   Iowa City, Iowa

University of Michigan Medical Center ⊙ ⊙ ⊙

http://www.med.umich.edu

The site offers information about the entire health system. The page for the University of Michigan Comprehensive Cancer Center is a major patient and professional resource. Information regarding patient referral, research programs, continuing education, news, treatment, clinical trials, seminars, and the facility is offered.

Research	Basic research is conducted in the areas of cancer genetics and virology, cancer cell biology, tumor immunology, and cancer pharmacology. Information about clinical research, prevention research, and grant opportunities is available. The Web site also gives access to the University of Michigan Human Breast Cell/Tissue Bank and Database.
Patient Resources	An exhaustive set of patient resources covers topics such as nutrition, clinical trials, patient seminars, maps, prevention, treatment, and research. A University of Michigan Cancer Information Line serves the Midwest region of the United States and offers information from healthcare professionals to patients about prevention, risk reduction, warning signs, detection methods, treatment options, support services, and clinical trials.
Location	Ann Arbor, Michigan, NCI-designated

University of Minnesota Cancer Center ⊙ ⊙ ⊙

http://www.cancer.umn.edu

Patient services for the Cancer Center are largely provided by University of Minnesota physicians and the Fairfield University Medical Center. There are details of outreach activities, research, clinical care programs, news, referrals, consultations, seminars, events, and contacts. A portion of the site is dedicated to nutrition and cancer.

Research	Programs of research are in prevention and etiology, cancer genetics, cell biology and metastasis, immunology and transplant biology, and therapy. Web pages for each program provide information about investigators and individual studies.
Patient Resources	There is information about outreach activities such as the Minnesota Colorectal Cancer Initiative, the Familial Cancer Clinic, and the Cancer Center Seminars Series. There are descriptions of services and of nutrition and cancer for patients.
Location	Minneapolis, Minnesota, NCI-designated

University of North Carolina Hospitals ⊚ ⊚ ⊚

http://cancer.med.unc.edu

The Web site for the UNC Lineberger Comprehensive Cancer Center offers an introduction, a virtual tour of the facility, patient resources, access to multidisciplinary clinics, access to research information, and contact listings.

Research | Listings of specific research protocols, facility profiles, and education opportunities are offered.

Patient Resources | This section provides details of treatments, clinics, support groups, individual cancers, clinical trials, and links to other information sources.

Location | Chapel Hill, North Carolina, NCI-designated

University of Pittsburgh
Medical Center (UPMC) Presbyterian ⊚ ⊚ ⊚

http://www.upmc.edu

The main page offers UPMC health, home care, CME, employment, residency, and directories information. The Web page for the University of Pittsburgh Cancer Institute provides cancer, facility, program, news, and other useful information. There are clinical and research images, a University of Pittsburgh Cancer Institute (UPCI) Scientific Report, and one can conduct a UPCI protocol or people search.

Research | Programs are conducted for Behavioral Medicine and Oncology; Biological Therapeutics; Cancer Epidemiology, Prevention and Control; Cancer Genetics; Immunology; Molecular and Cellular Oncology; Molecular Therapeutics and Drug Discovery; and Molecular Virology. In addition, there are a number of programs for the study of specific cancers.

Patient Resources | The UPCI Cancer Information and Referral Service provides information about early detection, prevention, diagnosis, clinical research studies, treatments, psychological support, education programs, and community resources and services. There are also links to other information sites.

Location | Pittsburgh, Pennsylvania, NCI-designated

University of South Carolina
Norris Comprehensive Cancer Center ⊚ ⊚ ⊚

http://ccnt.hsc.usc.edu

The Web site offers information about individual hospital and special program departments, clinical trials, correspondence, current events, and links. There are details of publications, basic research, employment opportunities, locations, cooperative groups, continuing education conferences, and disorders.

Research	There are brief descriptions of clinical trials, basic research, and translational research. One can search for open protocols by number or by anatomical site of disease.
Patient Resources	For each department within the Center, details regarding services offered, treatments, and faculty are provided. There is also information about individual cancers and support groups.
Location	Los Angeles, California, NCI-designated

University of Virginia Health Sciences Center ⊙ ⊙ ⊙

http://www.med.virginia.edu

The Web site's main page offers Center-wide general, health, and patient care information, education and research, and information technology material. Extensive information for each of these topics is supplied with links to various schools, departments, clinics, and other health centers. The Welcome Page for The Cancer Center at The University of Virginia provides information about the center, services, physicians, and other Internet cancer resources. One can seek a second opinion, view clinical trials, and obtain information about the treatment teams and disorders treated.

Research	Extensive information is provided concerning research in immunology, clinical oncology/developmental therapeutics, endocrinology, cell signaling and metastasis, and cell surfaces.
Patient Resources	Patient information services are offered for health education, complimentary therapies, counseling, genetics counseling, screening and prevention, clinical psychology, and spiritual care. There are online books, information documents, procedure information, and links lists. There is also an on site patient information library. Pages for Illness-Specific Teams have information about individual disorders.
Location	Charlottesville, Virginia

University of Washington Medical Center (UWMC) ⊙ ⊙ ⊙

http://www.washington.edu/medical

The site offers access to all University of Washington divisions and the University of Washington Medical School as well as to all Medical Centers and Clinics. The main page provides referral, continuing education, medical services, and UWMC facilities information. The UWMC Cancer Center has specialty clinics for a variety of individual cancers and the Web site has information about treatment, surgery, research, genetics, staff, services, diagnosis, and staging for each disorder serviced at each clinic.

Research	Individual research projects are detailed for each clinic. In addition, one may search the University of Washington Medical School Web site for basic science research.

Patient Resources Information about the facility, appointments, directions, treatment options, support groups, home care, and patient housing is available. In addition, there are basic cancer facts, pamphlets and brochures, links lists, and documents that cover coping with cancer. An on-site UWMC Cancer Patient Library offers books and other resources for specific information on aspects of individual cancers.

Location Seattle, Washington

University of Wisconsin Hospital and Clinics ◎ ◎ ◎

http://www.medicine.wisc.edu/sections

The Web site offers information about the University of Wisconsin Department of Medicine. There are links to each of the 16 clinical sections of the department. The page for the oncology programs provides details of the BMT, Hematology, and Medical Oncology Sections, affiliations, special services, referral information, locations, and of related resources at the University of Wisconsin Comprehensive Cancer Center.

Research Research programs at the University of Wisconsin Comprehensive Cancer Center consist of the Breast Cancer Program; Cancer Control Program; Cell Adhesion and Signaling Program; Ocular Tumor Program; Developmental Therapeutics Program; Urologic Oncology Program; Immunology and Biological Therapeutics Program; Pediatric Oncology Program; and Radiation Oncology and Physics Program.

Patient Resources The Cancer Connect program allows patients to pose specific questions to professionals. There are links and details of support groups, prevention, screening, diagnosis and treatment, symptoms, clinical trials, and community resources.

Location Madison, Wisconsin, NCI-designated

Vanderbilt University Hospital and Clinic ◎ ◎ ◎

http://www.mc.vanderbilt.edu/health/hospitals/main_hospital.html

The site specifically provides information for Vanderbilt University Hospital but also provides links to schools, the Vanderbilt University Medical Center and related clinics, and patient care facilities. The page for the Division of Hematology and Oncology offers details related to training programs, faculty and staff, conferences, research programs, clinical programs, publications and references, a bulletin board, and links.

Research Research programs are an extension of the Vanderbilt-Ingram Cancer Center (VICC). Programs of research include: Signal Transduction and Cell Proliferation; Host-Tumor Interactions; Gastrointestinal Cancer; Cancer Genetics; Breast Cancer; Cancer Prevention and Control; and Experimental Therapeutics. There are investigator listings, news, and summaries of each program.

Patient Resources The site for the VICC offers detailed and thorough information about cancer, prevention, specific types of cancer, support services, community events, clinical trials, programs available, contacts, and directions.

Location Nashville, Tennessee

Vermont Cancer Center (VCC) ⊚ ⊚ ⊚

http://www.vtmednet.org/vcc/index.html

The Center is a component of the University of Vermont College of Medicine. There are facts about VCC and its facilities and details including locations, affiliated organizations, programs and services, members, research, clinical care, and current happenings.

Research Research programs include Cancer Prevention and Control; Cell Signaling and Growth Control; Clinical Research; and Genome Stability and Expression. Web pages for each program offer information concerning members, goals, cancer focus, program elements, and accomplishments.

Patient Resources There is an overview of the care offered by VCC and a list of clinical trials. There is a directory of support groups and a patient newsletter. For information about cancer and disorders, there is a list of select links.

Location Burlington, Vermont, NCI-designated

Yale-New Haven Hospital ⊚ ⊚ ⊚

http://www.ynhh.org

Yale-New Haven Hospital is staffed by faculty from the Yale University School of Medicine. The hospital houses the clinical services section of the Yale Cancer Center. The Web site offers information about services offered, facilities, staff, and other hospital resources. Information about other facilities of Yale-New Haven Health is also offered. The site for the Yale Cancer Center details research, clinical trials, directories, and cancer information.

Research Research information is detailed at the site for the Yale Cancer Center. Major programs of research are in Breast Cancer; Cancer Genetics; Cancer Prevention and Control; Cell Biology; Developmental Therapeutics; Genetic Therapy/Medical Oncology/Hematology; Gynecologic Oncology; Immunology; Lymphoma; Molecular Oncology and Development; Molecular Virology; Stem Cell Biology and Transplantation; and Therapeutic Radiology. Specific program information and faculty and contact listings are provided.

Patient Resources The Center provides a number of education and patient service programs and support groups. The hospital features a Cancer Genetic

Counseling Service and the site provides lists of informational resources.

Location   New Haven, Connecticut, NCI-designated

8.4 State Cancer Societies

American Cancer Society (ACS):
Directory of State Cancer Societies ◎ ◎ ◎
http://www.cancer.org

A scroll-down menu of state listings in the upper right hand corner of this home page
of the American Cancer Society enables the visitor to locate state cancer societies,
including their individual home pages, programs, resources, and addresses.

8.5 Selected Medical School Oncology Departments

Boston University Cancer Research Center
http://www.bumc.bu.edu/Departments/HomeMain.asp?DepartmentID=109

Case Western Reserve University Cancer Center
http://mediswww.meds.cwru.edu/dept/cancer/trainprog/trainprog.html

Columbia University Department of Radiation Oncology
http://cpmcnet.columbia.edu/dept/radoncology

Duke University Department of Radiation Oncology
http://www.duke.edu/deptdir/Radiation_Oncology.html

Emory University Department of Hematology Oncology
http://www.emory.edu/WHSC/MED/HEMONC/

Emory University Department of Radiation Oncology
http://www.emory.edu/WHSC/MED/RADONC

Harvard University Department of Radiation Oncology
http://www.hmcnet.harvard.edu/temp/radonc.html

Indiana University, Indianapolis, Department of Radiation Oncology
http://www.radonc.iupui.edu

Johns Hopkins Oncology Center
http://www.hopkins.cancercenter.jhmi.edu

Johns Hopkins University Pediatric Neuro-Oncology Group
http://www.med.jhu.edu/pno

Mayo Medical School Department of Oncology
http://www.mayo.edu/cancercenter

Mount Sinai School of Medicine, The Derald H. Ruttenberg Cancer Center
http://www.mssm.edu/cancerctr

New York University Department of Radiation Oncology
http://www.med.nyu.edu/radonc/nyurad.html

Stanford University Department of Radiation Oncology
http://www-radonc.stanford.edu

Stanford University Division of Oncology
http://www.med.stanford.edu/school/Oncology/index.html

Tufts University Department of Radiation Oncology
http://www.tufts.edu/med/dept/clinical/radonc.html

University of Alabama, Birmingham, Department of Radiation Oncology
http://main.uab.edu/uasom/show.asp?durki=3976

University of Alabama, Birmingham, Division of Hematology and Oncology
http://www.dpo.uab.edu/cgi-bin/bp/query.cgi?key=JCBTVFTF

University of California, Los Angeles, Department of Hematology/Oncology
http://www.medsch.ucla.edu/

University of California, San Diego, Cancer Center
http://medicine.ucsd.edu/somdepts.htm#Cancer

University of California, San Diego, Department of Medicine Division of Hematology/Oncology
http://orpheus-1.ucsd.edu/hemonc/index.html

University of California, San Diego, Department of Radiology Division of Radiation Oncology
http://medicine.ucsd.edu/somdepts.htm#Radiology

University of California, San Francisco, Radiation Oncology
http://itsa.ucsf.edu/~radonc

University of California, San Francisco,
Department of Medicine, Division of Hematology/Oncology
http://medicine.ucsf.edu/divisions/

University of Chicago Department of Medicine, Division of Hematology/Oncology
http://www.uchospitals.edu/areas/medicine.html#hemonc

University of Chicago Department of Radiation and Cellular Oncology
http://www.radonc.uchicago.edu

University of Cincinnati
Department of Internal Medicine, Division of Hematology and Oncology
http://www.med.uc.edu/departments/displaydivisionshell.cfm?divisionid=26

University of Cincinnati Department of Surgery, Division of Surgical Oncology
http://www.med.uc.edu

University of Colorado Health Sciences Center
Department of Medicine, Division of Medical Oncology
http://www.uchsc.edu/sm/sm/divmedon.htm

University of Florida Department of Medicine, Division of Hematology/Oncology
http://www.med.ufl.edu/med/divisions.html

University of Florida Department of Radiation Oncology
http://www.med.ufl.edu/comdir.html#RadOn

University of Iowa Division of Hematology, Oncology, and Blood & Marrow Transplantation
http://www.med.ufl.edu/med/divisions.html

University of Massachusetts, Worcester, Cancer Center
http://www.umassmed.edu/internalmed/divisions/hema_oncology/

University of Miami Department of Medicine, Division of Hematology/Oncology
http://www.med.miami.edu/med/divisions/divisions.html

University of Miami Department of Radiation Oncology
http://www.med.miami.edu/guide/radionc.htm

University of Michigan, Ann Arbor, Department of Radiation Oncology
http://www.med.umich.edu/radonc

University of Michigan Division of Hematology and Oncology
http://www.med.umich.edu/intmed/hemeonc/

University of North Carolina
Department of Pediatrics, Division of Pediatric Hematology/Oncology
http://cancer.med.unc.edu/pediatrics/

University of North Carolina Department of Radiation Oncology
http://www.med.unc.edu/wrkunits/2depts/radonc

University of Pennsylvania Department of Pediatric Oncology
http://health.upenn.edu/poncol

University of Pennsylvania Department of Radiation Oncology
http://www.xrt.upenn.edu

University of Pennsylvania Hematology/Oncology Division
http://www.med.upenn.edu/~hematol/

University of Rochester Department of Hematology and Oncology
http://www.urmc.rochester.edu/cancercenter/hemeonc.html

University of Rochester Department of Radiation Oncology
http://www.rochester.edu/SMDBulletin/Departments/onc.html

University of Southern California Department of Oncology
http://www.usc.edu/schools/medicine

University of Southern California Department of Radiation Oncology
http://www.usc.edu/schools/medicine

University of Texas Southwestern Medical Center, Dallas,
Harold C. Simmons Comprehensive Cancer Center, Hematology/Oncology
http://www.swmed.edu/home_pages/cancerctr/bios/rutherfo.htm

University of Utah Department of Radiation Oncology
http://www.med.utah.edu/radoncol

University of Washington Department of Medicine, Division of Oncology
http://depts.washington.edu/oncology/

University of Washington Department of Radiation Oncology
http://www.washington.edu/medical/som/depts/oncology/index.html

University of Wisconsin, Madison,
Department of Medicine, Division of Hematology, and Medical Oncology
http://www.medicine.wisc.edu/sections/heme/

Washington University, St. Louis,
Department of Internal Medicine, Division of Hematology/Oncology
http://tollefsen.wustl.edu/heme/index.html

Yale University Cancer Center
http://info.med.yale.edu/ycc

Yale University Department of Internal Medicine, Division of Medical Oncology
http://info.med.yale.edu/intmed/

9. DISEASES

9.1 **Bone and Soft Tissue Sarcomas**

General Resources

American Academy of Orthopedic Surgeons (AAOS) ◎ ◎ ◎
http://www.aaos.org

The site for this professional organization provides information about most orthopedic issues for professionals and the public. Public information about the AAOS, disorders, and prevention is offered. For professionals, there are details on the AAOS Annual Meeting, links to other sites, and discussions of current legislative issues. A restricted section for AAOS members provides information about specialty societies, research, member directories, AAOS services, outcomes assessment, educational resources, discussion groups, and AAOS archives. Membership information is provided. An Orthopedic Yellow Pages section provides listings of clinical product suppliers, firms, office suppliers, and more.

Bonetumor.org ◎ ◎ ◎
http://www.bonetumor.org

This educational Web site has sections for patients and for physicians. The physicians' section provides an Online Atlas of Bone Tumors and Bone Cancer that features clinical, radiological, pathological, and surgical characteristics. There is also a case of the month and information about Tumor Mimics, Web resources, surgery, Metastatic Bone Tumors and Cancers, Bone Lesions from Metabolic Disease, and treatment options. One can also test his or her diagnostic talents via an online quiz. For patients, there is information about alternative treatments, surgery, metastatic tumors, and information about individual tumor types.

Center for Orthopedic Oncology and Musculoskeletal Research ◎ ◎ ◎
http://www.sarcoma.org

An information resource, the site offers information about Orthopedic Oncology, publications, fellowships, research at the Center, news, staff, and education. There are 19 captioned slide show presentations of surgical techniques, principles, and morphologic and radiographic features, links, and a list of contacts. A restricted section for patients and physicians offers online consultation.

Indiana University School of Medicine
Bone Cancer Research Fund ⊚ ⊚

http://www.medlib.iupui.edu/bcr

This site offers details of current research at the University, future research, investigators, and a large listing of technical papers. For patients, there is a series of information documents that cover tumors, procedures, and sarcoma details. The site also offers a newsletter.

Johns Hopkins Musculoskeletal Oncology Unit ⊚ ⊚

http://www.path.jhu.edu/mou.html

This site provides descriptions of services offered, faculty, consultation arrangements, research, surgical treatments, and diseases. For patients, the site supplies an online chat room.

Madison Research Group (MRG) ⊚ ⊚ ⊚

http://www.mrgx.com

The primary focus of MRG research is in the area of childhood osteosarcoma. The MRG Web site offers details on occurrence, inherited osteosarcoma, treatment, molecular biology, and on other bone cancers. There is a glossary of osteosarcoma research as well as research and other information on the p53 gene and osteosarcoma, Rb gene and osteosarcoma, and TGF-beta and osteosarcoma. Some information is patient friendly and there is a links section.

Orthopedic Research Society (ORS) ⊚ ⊚ ⊚

http://www.ors.org

Goals of the ORS are to support and promote research in the areas of orthopedic surgery and muskuloskeletal diseases and injuries. The site offers details of seminars, announcements, news, membership, abstracts, directors, and World Health Organization (WHO) initiatives. There is an online discussion group, a newsletter, and a link to the *Journal of Orthopedic Research*. There are links to relevant sites and to specific resources for researchers.

Wheeless' Textbook of Orthopedics ⊚ ⊚ ⊚

http://www.medmedia.com

From the Main Menu, one is given access to all sections of the Textbook and hundreds of topics are discussed. The section on Bone Tumors (direct link: http://www.medmedia.com/o6/136.htm) is extensive and provides details of biopsy, chemotherapy, radiologic and histologic features, location, metastatic tumors, and staging. Information concerning osseous, cartilaginous, fibrous, reticuloendothelial, and vascular tumors, as well as tumors of unknown origin, is given. Comprehensive sections for other orthopedic tumors and sarcomas are also available.

Sarcomas

British Columbia Cancer Agency:
Bone and Connective Tissue Sarcomas ⊙ ⊙ ⊙
http://www.bccancer.bc.ca/cid/03.html

This Canadian site provides details on symptoms, signs, etiology/risk factors, diagnosis, and staging information related to bone and connective tissue sarcomas. Specific sarcomas of the bone, bone marrow, and cartilage; and soft tissues sarcomas are discussed at the site, including osteosarcoma, Ewing's sarcoma, chondrosarcoma, malignant fibrous histiocytoma of the bone, chordoma, fibrosarcomas, liposarcomas, rhabdomyosarcomas, leiomyosarcomas, angiosarcomas and lymphangiosarcomas, synovial cell sarcomas, and malignant fibrous histiocytoma. General information on anatomy and normal function of each affected area and statistics on each disease are also available.

European Intergroup Cooperative
Ewing's Sarcoma Study (EICESS) ⊙ ⊙
http://www.staff.ncl.ac.uk/s.j.cotterill/eicess.htm

The EICESS site offers information about the group, Ewing's Sarcoma of Bone, trials, and about participating groups. There are also links to other Web sites concerning the aforementioned topics.

Ewing's Sarcoma Support Group Resources Page ⊙ ⊙
http://www.diverstech.com/ewings.htm

This patient site offers an organized collection of links to other sites and information pages. Links are organized under these topics: Clinical Trials; Mailing Lists; Oncology; Bone Marrow and Stem Cell Transplants Information; Associations; Ewing's Sarcoma Patient Pages; Research Sites; Alternative and Complimentary Therapies; and more.

Intergroup Rhabdomyosarcoma Study Group (IRSG) ⊙ ⊙ ⊙
http://rhabdo.org

IRSG is a coalition of academic institutions and treatment centers that is funded by the National Cancer Institute that conducts clinical trials for the treatment of rhabdomyosarcoma. Its Web site provides information about the group, clinical trials, the disorder, and announcements. A section geared towards health professionals details citations, abstracts, and information about tumor cell lines. A links section for patients provides additional sources of information.

Kaposi's Sarcoma ⊙ ⊙ ⊙

http://www.thebody.com/treat/kaposis.html

As a section from the Web site for The Body: An AIDS and HIV Information Resource, this site provides a collection of medical and other articles, treatment options, research, pharmacology, and more on the subject of Kaposi's Sarcoma.

Kristen Ann Carr Fund Sarcoma Forum ⊙ ⊙ ⊙

http://www.sarcoma.com

The Kristen Ann Carr site offers patient and family support and disorder information. There is information concerning news and events and details of the organization's wish fulfillment program. The Post-Treatment Resource Program provides practical, psychological, social, and existential education and support information.

Leiomyosarcoma ⊙ ⊙

http://userwww.sfsu.edu/~donmillr

This patient education site provides danger, treatment, prognosis, malignancy, recurrence, survival rate, staging, and more information about leiomyosarcoma and soft tissue sarcoma. There is general cancer information, references, and an online test.

Leiomyosarcoma of the Head and Neck ⊙ ⊙ ⊙

http://www.bcm.tmc.edu/oto/grand/7893.html

This is a page from the Web site provided by Baylor College of Medicine's Department of Otorhinolaryngology and Communicative Sciences. It details incidence and differentiating characteristics and provides a case presentation of Leiomyosarcoma.

OncoLink: Adult Sarcomas ⊙ ⊙ ⊙

http://www.oncolink.upenn.edu/disease/sarcoma1

General resources on cancer and symptom management resources are available from this informative site, as well as information specific to sarcomas in adults. The site provides links to a list of clinical trials at the University of Pennsylvania related to adult sarcomas, pediatric sarcoma information, answers to Frequently Asked Questions related to sarcomas, online support groups, articles describing treatment advances, and other information resources for patients and professionals. The site also offers a link to the National Cancer Institute CancerLit network, automatically returning article citations related to soft tissue/rhabdomyosarcomas.

OncoLink: National Cancer Institute Fact Sheet: Questions and Answers about Soft Tissue Sarcomas ⊙ ⊙ ⊙

http://www.oncolink.upenn.edu/pdq_html/6/engl/600612.html

Soft tissue sarcomas are described at this site, which is directed at both professionals and the general public. A fact sheet includes a definition of soft tissue and soft tissue sarcomas, and a discussion of possible causes, including genetics and occupational exposure to certain chemicals. The site also describes common body sites for these tumors, percentage of cancer cases diagnosed as sarcomas, symptoms of sarcomas, diagnosis, and treatment. Tables list all types of soft tissue sarcomas found in adults and children by affected area. National Cancer Institute contact details are available for additional information, and users can also find suggested Web addresses for educational resources.

Osteosarcoma ☉ ☉ ☉

http://www.med.ufl.edu/medinfo/ortho

A tutorial from the University of Florida College of Medicine offers detailed text and images that concern osteosarcoma. Details of definitions, demographics, clinical presentations, natural history, radiographic features, imaging studies, gross features, microscopic features, treatment, example cases, and a self-examination are included in the tutorial.

Progress in the Systemic Treatment of Advanced Soft-Tissue Sarcomas ☉ ☉ ☉

http://www.moffitt.usf.edu/cancjrnl/v5n1/article4.html

The H. Lee Moffitt Cancer Center offers research findings suggesting that a combination therapeutic regimen of chemotherapy, radiation, and surgery may be more effective than chemotherapy alone in the treatment of advanced soft tissue sarcomas. The article provides background information and statistics on soft tissue sarcomas, and a description of conventional chemotherapy, factors affecting chemotherapy response, current investigational efforts, the proposed integration of chemotherapy, radiation, and surgery, and two illustrative case studies.

Sarcoma Foundation ☉

http://www.sarcomafoundation.com

The organization provides patient information and funds research. The Web site offers a number of links to disorder and support sites and documents. Contact listings for more details is provided.

Soft-Tissue Sarcoma of the Extremities and its Mimics: Clinicopathologic and MR Imaging Features ☉ ☉ ☉

http://rpiwww.mdacc.tmc.edu/se/sts

This professional tutorial is provided by the Levit Radiologic Pathologic Institute of the M.D. Anderson Cancer Center. There are multiple sections with images, text descriptions, and patient studies. Section topics include general characteristics, post-chemotherapy/radiation therapy, MR imaging, post surgical fluid collections, post-surgical appearance of extremity sarcoma, and more.

Staging, Pathology, and Radiology of Musculoskeletal Tumors ◎ ◎ ◎

http://dev.newc.com/sarcoma/html/body_ch3.html

Chapter Three of Paul Sugarbaker and Martin Malawer's book, *Musculoskeletal Surgery for Cancer,* Principles and Techniques, is available online, providing information for health professionals on staging, pathology, and radiology of muskuloskeletal tumors. Detailed descriptions of clinical, radiographic, and pathological characteristics are presented for each type of tumor. The natural history and biology of bone and soft tissue tumors and metastasis is outlined, followed by a discussion on different types of soft tissue sarcomas. References at the end of the chapter provide further information sources (books and articles) on the various subjects discussed in the chapter.

University of Newcastle upon Tyne: The Sarcoma Page ◎ ◎ ◎

http://www.ncl.ac.uk/child-health/guides/clinks2c.htm

The University of Newcastle offers a guide to cancer resources including bone cancers and soft tissue sarcoma. There are 84 links to bone cancers, which include general resources, Ewing's sarcoma, osteosarcoma, chondrosarcoma, and other bone tumors. In addition, there are 53 links to soft tissue sarcoma sites, including general resources, childhood soft tissue sarcoma, adult soft-tissue sarcoma, and Kaposi's Sarcoma. The general resources link for soft tissue sarcoma includes an OncoLink menu for Sarcoma. Both bone cancer and soft-tissue sarcoma sites contain separate information sections for health professionals.

9.2 Bone Marrow Failure and Transplant

General Resources

American Society for Blood and Marrow Transplantation (ASMBT) ◎ ◎ ◎

http://www.asbmt.org

The ASMBT is a professional association for researchers and clinicians that seeks to foster research, represent physicians, establish clinical standards, promote communications, provide accreditation programs, and provide recommendations for insurance reimbursement. Information about the society's meetings, directors, membership, policy, and contacts is provided. Reviews and informative documents are also provided. There is a link to *Biology of Blood and Marrow Transplantation;* this journal publishes research, reviews, commentaries, news of the ASMBT, and more.

American Society of
Transplant Surgeons (ASTS) ⊙ ⊙ (fee-based)

http://www.asts.org

The ASTS Web site offers information about its committees, bylaws, membership, meetings, fellowship accreditation, awards, and an ethics section to aid in clinical decision making. A substantial portion of the site has restricted access for members, and these sections offer a journal, a member directory, conference rooms for discussion, and organization reports. An online membership application is required.

American Society of Transplantation (AST) ⊙ ⊙

http://www.a-s-t.org

The professional Society serves physicians and scientists and promotes research, patient care, advocacy, and education. Information concerning bylaws, CME, meetings, ethics, officers, membership, job postings, publications, and certification is provided. A restricted section for members provides committee reports, slide lectures, a newsletter, CME transcripts, and a member directory. Preregistration for meetings is also possible via the site.

Blood and Marrow Transplant Newsletter ⊙ ⊙

http://www.bmtnews.org

The newsletter's Web site serves as its online version. There are listings of news and current events, links to a variety of publications, support details, and contact lists.

Bone Marrow Foundation (BMF) ⊙ ⊙ ⊙

http://www.bonemarrow.org

This nonprofit organization provides education, financial assistance, and support to patients and their families. Financial support comes in the form of grants to cover search, procedure, and other indirect costs. The BMF Web site provides a password protected support line and an expert question/answer forum. Registration materials are available online. There are full descriptions of all services offered and there is information available about other organizations, offline references, a donor registry, and insurance problems.

Bone Marrow Transplant (BMT) Information ⊙ ⊙ ⊙

http://www.bmtinfo.org

This highly informative site provides information to patients, donors, and physicians. Information regarding the diseases that require BMT, and regarding transplant topics is provided. The Physician's Corner provides physicians and other medical specialists an opportunity to ask BMT specialists specific questions and also displays the most recent questions and answers. One can also download an application for a preliminary donor search.

Bone Marrow Transplantation
Branch of the Health Resources and Services Administration ⊙ ⊙ ⊙
http://www.hrsa.dhhs.gov/osp/dot/bone.htm

This branch oversees the National Marrow Donor Program (NMDP) and its site provides information for professionals. Information about the branch and its staff, health history guidelines, diseases treatable by BMT, and considerations when choosing a BMT provider are offered. There is also a list of NMDP links. A Newsletter Resource Directory contains a large number of links regarding transplant information, support, and fundraising/financial aid. It points to other sites with information on general cancer information and support, and sites covering specific diseases, including anemias, brain tumors, breast cancer, leukemia, lymphoma, multiple myeloma, myelodysplasia, and other disorders. Support for patients with insurance questions can also be found here.

CenterSpan ⊙ ⊙ ⊙
http://www.centerspan.org

A comprehensive professional resource for transplant information, the site features TNN, the Transplant News Network, for the latest news. One can view abstracts online and participate in e-mail discussions with colleagues. Information about registries, employment opportunities, publications, and fellowships is provided along with many links.

Columbia Presbyterian Medical Center:
The Nuts and Bolts of Bone Marrow Transplants ⊙ ⊙ ⊙
http://cait.columbia.edu:88/dept/medicine/bonemarrow/bmtinfo.html

Bone marrow transplant information is available at this site, including a description of bone marrow and diseases treated with bone marrow transplants. The site explains why transplants are performed, different types of transplants, preparation for the transplant, bone marrow harvesting, the transplant procedure, engraftment, recovery, handling emotional stress, and life after the transplant. Information is targeted to patient and caregiver audiences.

Emory School of Medicine
Department of Pediatrics Division of
Hematology/ Oncology and Bone Marrow Transplantation ⊙ ⊙
http://wwwph1.cc.emory.edu/PEDS/HEMONC

This Web site provides information about clinical programs, training programs, research activities, and faculty. Disease and treatment protocols are provided along with descriptions of bone marrow transplantation. There is a pediatric BMT priority list, and a list of pediatric BMT protocols.

European Group for Blood and Marrow Transplantation (EBMT) ◉ ◉
http://www.bmdw.org/EBMT

The EBMT Web site provides information about the group, ongoing trials, group members, and EBMT publications. A link for a publication search service is also provided.

Gift of Life Foundation ◉ ◉ ◉
http://www.giftoflife.com

A marrow donor recruitment organization and registry, this nonprofit organization maintains "a database of 32,000 donors not found elsewhere" and has a donor file published with Bone Marrow Donors Worldwide. An online search system is available to physicians, transplant center search coordinators, and registry search coordinators. The search area has restricted access and an online application is provided. Other information provided concerns special articles, links, and general patient and donor information.

National Bone Marrow Transplant Link ◉ ◉
http://comnet.org/nbmtlink

This site offers informational resources on bone marrow transplantation to better educate patients and their families. Topics covered are BMT definitions, stem cell transplants, bone marrow donation, and a stem cell transplant guide for breast cancer patients.

National Foundation for Transplants (NTF) ◉ ◉
http://www.otf.org

The organization provides financial support services for patients. An overview of the organization is provided along with grant, support, and assistance information.

National Transplant Assistance Fund ◉ ◉ ◉
http://www.transplantfund.org

The organization provides financial assistance to those in need of tissue and organ transplants. The site serves as a resource of information about the organization and its services. Transplant-related materials for professionals to provide to patients are offered along with an FAQ section, newsletter, and substantial patient information. Transplant centers, insurance topics, and contact addresses are listed.

Ohio University Health Sciences Center Columbia
Presbyterian Blood and Marrow Transplant Program ⊙ ⊙

http://w3.ouhsc.edu/hemaonco/bbmt.htm

The program site provides information about the organization's history, facilities, staff, support group, and referrals. Professional resources include a statistics section that offers many distributions and plots concerning autologous and allogenic transplants. The Referrals section discusses treatment protocols and clinical trials available.

Stem Cell Transplant: A Companion Guide
for Breast Cancer Patients ⊙ ⊙ ⊙

http://comnet.org/nbmtlink/breastcancerstemcellguide.html

This site aims to educate breast cancer patients and families about stem cell transplants, and includes a resource listing and glossary of terms, updates and new developments related to treatment, and a detailed description of all aspects of the transplant procedure. Suggestions on coping with emotional issues are also available for patients and families. Visitors can also order print copies of the Companion Guide and other publications from the site.

Stepping Stones ⊙ ⊙

http://www.stepstones.org

Stepping Stones is a New Hampshire-based support group for those who have undergone BMT that allows for sharing of information and a network of support. There is information about group meetings, a newsletter, and off-site services. Information about BMT and referrals is provided at the site along with complimentary therapy information and relevant links to BMT and cancer-related sites.

Transplant Pathology Internet Services (TPIS) ⊙ ⊙ ⊙

http://tpis.upmc.edu

This site serves as a tool for information exchange and as an educational resource for physicians and researchers. Many aspects of organ and tissue transplant are discussed at this site with an emphasis on pathology. Services offered are an electronic forum, synchronized slide shows with audio, a consult corner for posted cases, a self-test, and more.

TransWeb ⊙ ⊙ ⊙

http://www.transweb.org

A comprehensive Internet resource that provides both basic and in-depth information regarding transplants of all kinds, the site boasts having 10,000 items for donors, recipients, and professionals. The Reference Desk provides articles, audio, books, journals, links, maps, videos, newsletter, and more. Multimedia learning tools for patients and a major news section for professionals are available.

University of Colorado Health Sciences Center: Bone Marrow Medical Terms Glossary ◎ ◎
http://www.uchsc.edu/uh/marrow/www/overview/terms.htm

Definitions of medical terms related to bone marrow transplants and the medical conditions sometimes requiring this therapy are presented at this site. Forty-one definitions are available, and terminology is targeted to patients and nonprofessionals.

Donor Registries

American Bone Marrow Donor Registry (ABMDR) ◎ ◎
http://www.abmdr.org

The ABMDR Web site provides information about the registry for patients, donors, and families. There is an FAQ section, cost and risk information, and procedural descriptions. The society seeks to minimize costs, provide advocacy, coordinate requests, maintain confidentiality, and to maintain records.

Anthony Nolan Bone Marrow Trust ◎ ◎
http://www.anthonynolan.com

This U.K. service serves to match bone marrow donors with patients, worldwide. In addition, the organization operates a testing laboratory and research institute. Information for patients and donors is provided along with research laboratory information. The research institute seeks to develop and maintain an HLA sequence database and has research groups devoted to Immunotherapy, human leucocyte antigens (HLA), graft vs. host disease, HLA informantics, molecular immunobiology, and allorecognition.

Asian American Donor Program ◎
http://www.nonprofitadmin.com/aadp

This organization serves to make donors available for patients. Donor information, news, event schedules, and registration information are available.

Asians for Miracle Marrow Matches ◎ ◎
http://www.ltsc.org/a3m/a3m.html

A donor registry that serves the Asian and Pacific Islander communities, the organization registers donors for the National Marrow Donor Program (NMDP) and assists donor and transplant centers. The site offers basic information and support for patients, provides a monthly newsletter, and lists national registries, Asian registries, and donor centers.

Bone Marrow Donors Worldwide (BMDW) ◎ ◎ ◎

http://www.bmdw.org

BMDW is a comprehensive resource that seeks to collect human leucocyte antigens (HLA) phenotypes of donors and cord blood units and to coordinate distribution. A list of participating registries and nonparticipating registries is offered along with general information, links, staff, and address information and news. For professionals, information about the HLA system and events is provided. Restricted access exists for professionals to information about online match programs, search advice requests, lists of registry fees, updates, the BMDW Internet manual, and survey results. One can contact BMDW for access or download application materials directly from the site. For nonprofessionals, information about donations and BMDW procedures is offered.

International Bone Marrow and Cord Blood Donor Search ◎ ◎ ◎

http://www.crir.org

This site is a resource for patients and physicians to search for bone marrow or cord blood donors. Information about the organization's mission is provided along with donor bank listings, contact information, and physician's forms.

National Marrow Donor Program (NMDP) ◎ ◎ ◎

http://www.marrow.org

The mission of the program is to promote the transplant of hematopoetic stem cells and it does so via the NMDP registry, education, research, awareness, and through patient support. The site provides a tremendous amount of information concerning donation, therapy, financial issues, and news. There is a professional section of the site that provides announcements of conferences, grants, employment opportunities, and news.

Unrelated Bone Marrow Donor Registry ◎

http://srv02.anaserve.com/~lori

Supplied by the Canadian Red Cross, this site offers information about the registry and general donor information. Contact information is supplied concerning the data bank itself and search information.

World Marrow Donor Association (WMDA) ◎ ◎

http://www.bmdw.org/WMDA

WMDA is a professional organization whose mission is to promote information exchange and to develop standards for the exchange of hematopoietic stem cells, internationally. The WMDA Web site provides extensive membership information, house rules, numerous reports of the Association's guidelines, and online access to minutes from past meetings.

Graft versus Host Disease

Graft versus Host Disease ◉ ◉
http://ww2.med.jhu.edu/cancerctr/hematol/gvh.htm

From the Johns Hopkins Oncology Center, this page provides a description of GvHD, along with relevant services available at the center, therapy highlights, and a listing of clinical protocols that are available.

Graft versus Host Disease Web Site ◉ ◉
http://www-perso.infini.fr/gvhd/us/general_us/frameset1_us.html

Here, a medical file to physicians is available by filing an online form. Also, there is offline reference information and links to relevant sites and newsgroups. French users can link to a mirror site in their native language.

9.3 **Breast Cancer**

Advocacy

Men's Crusade Against Breast Cancer (MCABC) ◉ ◉ ◉
http://home.earthlink.net/~rkupbens/mcabc

A nonprofit organization that is affiliated with the Lombardi Cancer Center at Georgetown University Hospital in Washington, D.C., MCABC provides support for men and their families and promotes research. The MCABC site offers statistics, articles, a list of current activities, family guides, and information about how to join. In addition, a listing of other online and offline resources is supplied.

National Breast Cancer Coalition (NBCC) ◉
http://www.natlbcc.org

This advocacy organization is focused on influencing legislation to increase appropriations for research, to increase women's access to treatment, and to increase activist impact. Its site provides information about the society, its legislative activities, and news. Educational programs include congressional and state forums, media workshops, and clinical trials projects.

Education and Support

Breast Cancer Center ⚙ ⚙
http://www.patientcenters.com/breastcancer

This site is aimed at providing a resource for those with metastatic breast cancer—individuals who have been initially diagnosed with Stage IV cancer or who are facing a recurrence. The site provides excerpts from current books, journals, and other media, updated monthly, plus general reference material on metastatic breast cancer. The articles section, for example, has included articles ranging from what is metastatic cancer and standard treatments to how humor helps cancer patients cope. The general resources section contains both general information, plus specific sections on emotional support, research, dying and hospice care, coping with treatment, advocacy, and a very thorough glossary of terms used in the diagnosis and treatment of metastatic breast cancer.

Breast Cancer Glossary ⚙ ⚙
http://www.cancerhelp.com/ed/glossary.htm

There are hundreds of specialized terms associated with breast cancer, including treatment names, procedures, hormones and glands, chemical agents, side effects, and many more. This glossary begins with such terms as abscess, acini, adenocarcinoma, adjuvant treatment, alkylating agents, and alopecia, and continues through the alphabet. Patients and family members will find this to be a convenient reference as they come into contact with many new breast cancer terms. The glossary was developed by the site sponsor, EduCare, Inc.

Breast Cancer Information Service (BCIS) ⚙ ⚙
http://trfn.clpgh.org/bcis

The Breast Cancer Information Service (BCIS) is a joint project of the Pittsburgh Breast Care Test Coalition, an umbrella organization of healthcare providers, women's groups, and individuals. The site provides information about diagnosis, treatment, prevention, support, and insurance issues concerning breast cancer. It is particularly user-friendly for those new to the World Wide Web, offering a navigation page with information on getting around the site and an online tutorial that goes into more detail. Hot News and New Additions pages keep the material current. BCSI also hosts a chat room the first Monday of each month and lists a calendar of events. The site is hosted by Three Rivers Free-Net, a community-based network in Pittsburgh.

Breast Cancer Resource Center ⚙ ⚙ ⚙
http://members.aol.com/healwell/breast.htm

A comprehensive online resource for breast cancer information for professionals and patients, the site provides links to a variety of medical sites and sites devoted to breast cancer. Search engines are also provided for searching specialized medical directories, the Web, and bookstores for relevant information. Information directly from the site refers to diagnosis, self-examination, mammography and pregnancy, and general information. Message boards are available for patients to share information.

Breast Health—Your Decision   ◉ ◉ ◉

http://www.tricaresw.af.mil/breastcd/hospital/read_the_book/toc.htm

An online breast health book, the site displays a table of contents with 21 chapters. Topics include breast anatomy and changes of the breast; breast cancer statistics; risk factors; genetics; screening; diagnostics; palpable breast abnormalities; pathology of breast cancer; staging and patterns of spread; predictors of outcome; treatment overview; local/regional therapy of invasive breast cancers; and surgical and radiation treatments including chemotherapy; breast reconstruction; follow-up issues; nursing issues; and alternative medicine.

Canadian Breast Cancer Network (CBCN)   ◉ ◉ ◉

http://www.cbcn.ca

The CBCN provides a voice for patients, promotes education and awareness, and offers support information. An Information Center offers a newsletter, news releases, current issues papers, events listings, and an "ABCs" kit for patients that offers information about linking patients, a catalog of resources and reproducible handouts, and forms. A Support Groups section allows the user to perform a search of local groups by city. There is an extensive and well-organized links section for patients and professionals.

Dr. Mary Jo Nugent Breast Cancer Foundation   ◉ ◉

http://www.xensei.com/users/mjinfo

The Dr. Mary Jo Nugent Breast Cancer Foundation provides financial assistance to disadvantaged patients and funds awareness, education, and research. The Foundation's Web site includes a newsletter, a member directory, a statement on its funding policy, and links to other U.S. breast cancer-related Web sites.

Gillette Women's Cancer Connection   ◉ ◉

http://www.gillettecancerconnect.org

This site offers extensive psychological and other support information for women with breast cancer and their families and friends. Information about breast cancer is provided through a free brochure and book list of printed resources. The site also provides a searchable database of local support groups. Also found on the site is an online registration for "Connecting to Wellness" seminars, support group chats, and a message board.

How Breast Cancer is Diagnosed ◎ ◎

http://mammary.nih.gov/reviews/tumorigenesis/Fischer001/index.html

This thorough site provides a detailed text description of methods of breast cancer diagnosis along with many images. Literature cited, a glossary of terms, and a self-test are provided as well.

National Alliance of
Breast Cancer Organizations (NABCO) ◎

http://www.nabco.org

The National Alliance of Breast Cancer Organizations (NABCO) is a network of breast cancer organizations that provides information, assistance, and referral to anyone with questions about breast cancer. NABCO also acts as a voice for the interests and concerns of breast cancer survivors and women at risk. Resources found at its Web site include fact sheets about breast cancer in the U.S., how to get a low-cost mammogram, getting the best mammogram, abnormal mammograms, plus information on joining a clinical trial, clinical trial basics, and a directory of breast cancer trials. In addition, there is a very useful search tool that will locate a nearby support group by state.

National Lymphedema Network (NLN) ◎ ◎ ◎

http://www.lymphnet.org

The NLN site provides education and information to patients and healthcare professionals. Included in this site are descriptions of lymphedema, which include lists of many of the primary and secondary causes of lymphedema. Also provided is information regarding support groups, resources, guidelines, conferences, and the NLN newsletter. The site details the newsletter and publication and videotape educational materials offered. A question/answer database chronicles questions and answers from 1996 on.

Y-Me National Breast Cancer Organization ◎ ◎ ◎

http://www.y-me.org

The Y-Me National Breast Cancer Organization was founded in 1978 by two breast cancer patients to provide information and support to patients, their families, and friends. Its site provides information in both English and Spanish about the organization, its chapters, general facts for patients, FAQs (frequently asked questions), access to the organization's newsletter, and information about offline resources such as a current calendar of its monthly open door education and support groups held throughout the country, early detection workshops, peer support programs, wig and prothesis bank, and teen program. There is a section devoted to males with the disorder. The site also lists the 800 numbers for their 24-hour toll-free hotlines and links to other resources.

Male Breast Cancer

Breast Cancer in Men ⚙ ⚙ ⚙
http://interact.withus.com/interact/mbc

This site specializes in providing information about breast cancer in males. Physician information comes in the form of a large list of medical references that point the user toward reviews, other Web sites, research information, and to recent news. General information is provided to patients such as incidence, risk factors, and treatment. Support resources and a Frequently Asked Question (FAQ) section are also provided.

Male Breast Cancer ⚙ ⚙
http://www.surgery.uiowa.edu/surgery/oncology/malebreastcancer.html

This information page related to male breast cancer includes discussions of causes, genetics, symptoms, staging, hormonal influences, reconstruction surgery, and relation to gynecomastia. A text description is provided with lists of offline references for more detailed information.

Prevention and Treatment

Breast Cancer Answers ⚙ ⚙ (some features fee-based)
http://www.medsch.wisc.edu/bca

This site is provided by the University of Wisconsin Comprehensive Cancer Center (UWCCC). It provides information about clinical trials, research results, breast cancer treatment provided by the UWCCC, and frequently asked questions. For patients, there is a section detailing general questions they should ask their doctor. There is also a restricted section for UWCCC patients and families that allows for specific questions to be asked.

Breast Cancer Resources ⚙ ⚙
http://www.bcresources.org

This site has sections for patients, medical professionals, and support. Also offered are news, alternative treatment, and second opinion resources for professionals, which come in the form of articles, clinical trials listings, government resources, and test resources. For patients, there is breast education, diagnosis, treatment, and post treatment information. The support section provides information concerning support groups, advice, and chronic illness.

Breast Cancer Society of Canada ⊙ ⊙

http://www.bcsc.ca

This society funds breast cancer research and provides information concerning detection, prevention, and treatment of breast cancer. Included are questions patients should ask their doctor, details about the society, information about research the society funds, FAQs, recent news, contact, and location information.

Breast Cancer Updates ⊙ ⊙ ⊙

http://www.pgh.auhs.edu/bfisher

This is a private site from a professor in the Department of Surgery at the University of Pittsburgh. It offers continually updated, clinically relevant links to breast cancer news and reviews concerning prevention, chemotherapy, surgical approaches, clinical trial news, and recent medication information.

Breast Clinic ⊙ ⊙ ⊙

http://www.thebreastclinic.com

This comprehensive site supplies detailed information concerning symptoms, investigations, screening, risk factors, benign disease, surgery, adjuvant therapy, and staging. Explanations are thorough and text descriptions are linked to definitions and information pages. Links to related sites, an FAQ section, and contact information are also supplied.

BreastCancer.net ⊙ ⊙

http://www.breastcancer.net

This news site supplies very current information on breast cancer topics in recent and archived news articles. Late-breaking stories on breast cancer are posted on the home page. Activate the link "Newsroom" and you can reach 1,500 more articles. Support and treatment are other useful links on the site, plus there is a link to other important Internet sites relating to breast cancer.

BreastCancerinfo.com ⊙ ⊙

http://www.breastcancerinfo.com

Breast Cancer Info is a service of the Susan G. Komen Breast Cancer Foundation. The Foundation's mission is to eradicate breast cancer as a life threatening disease by advancing research, education, screening, and treatment. The site gives information on breast health with in-depth links to living with breast cancer, treatment options, facts and figures, taking charge of your health, news and events, and Komen affiliates by area. There is also a link to "Race for the Cure," the Foundation's annual fundraiser held in 98 cities throughout the U.S.

BreastDoctor.com: Information on Breast Cancer and Breast Cancer Treatment ◎ ◎

http://www.breastdoctor.com

Visitors to this site can access a physician directory, recommend a doctor, participate in online chat forums, and search the site for specific information. Physicians can add their name to the directory. The site offers detailed discussions of breast anatomy, benign breast disease, and an overview of breast cancer. Breast cancer information includes discussions of different forms of the disease, staging and treatments, sentinel lymph node surgery and lymphatic mapping, surgery, new biopsy techniques, chemotherapy, reconstructive surgery, risk factors, mammograms and other X-ray tests, breast self-examination and clinical exams, and breast disease in men.

Cancer Research Foundation of America (CRFA) ◎ ◎

http://www.preventcancer.org

The Cancer Research Foundation of America seeks to prevent cancer through funding research and providing educational materials on early detection and nutrition. The women's health section on its site menu starts with a questionnaire about your healthcare. The site offers general information on the foundation's other programs, including Buddy Check, a comprehensive breast health program, the George Washington University Mammovan (bringing mammography into the community, and its breast health education program for Spanish-speaking women).

Inflammatory Breast Cancer (IBC) ◎

http://www.bestiary.com/ibc

A page specifically for patients with IBC, this site offers a description of the disease including its symptoms, journal articles and abstracts, and information on nonmedical treatment and for caregivers. The site also includes encouraging stories of IBC survivors, treatment, questions to ask your doctor, and other patient issues. One can subscribe to the IBC mailing list which entitles members to search its archives.

INFO Breast Cancer ◎ ◎

http://www.intranet.ca/~stancar

This site created by a breast cancer survivor offers many useful resources to patients and others searching for breast cancer resources on the Internet. Detailed information is available on diagnostics, treatments, breast self-examination, lymphedema, menopause, osteoporosis, and nutrition. Suggested publications are listed as well as links to other breast cancer sites, breast cancer news sites, health information sites, pharmaceutical information sites, and media sites for general news items.

OncoLink: Breast Cancer General Information ◎ ◎ ◎

http://www.oncolink.upenn.edu/disease/breast

OncoLink was developed by University of Pennsylvania cancer specialists interested in helping patients, families, health professionals, and the general public find cancer-related information at no charge. This informative section of the larger OncoLink site offers comprehensive information about breast cancer, including an overview and discussions of screening, risk factors and prevention, treatment options, genetics, support, hormones, and other topics. Visitors can also find answers to Frequently Asked Questions and news stories related to breast cancer. General cancer resources include psychosocial support information, news, clinical trials resources, links to global sources for information, conference and meeting announcements, information on financial issues, and book reviews.

Pathologia Paldlon ◎ ◎ ◎

http://www.erinet.com/fnadoc/index.htm

This user-friendly site developed by Pat Connelly, a private physician, provides detailed information on breast cancer prevention, causes, and treatment. The site is organized as a detailed information page with hyperlinked text to term definitions, resources, and to related sites about breast and lung cancer. The site visuals include: photographs of tumors, before and after photographs of breast reconstruction surgery, mammograms, and images of surgical procedures and instruments used. Nearly 100 pages of technical information is available for the site visitor, but it is clearly presented and easily understood by the lay person. A family profile written by Dr. Connelly adds an especially human note to the page.

Plastic Surgery Information Service: Breast Reconstruction Following Breast Removal ◎ ◎

http://www.plasticsurgery.org/surgery/brstrec.htm

This is a page from the Web site provided by The American Society of Plastic and Reconstructive Surgeons and Plastic Surgery Educational Foundation. Included is information for patients and professionals about types of surgery offered, planning the surgery, mastectomy, follow-up, and more. There are before and after diagrams and one can also search the site and locate a surgeon.

Professional/Clinical Resources

Breast Cancer: Molecular Aspects ◎ ◎

http://www.geocities.com/HotSprings/Spa/3430/intro1.htm

This creative site is informative, and welcomes the user to each new page with a musical piece. It is dedicated to providing information concerning breast cancer metastasis. It provides information about bone formation and about molecular actors involved in breast cancer dissemination. In addition, the site provides access to selected papers from 1999 to the present that cover estrogen receptors and breast cancer, breast cancer and gene therapy, and breast cancer metastasis.

Breast Cancer Online ◎ ◎ ◎ (free registration)
http://www.bco.org

This is an educational resource solely for professionals that provides news, symposia information, access to medical databases, articles, reviews, and case studies. In addition, access to multiple choice tests is provided. The site is geared toward professionals and requires a one-time free registration.

Breast Net ◎ ◎
http://www.bci.org.au

Provided by New South Wales Breast Cancer Institute, Australia, Breast Net provides information to the general public, patients, and physicians. An informative set of links is provided to individual case studies where the entire histories of cases are followed and, in some cases, diagnostic pictures are supplied. Access to data, research publications, and to current research projects is also given. Available to patients are general information resources and descriptions of research and clinical care available at the Institute.

Doctor's Guide to Breast Cancer Information ◎ ◎ ◎
http://www.pslgroup.com/BREASTCANCER.HTM

This detailed Web site is a guide to physicians, patients and family members to hundreds of links of up-to-date medical news and information concerning breast cancer and other breast-related disorders. The links are presented in an organized fashion under topics such as current content, medical news and alerts, general information, discussion groups, and related sites.

Online Management of Breast Diseases ◎ ◎ ◎
http://www.breastdiseases.com

A reference site that offers a huge amount of information for healthcare providers, the site is divided into patient and physician sections. The physicians section offers detailed explanations of patient evaluation, the high-risk patient, examinations, anatomy, surgical office management, imaging modalities, diagnostic techniques, pathology, surgical assessment, surgical control, reconstruction options, radiotherapy, and more. Information provided covers psychological support of the patient and hereditary breast cancer and genetic counseling. Explanations are in the form of text with images and figures provided when necessary. The patient section provides information about the disorder along with detailed explanations of treatments available, questions to ask their doctors, and follow-up care.

WebPath: Breast Pathology ○ ○ ○

http://www-medlib.med.utah.edu/WebPath/ORGAN.html#1

WebPath is an Internet Pathology Laboratory for Medical Education. This page comprises the Breast Pathology index and includes 47 continually updated images of the male and female breast. In addition, there is a text tutorial that offers a myriad of details concerning breast cancer, links to images, and definitions.

Research and Funding

Susan G. Komen Breast Cancer Foundation ○ ○

http://www.komen.org

Most people know the Susan G. Komen Breast Cancer Foundation through its "Race for the Cure," the largest series of 5K races throughout the U.S. On average, over 700,000 participants race to raise funds for both national research efforts and local breast cancer initiatives. The Foundation is the largest private funder of research dedicated solely to breast cancer in the nation and its mission is to eradicate breast cancer as a life-threatening disease by advancing research, education, screening, and treatment. The Foundation's Web site is a comprehensive resource for patients that provides educational information, news, and treatment information. The site also lists the Foundation's Helpline, an 800 number for information about breast cancer concerns, information, and support.

Surgical Procedures

Imaginis.net: Lumpectomy ○ ○ ○

http://www.imaginis.net/breasthealth/lumpectomy.html

Provided by Imaginis.net, this site provides an overview of the lumpectomy procedure. There are also discussions of the following topics: determining candidacy for lumpectomy, the lumpectomy procedure, radiation therapy after lumpectomy, and auxillary node dissection. There are also links to additional resources and references.

Imaginis.net: Mastectomy ○ ○ ○

http://www.imaginis.net/breasthealth/mastectomy.html

Provided by Imaginis.net, this site provides patient information about mastectomy. Topics discussed include what is mastectomy, auxillary node dissection, sentinel lymph node biopsy, choosing mastectomy as breast cancer treatment, mastectomy and breast reconstruction, before surgery, the mastectomy procedure, after surgery, and the recurrence of breast cancer. The site also provides links to additional references and resources.

Tutorials

Benign Breast Disease and Breast Cancer Tutorial ⊙ ⊙ ⊙
http://www.surgery.wisc.edu/wolberg

This online tutorial is aimed towards teaching third-year medical students, although links and information are provided for medical practitioners. This thorough tutorial is provided by William H. Wolberg, M.D. and provides written description, figures, tables, terminology definitions, histology photographs, and links to references. Subcategories include self-help, case management, adjunctive chemotherapy, diagnosis and prognosis, genetic considerations, breast anatomy, physiology, examination, and postmenopausal hormonal replacement.

Biology of the Mammary Gland ⊙ ⊙ ⊙ (some features fee-based)
http://mammary.nih.gov/Atlas

Sponsored by the National Institutes of Health, this page provides a tremendous number of detailed educational resources to professionals. The site is organized into six educational categories: Experimental Models, Reviews, a Histology Atlas, Tools and Technologies, and the Mammary Genome Program. Reviews are offered on development, function, tumorgenesis, and gene expression. Experimental models to study mammary gland development, physiology, and tumorgenesis are offered, and these cover natural mutants, transgenic, and gene deletion models to study development, physiology, and cancer. The Histology Atlas is interactive and provides video lectures and images. Written information and video and slide clips are offered as tools to study animal, histological, and molecular techniques. The Mammary Genome Program link offers cDNA libraries and microarrays, reference genes, and cancer models, but has restricted access.

Breast Diseases ⊙ ⊙
http://mystic.biomed.mcgill.ca/MedinfHome/
MedInf/Breastcourse/htmltext/home/BreastHome.html

Provided by the McGill University faculty department, this site offers a teaching aid geared toward third-year medical students. There are thorough explanations of anatomy, physiology, pathology, radiology, management, risk assessment, tumor/nodes/metastases (TNM) classification, surgery, and more in this online teaching tool. A case presentation is also provided.

9.4 **Carcinoid Cancer**

General Resources

Cancer BACUP: Carcinoid Tumors ◉ ◉
http://www.cancerbacup.org.uk/info/carcinoid.htm

This fact sheet describes all carcinoid tumors, including discussions of typical locations, causes, signs and symptoms, carcinoid syndrome, and details of diagnostic tests and therapies. Visitors can also find links to information on many other types of cancers.

Carcinoid Cancer Foundation ◉ ◉ ◉
http://www.carcinoid.org

The nonprofit organization was chartered by the state of New York and promotes research and education. The site offers information about research, the disorder, treatments, references, and support. There are reviews, links, articles, and contact listings.

Carcinoid Cancer Internet Mailing List ◉
http://www.acor.org/listserv.html?to_do=interact&listname=CARCINOID

Instructions for joining this mailing list are provided at the site. Postings to the e-mail list are archived and searchable at the site. All postings are related specifically to carcinoid cancer.

National Carcinoid Support Group (NCSG), Inc. ◉ ◉ ◉
http://members.aol.com/thencsg

The NSCG is a peer support group that provides detailed information about disorders, causes, liver embolization, treatments, news sources, current research, and contacts. The site also sponsors a carcinoid newsletter, lists cases/testimonials and has information about carcinoid conferences.

Virtual Hospital: Lung Tumors ◉ ◉ ◉
http://australia.vh.org/Providers/Textbooks/LungTumors/TitlePage.html

Carcinoid tumors of the lung are described at this site, including a general discussion of tumor type and prognosis, gross appearance, and microscopic features. Information is technical and meant for health professionals or students. A bibliography of information sources is available.

9.5 **Cutaneous (Skin) Cancer**

General Resources

American Academy of Dermatology (AAD) ◎ ◎ ◎
http://www.aad.org

The AAD site includes patient information, a referral service, and a link to the society's official journal. There is a link to a special physician and patient education section that provides information that concerns melanoma. A professional section details, news, AAD information, a virtual exhibit hall, meetings information, residents news, a marketplace, and more.

American Society for Dermatologic Surgery (ASDS) ◎ ◎
http://www.asds-net.org

The ASDS provides information regarding all skin disorders including cancer. It includes information about ASDS, patient education materials, news, and continuing education.

An Introduction to Skin Cancer ◎ ◎
http://www.maui.net/~southsky/introto.html

This page provides general information about skin cancer. There are links to news sources and public-oriented science articles. The Resources Section provides a number of links to fact sheets, medical reviews, and studies for more detailed and scientific resources concerning skin cancer.

Cancer BACUP: Understanding Skin Cancer ◎ ◎ ◎
http://www.bacup.org.uk/info/skin.htm

This site offers a discussion of cancer, the morphology of the skin, causes of skin cancer, and diagnosis of basal cell and squamous cell carcinomas. Treatments described include surgery, radiotherapy, and chemotherapy. Visitors can also access information on common follow-up care, current research and clinical trials, emotions and cancer diagnosis, recommended reading, and find links to useful organizations.

Centers for Disease Control and Prevention (CDC): Skin Cancer Prevention and Early Detection ◎ ◎ ◎
http://www.cdc.gov/cancer/nscpep/skin95.htm

The Centers for Disease Control and Prevention presents this site in an effort to raise public awareness of skin cancer. Statistics and symptoms associated with squamous cell skin cancer, basal cell skin cancer, and malignant melanomas are offered at the site, as well as discussions of risk groups, prevention, CDC program activities related to prevention, state and federal partnerships, and professional education activities. The site also describes activities of the Anti-Cancer Council of Victoria in Australia, a leader in efforts aimed at prevention and early detection.

DermaGraphix ⚙ ⚙ ⚙

http://www.dermagraphix.com

DermaGraphix provides information about a network of comprehensive Mole Mapping Systems for the ultimate goal of early skin cancer detection. There are also details of medical research and treatment options. The site functions as a forum for professional information exchange, offers links, provides body maps, and offers information about self-examination for patients.

Dermatologic Image Database ⚙ ⚙ ⚙

http://tray.dermatology.uiowa.edu/DermImag.htm

Designed for physicians, this site offers a tremendous number of images relating to all aspects of dermatology. Included are numerous pictures of different types of melanoma. The images are organized alphabetically and thus, are very easy to find and open.

Increased Exposure to UV-B Radiation Due to Stratospheric Ozone Depletion ⚙ ⚙ ⚙

http://www.ciesin.org/TG/HH/ozhlthhm.html

This is a continually updated page from the Web site from the Center for International Earth Science Information Network at Columbia University. The page provides overview information and offers links to a more detailed description of the topic as well as to dozens of in-depth essays covering the key health effects of Ultraviolet-B radiation exposure.

Skin Cancer Zone ⚙ ⚙ ⚙ (fee-based)

http://www.melanoma.com

Skin Cancer Zone is provided by the Schering Plough Corporation and is divided into sections for consumers and for healthcare professionals. The healthcare professional's section provides access to all of the professional education material on the Schering Web sites. Included in this section are pharmaceutical details, patient education aids, case studies, and more. Entry to this section requires a password or requires that physicians enter their DEA number. The consumer's section provides skin safety and treatment information, skin cancer facts, activities, and access to educational resources.

Sun Damage and Prevention ◉ ◉

http://telemedicine.org/sundam2.4.1.html

For patients and professionals, this site chronicles the subacute chronic and immunologic effects of UV radiation, carcinogenesis, melanoma formation, the melanoma action spectrum in animals and human beings, and UV and nonmelanoma skin cancer. For patients, information regarding sun protection strategies is provided.

Basal Cell and Squamous Cell Carcinoma

Basal Cell and Squamous Cell Cancer ◉ ◉

http://www.jas.tj/skincancer/bc_sc.html

Causes, signs and symptoms, increased risk groups, and any health problems associated with basal cell and squamous cell cancers are discussed at this site. The site also describes estimated risks of the cancer spreading beyond the site of growth and symptoms after surgical removal requiring medical attention.

Basal Cell Carcinoma ◉

http://www.k-Web.co.uk/charity/wct/wctno28.html

This is an information page with many images. Treatment, prevention, and warning signs are discussed.

HealthGate.com: Basal-Cell Skin Cancer ◉ ◉

http://www.bewell.com/sym/sym431.asp

Information about basal-cell skin cancer is presented here, including a definition, body parts involved, sex or age most affected, signs and symptoms, causes, increased risk factors, prevention, diagnostic measures, appropriate healthcare, possible complications, and probable outcome. Suggested home treatments after surgical removal of a growth are also available.

HealthGate.com: Squamous-Cell Skin Cancer ◉ ◉

http://www.bewell.com/sym/sym432.asp

The site presents patient information about squamous-cell skin cancer, including a definition, body parts involved, sex or age most affected, signs and symptoms, causes, increased risk factors, prevention, diagnostic measures, appropriate healthcare, possible complications, and probable outcome. Suggested home treatments after surgical removal of a growth are also available.

Cutaneous T-Cell Lymphoma

Cutaneous T-Cell Lymphoma—Mycosis Fungoides ◎ ◎
http://www.acor.org

A mailing list information and support resource for patients with CTCL-MF. Membership, contact information and instructions are provided.

Lymphoma Information Network: Cutaneous T-Cell Lymphoma, Mycosis Fungoides, and Sezary Syndrome ◎ ◎ ◎
http://www.lymphomainfo.net/nhl/types/ctcl-mf.html

This site defines cutaneous T-cell lymphoma, mycosis fungoides, and Sezary syndrome, offering information on diagnosis, staging, and treatment of this rare lymphoma. Visitors to the site can also access links to useful Web resources related to the disease, including mailing lists, general information sites, visual aids, organizations, and other sites of interest.

National Cancer Institute (NCI): Cutaneous T-cell Lymphoma ◎ ◎ ◎
http://rarediseases.info.nih.gov/clinpdq/soa/Cutaneous_T-cell_lymphoma_Physician.html

Cutaneous T-cell Lymphoma, mycosis fungoides, and the Sezary syndrome, and rare neoplasias of malignant T-lymphocytes are discussed at this site. Resources are technical in nature, and include general information, cellular classification, staging information, a treatment option overview, detailed descriptions of each stage of the disease, and information on treatment of recurrent cases of cutaneous T-cell lymphoma.

Melanoma

Melanoma and Related Cancers of the Skin—MARCS LINE ◎ ◎
http://www.k-Web.co.uk/charity/wct/marcsline/marcshome.html

This site provides information about melanoma, basal cell carcinoma, squamous cell carcinoma, and other skin cancers. Information about causes, treatment, and prevention is provided along with pictures.

Melanoma and Skin Cancer Research Institute ◎ ◎
http://www.med.usyd.edu.au/medicine/melanoma

This institute is at the University of Sydney and offers information about melanoma types, prevention, treatment, Institute research, products, and events. There are links to The Melanoma Foundation and to The Sydney Melanoma Unit.

Melanoma Diagnosis ◎ ◎ ◎

http://matrix.ucdavis.edu/tumors/new/tutorial-intro.html

This is a page from the Matrix Dermatology Resources site supplied by the University of California Davis. The page begins an entire section of the site that is dedicated to teaching the user the differential diagnosis of pigmented skin lesions. There are 37 text files and 243 images. The educational materials are arranged in a presentation format.

Melanoma FAQ ◎ ◎

http://westbyserver.westby.mwt.net/~ctustis/melfaq.html

This site is a comprehensive educational and informational source of melanoma information. The site provides text answers to common questions and descriptions about melanoma. In addition, there are listings of other Internet information sources, cancer support mailing lists, and listings of offline information sources.

Melanoma.net ◎ ◎

http://www.melanoma.net

This informative site of more than 100 pages offers educational information to patients and physicians. Information covers all aspects of melanoma from basic information and diagnosis to surgery. There is also a physician referral service that enables the user to search for a local practitioner of surgery, oncology, or dermatology. Information about joining the physician's referral service is supplied.

Melanoma Patient's Information Page (MPIP) ◎ ◎ ◎

http://www.mpip.org

A well-organized site, MPIP provides online patient education guides, recommended readings, news, clinical trials information, articles, a physician referral service, and therapy and support information. In addition, there are staging and prognostic calculators. The comprehensive abstract, article, and clinical trial details may be of use to professionals as well.

Melanoma Research Foundation ◎ ◎

http://www.melanoma.org

This site is provided by a California-based foundation providing grants directly to melanoma researchers. Information about current research projects, foundation sponsored research awards, the Foundation's newsletter, and contacts is provided. In addition, there is a link to a patient-oriented information page.

Melanoma Research Project ◎ ◎ ◎

http://www.melresproj.com

This comprehensive site is oriented towards professionals and provides a tremendous amount of information about malignant melanoma and cutaneous cancers. Diagnosis, treatment options, follow-up, and research data information are provided. An Early Diagnosis Guide takes the user through the ABC&D steps to melanoma diagnosis, while the Clinic gives the user access to clinical melanoma presentations that provide images with text descriptions. A Workshop area allows the user to view symposia information on past, present, and future events. The site's text is available in both German and English.

Multidisciplinary Melanoma Program Home Page ⊙ ⊙ ⊙

http://p53.cancer.med.umich.edu/melanoma/melanoma.html

Provided by the University of Michigan, the site offers comprehensive information about the disorder. This information resource has articles, clinical trials information, staging information, educational resources, listings of physicians and scientists, and support group services that deal with melanoma. The educational resources offered are sunscreen information, common resources, a reading list, and links.

StopMelanoma.com ⊙ ⊙ ⊙

http://www.stopmelanoma.com

Dedicated to providing educational information about melanoma for patients, their families, and professionals, the site contains basic and support group information. Also, there are a large number of links that lead the user to other sites, information pages, and to select articles and reviews. The links are categorized under specific topics.

W.H.O. Melanoma Program ⊙ ⊙

http://www.who-melanoma.org

The official Web site of the World Health Organization's Melanoma Program, this group is a worldwide cooperative that spans 22 countries and is concerned with clinical research and pathology of melanoma. Provided is a list of participating institutions, trial information, minutes of past meetings, the group's newsletter, and a listing of upcoming events. There is also a link to the Web site of the World Health Organization.

William S. Graham Foundation for Melanoma Research, Inc. ⊙ ⊙

http://www.bfmelanoma.com

The Graham Foundation is a nonprofit organization that raises and provides funds for scientific research to ultimately find a cure for Malignant Melanoma. It also provides education in the areas of prevention and detection. The Foundation's Web site provides facts about the disorder and information concerning recipients of grants, fellowships, and of research equipment. Members of the Foundation's medical advisory committee determine grant eligibility, and contact information is provided.

9.6 Endocrine Neoplasms

General Resources

A Clinical Evaluation of
the Thyroid in Health and Disease ⊙ ⊙ ⊙
http://www.meddean.luc.edu/lumen/MedEd/medicine/endo/thyroid.htm

This site provides descriptions of the thyroid gland and of many aspects of thyroid gland disease. The main menu lists various conditions including thyroid malignancies. This link takes the user to a page of links to more than 20 documents that are rated as being for use by the student, resident, or attending. Contact information is also provided.

American Association of
Clinical Endocrinologists (AACE) ⊙ ⊙
http://www.aace.com

The AACE site offers organization, publication, clinical, education, research, events, and membership information. Clinical information is about all endocrine disorders including cancer. There are listings of regional meetings and clinical abstracts, calendars, and directories. A restricted access members area provides information about CPT coding, and legislative and socioeconomic issues, and a professional chat room.

EndocrineWeb.com ⊙ ⊙ ⊙
http://www.endocrineweb.com

The EndocrineWeb.com site provides information about all endocrine disorders and surgery. It also provides introductory, disorder, imaging, prognosis, chemotherapy, testing, and more information about pancreas, thyroid, adrenal, and parathyroid cancers.

M. D. Anderson Cancer Center: Section
for Neoplasia and Hormonal Other Disorders ⊙ ⊙ ⊙
http://endrcr06.mda.uth.tmc.edu

Details regarding the program, faculty, and contacts are supplied at this site. Educational materials provided concern a variety of endocrine cancers and related issues, problems in the management of endocrine neoplasia, and genetic testing for endocrine tumors. There are also links and a patient discussion forum.

Society for Endocrinology   ◎ ◎ ◎

http://www.endocrinology.org

Information for all aspects of endocrinology including cancer is available here. There are details of the Society, membership, its journals, conferences, events, grants, books, education, topical briefings, and training courses. In addition, *Endocrine-Related Cancer,* one of the Society's journals, details subscription criteria and includes some online articles.

Support Site for Endocrine Problems   ◎ ◎

http://members.aol.com/ThreePeb/title.html

This site for patients and family members offers disorder and support information for all types of endocrine tumors. Articles and details concerning other endocrine disorders are included.

Adrenal Cancer

Adrenal Neoplasms Patient/Family Resources   ◎ ◎

http://www.slis.ua.edu/cdlp/WebCoreAll/patientinfo/oncology/endocrine/adrenal.html

Links at this address provide visitors with access to patient information, documents, and fact sheets from the National Cancer Institute, OncoLink, and other sources.

OncoLink: Adrenocortical Carcinoma   ◎ ◎

http://www.oncolink.com/cancernet/99/apr/704120.html

This address contains four recent article citations with abstracts found through the CancerLit system specific to adrenocortical carcinoma. Users can also access other sections of the OncoLink site through this Web page.

OncoLink: PDQ Patient Statement—Adrenocortical Carcinoma   ◎ ◎ ◎

http://www.oncolink.com/pdq_html/2/engl/201198.html

Comprehensive information for patients on adrenal cancer is available at this address. The disease and normal morphology of the adrenal cortex are explained, and information is available on each stage, on treatments for the disease, and on treatments specific to each disease stage. Medical terms are linked to a glossary for clarification. Contact details are available for additional resources, and users can access additional OncoLink cancer information at the site.

UrologyChannel: Adrenal Cancer   ◎ ◎

http://www.urologychannel.com/adrenalcancer/index.shtml

Adrenal cancer is described at this site for patients and the general public, with a discussion of adrenal gland morphology, different malignancies of the adrenal gland (functional and nonfunctional), disease rates, typical staging definitions (no universal staging system has been developed), prognosis, and general treatment regimens.

Islet Cell Cancer

Johns Hopkins Medical Institutions: Pancreas
Cancer Web—Islet Cell/Endocrine Tumors of the Pancreas ⊚ ⊚ ⊚
http://128.220.85.41/MCGI/SEND^WEBUTLTY(704)/414384247

This site contains an excerpt of a book chapter, written by Dr. Charles Yeo of Johns Hopkins, describing neoplasms of the endocrine pancreas. Information is presented as useful to both physicians and patients. The chapter includes an introduction to the disease, and specific topics cover localization and staging, surgical exploration, insulinoma, gastrinoma, Vernor-Morrison syndrome, glucagonoma, somatostatinoma, and nonfunctional islet tumors. Reference citations are also available at the site.

National Cancer Institute (NCI): PDQ, Islet Cell Carcinoma ⊚ ⊚ ⊚
http://cancernet.nci.nih.gov/clinpdq/soa/Islet_cell_carcinoma_Physician.html

Physician resources on islet cell cancer from the National Cancer Institute are available at this site. A general discussion of the disease is followed by information on cellular classification, staging, and treatment options. The site also offers a treatment overview specific to each disease stage. Information is supported with academic article citations.

OncoLink: PDQ Patient Statement—Islet Cell Carcinoma ⊚ ⊚ ⊚
http://oncolink.upenn.edu/pdq_html/2/engl/200790.html

Islet call cancer and the normal function of islet cells are described for patients at this site. Stages of the disease and treatments are explained, and different treatments for each stage of the disease are listed. Users can also access additional OncoLink cancer resources through this site.

Parathyroid Cancer

MedNews/National Cancer Institute (NCI):
Parathyroid Cancer ⊚ ⊚ ⊚
http://www.meb.uni-bonn.de/cancernet/100541.html

Technical resources on parathyroid cancer for health professionals are available at this site. General information about the disease includes a discussion of statistics and risk groups, diagnosis, signs, and symptoms. Cellular classifications, staging definitions (localized and metastatic), an overview of treatment options, and treatment discussions specific to localized, metastatic, and recurrent parathyroid cancer are also presented at the site. All information is supported with references.

OncoLink: Parathyroid Cancer ◎ ◎

http://www.oncolink.com/cancernet/99/may/705140.html

Visitors to this address will find nine journal article citations and abstracts found through CancerLit, presenting recent research findings related to parathyroid cancer. Information is technical and meant for investigators and health professionals.

Pheochromocytoma

Diagnosis of Pheochromocytoma ◎ ◎ ◎

http://www.his.com/~graeme/pheo.html

This site offers a detailed and technical discussion with figures and images of plasma metanephrines in the diagnosis of pheochromocytoma. There are references, background details and links to other information pages.

MedNews/National Cancer Institute (NCI): Pheochromocytoma ◎ ◎ ◎

http://www.meb.uni-bonn.de/cancernet/102494.html

Professional resources on pheochromocytoma, a rare tumor of the chromaffin cells, are available at this site. Topics include familial pheochromocytoma and general information about the disease, statistics, associated diseases, diagnosis protocols, cellular classification, and disease classifications (no staging system is used). An overview of treatment options includes typical treatment regimens of localized benign pheochromocytoma, regional pheochromocytoma, metastatic pheochromocytoma, and recurrent pheochromocytoma. All information is supported with reference bibliographies.

OncoLink: Pheochromocytoma ◎ ◎

http://www.oncolink.upenn.edu/cancernet/99/june/706145.html

OncoLink lists titles and abstracts of recent articles at CancerLit related to pheochromocytoma. Publications listed are highly technical, and topics within this disease heading include case studies, laboratory diagnostics, observed complications arising from the disease, and treatment advances.

Pheonet ◎ ◎

http://www.dfc.unifi.it/pheo/pheonet.htm

An Italian Study Group on Pheochromocytoma provides information at their site regarding group objectives, previous studies, group members and entry, contacts and clinical discussion or consult.

Pituitary

National Institute of Neurological Disorders and Stroke (NINDS): Pituitary Tumors ◎ ◎ ◎
http://www.ninds.nih.gov/patients/Disorder/pituitar/pituitar.htm

This site describes abnormal growths in the pituitary gland and possible health problems associated with these growths. Resources are meant for patients and the general public, and include explanations of different tumor types, problems caused by functioning tumors, general health problems caused by all pituitary tumors, common treatments for these tumors, and general prognosis. Visitors can also access a related research article on the treatment of these tumors and contact details for organizations offering additional resources.

Pituitary Tumor Network Association ◎ ◎
http://www.pituitary.com

This nonprofit organization supports, encourages, and funds research. Information about many pituitary disorders is provided along with patient resources. There are links to the Association's magazine that provide information about medical advances and other in-depth articles. The physician's section provides information dealing with publication opportunities, an Internet referral program, and resource guide listings.

Thyroid Cancer

About.com: Thyroid Disease: Thyroid Cancer ◎ ◎
http://thyroid.miningco.com/health/thyroid/health/diseases/thyroid/msub2.htm

This site contains links to support organizations, conference information, general thyroid cancer information, and several sites offering information specific to medullary thyroid cancer, papillary thyroid cancer, follicular thyroid cancer, and anaplastic cancer. Links to several medical journal articles are also available. Sites are listed with short descriptions of resources found at the address.

American Association of Clinical Endocrinologists (AACE): Clinical Practice Guidelines for the Management of Thyroid Carcinoma ◎ ◎ ◎
http://www.aace.com/clin/guides/thycancer.html

Provided by the AACE and The American College of Endocrinology, this online form of the guide is a comprehensive multiple page document with figures and tables.

American Thyroid Association (ATA) ◉ ◉

http://www.thyroid.org

The official Web site of the ATA provides information about thyroid disease and thyroid cancer. The Site Menu provides links to information for patients, research, the ATA journal, announcements, the ATA newsletter, physician guidelines, and contacts.

Mapping of the Gene(s) Predisposing to Non-Medullary Thyroid Cancer ◉ ◉

http://www.geocities.com/ResearchTriangle/4485/fnmtc.html

Part of the Geocities Research Triangle, this site details the study protocol and provides contact information for joining the consortium. Information pertaining to the primary investigators and instructions for sample collection and shipment are also provided.

MedNews/National Cancer Institute (NCI): Thyroid Cancer ◉ ◉ ◉

http://www.meb.uni-bonn.de/cancernet/101252.html

Technical resources on thyroid cancer for health professionals are available at this site. General information about the disease includes a discussion of statistics and risk groups. Cellular classifications, staging information, an overview of treatment options, and treatment discussions specific to all stages of the disease are also presented. All information is supported with references.

OncoLink: Frequently Asked Questions About Head and Neck Cancer ◉ ◉

http://www.oncolink.upenn.edu/disease/headneck1/faq

This site lists answers to recent questions asked by both patient and physician visitors to OncoLink. Questions relate to head and neck cancers, including parotid cancer, salivary cancer, esthesioneuroblastoma, and adenoid cystic carcinoma. Questions on other issues, including complications of treatment and synthetic thyroid hormones are also answered.

Thyroid Cancer Home Page ◉ ◉

http://bjach.polk.amedd.army.mil/13/homepg.htm

This informational resource has consolidated PDQ information into a user-friendly forum. There are multiple pages of text and links and additional details about health-care administration.

Thyroid Cancer Resource Center ⊙

http://www3.cancer.org/cancerinfo/res_home.asp?ct=43

Provided by the American Cancer Society (ACS), the site provides information about causes, risk factors, prevention strategies, diagnostic techniques, and treatment. Access to ACS materials and publications is also provided.

Thyroid Foundation of Canada: Thyroid Cancer ⊙ ⊙ ⊙

http://home.ican.net/~thyroid/Guides/HG12.html

Information on thyroid cancer for the general public and patients is available at this site. Resources include background information about the disease, statistics, and prognosis, discussions of different types of thyroid cancers, and radiation exposure as a risk factor. Treatments described include surgery, radioactive iodine therapy, external radiation therapy, and post-treatment care. Answers to common questions and contact information for additional resources are also available.

University of Newcastle upon Tyne: Head and Neck Cancers ⊙ ⊙ ⊙

http://www.ncl.ac.uk/child-health/guides/clinks2h.htm

Links available at this address relate to head and neck cancers, presented as general resources, or resources specific to oral cavity, lip, and salivary gland cancer; larynx, hypopharynx, and oropharynx cancer; nasal, paranasal, and nasopharynx cancer; or parotid gland cancer. Short descriptions are provided of most listed sites, and resources for health professionals are labeled as such. Patient information resources, mailing lists, government information sources, support groups and organizations, online tutorials, and other educational resources are typical of the sites found through this address.

9.7 Gastrointestinal Tract Cancers

General Resources

American College of Gastroenterology (ACG) ⊙ ⊙ ⊙

http://www.acg.gi.org

The ACG offers professional and patient information regarding all aspects of GI disease. Patient education brochures and a special section for patients that provides colon cancer information are provided. The physician section provides publication, symposia, grants and awards, and clinical updates information. There is also a link to the *American Journal of Gastroenterology*. The members' section details ACG national affairs, legislative updates, and practice guidelines. Membership is multidisciplinary and guidelines are available at the site.

American Gastrointestinal Association (AGA) ◉ ◉

http://www.gastro.org

The site of the AGA primarily serves gastroenterologists and related professionals. There are details about sections, committees, documents, and courses that concern gastrointestinal oncology.

American Society for Gastrointestinal Endoscopy ◉ ◉ ◉

http://www.asge.org

The professional society for gastroenterologists, surgeons and other health professionals provides information about GI disease and the use of endoscopy. Information about endoscopy related to all GI disease, including cancer, is provided. Patient information comes in the form of educational documents that discuss upper endoscopy, flexible sigmoidoscopy, colonoscopy, and more. One can view an online database of clinical updates, policy and position statements, and patient care guidelines. There is a member section that has restricted access by password.

International Ostomy Association (IOA) ◉ ◉

http://www.ostomyinternational.org

This Web site provides information and a forum for patients. There is information about meetings, membership, regional events, local support and information organizations, and about care. A feature of the site is the global discussion forum where participants can post new questions or reply to those of others. There is an active forum as well as archives.

National Surgical Adjuvant Breast and Bowel Project (NSABP) ◉ ◉ ◉

http://www.nsabp.pitt.edu

The NSABP is a cooperative group that performs clinical trials in the areas of breast and colon cancer. The NSABP Web site provides a thorough description of the Project, an overview of protocols, news, contact information, a list of references, future meetings information, and online press releases. The Pathology Section details research activities, pathology section publications, the NSAPB tissue bank, and more.

Society for Surgery of the Alimentary Tract (SSAT) ◉ ◉ ◉

http://www.ssat.com

The SSAT, an organization dedicated to the alimentary tract, provides membership information, a directory, news, and a link to its official journal. Information concerning cancer and other diseases is offered. There are patient guidelines written in English, Spanish, and Japanese for the treatment of cancer of the colon or rectum, the surgical treatment of pancreatic cancer, and the management of colonic polyps and adenomas. An electronic abstract submission program is also offered.

United Ostomy Association (UOA) ◎ ◎ ◎

http://www.uoa.org

UOA is a nonprofit information and support organization for patients. The UOA Web site offers information about ostomy, local chapters, conferences, and links to related sites and distributors of ostomy equipment. There is also information about the local chapter visitor and support service where certified visitors are made available to patients in need. An FAQ and documents concerning insurance issues and rights are available along with links to special committees for parents of ostomy children and for gay and lesbian ostomates.

Colorectal Cancer

3D Virtual Colonoscopy ◎ ◎ ◎

http://www.cs.sunysb.edu/~vislab/projects/colonoscopy/colonoscopy.html

This page is provided by the Web site of the Computer Science Department at the State University of New York. Offered is a virtual image that was created from multiple CT scans and patient data that takes the user through a tour of the colon. Currently, there are two animations; the first is a flythrough of a plastic pipe with three simulated tumors and the second is a flythrough of the colon of the human. News, related publications, contacts, and sample images are also offered at the site.

American Society of
Colon and Rectal Surgeons (ASCRS) ◎ ◎ ◎

http://www.fascrs.org

The ASCRS provides information about many colon and rectal disorders and their relation to surgery. Information available at the site concerns the ASCRS council, committees, research, residency programs, core subjects, a practice registry, and regional societies. One can locate a colorectal surgeon and find general patient information via the site. The Practice Parameters section features documents devoted to the treatment of rectal carcinoma and detection of colorectal neoplasms. The documents are quite detailed and come with extensive information concerning supporting documentation.

Cleveland Clinic Foundation:
Center for Colon Cancer and Polyps ◎ ◎

http://www.clevelandclinic.org/gastro/colon/colon.html

This site provides information for patients and physicians. Patient sections provide general information, an FAQ area, screening and treatment information, and lists of patient education programs, and support groups. For professionals, information concerning the Center and its medical genetics program, registries, contacts, reference documents, and physician education programs is provided.

Colon Cancer Alliance (CCA) ○ ○ ○

http://www.ccalliance.org

A support, education, and advocacy organization for patients, the CCA provides survivor stories, a buddies program, clinical trials information, and an online chat service. Information offered concerns the disorder, a question and answer forum, and links. There are also pages of news, current activities, and screening fact sheets. Membership is free and materials are available.

Colon Connections ○ ○ ○

http://rattler.cameron.edu/colon

This frequently updated site provided by Cameron University has a large number of links to information pages and other sites that deal with colon cancer. Resources are provided for patients and professionals. Links are broken down by topics such as news, abstracts, screening, hereditary, alternative treatment, images, and journals.

Colon Polyps & Colon Cancer ○ ○

http://www.maxinet.com/mansell/polyp.htm

A board certified gastroenterologist is responsible for this site which serves as a professional reference tool that can also be used by patients. Topics discussed include colonoscopy, flexible sigmoidoscopy, staging, barium enema, treatment, prognosis, and Duke's Classification. An extensive list of references is provided.

Colorectal Cancer Association of Canada (CCAC) ○ ○ ○

http://www.ccac-accc.ca

The CCAC organizes educational and support activities for patients, and this information is provided with membership information, links, and news. The information program supplies updates about the disorder, treatment risks or benefits, and research and clinical trials news.

Colorectal Cancer Homepage ○ ○ ○

http://home.swipnet.se/~w-15548

This physician-led site has basic information for patients. Detailed information about treatment options are available, as well as a number of links geared towards both professionals and patients.

Colorectal Forum ○ ○ ○ (fee-based)

http://www.colorectal-forum.org

A vast number of educational resources for professionals can be found here. The site is updated by an editorial board of experts and provides current news, symposia information, patient management recommendations, articles, visual images, publication reviews, and a discussion forum. Site entry requires a password and online registration is provided.

Dad's Colon Cancer Pages ◎ ◎ ◎
http://members.tripod.com/~cancer49

This personal Web site offers a tremendous amount of references and educational information. The table of contents lists 50 categories and within each category there are dozens of links to other sites and information pages. Very basic as well as in-depth information is provided in this organized Web site. Links postings are dated and the site is updated frequently.

Hereditary Colon Cancer ◎ ◎ ◎
http://www.mdanderson.org/~hcc

A newsletter and information page supplied by The University of Texas M.D. Anderson Cancer Center, this professionally-oriented page offers general information, access to current and archived newsletters, a list of registries, and contact information.

International Collaborative Group of Hereditary Non-Polyposis Colorectal Cancer (ICG-HNPCC) ◎ ◎ ◎
http://www.nfdht.nl

This technical resource provides general information about the collaborative group, a mutation database, meeting reports and registration information, clinical guidelines, and links. There is a complete list of members and a service that allows the user to calculate probability mutation via downloadable software.

Johns Hopkins Colon Cancer Center ◎ ◎ ◎
http://www.med.jhu.edu/cancerctr/colon/main.htm

Provided by The Johns Hopkins Oncology Center, this site offers study, center, hereditary colon cancer, research, news, colon and rectal, diagnosis, and treatment information. There is a description of the anatomy of the colon and rectum, a colon and rectum classification section, and symptoms lists.

Lower Your Risk of Colon Cancer ◎ ◎ ◎
http://www.hsph.harvard.edu/colonrisk

Established by the Harvard Center for Cancer Prevention, this site offers detailed information for patients about colon cancer, treatments, procedures, tests, and the Center. Featured is a colon cancer risk index that calculates one's risk for the disorder via a question and answer session.

Medicine Online: Colon Cancer Information Library ◉ ◉
http://www.meds.com/colon/colon.html

The site provides professional and patient information and links to relevant sites. Professional resources concern screening reviews, therapy, heredity, and more. Patient information concerns colonoscopy, clinical trials listings, and general information.

National Colorectal Cancer Action Campaign ◉ ◉
http://www.cdc.gov/cancer/screenforlife

The Center for Disease Control (CDC) site details its action campaign, provides basic information, offers CDC prevention and control initiative information, and contains useful links.

Esophageal Cancer

Esophageal Carcinoma ◉ ◉ ◉
http://www.vh.org/Providers/Textbooks/
EsophagealCarcinoma/EsophagealCarcinoma.html

The University of Iowa's Virtual Hospital offers this site on Esophageal Carcinoma. The Table of Contents includes the following: Background, Risk Factors, Anatomy, Normal Histology, Squamous Cell Carcinoma (Epidermoid Carcinoma), Adenocarcinoma Symptoms of Esophageal Carcinoma, Diagnosis, Staging, Survival, Treatment, and Curative Treatment. Subtopics are also listed for some of these topics.

HealthTouch Online: Esophageal
Cancer Treatment and Treatment Side Effects ◉ ◉ ◉
http://www.healthtouch.com/level1/leaflets/nci/nci048.htm

Information from the National Cancer Institute on esophageal cancer and treatment for patients and non-professionals is presented here. Treatment options are discussed, including a list of important questions patients should ask. Planning of treatment, treatment methods, clinical trials, and side effects are explained, including suggestions for patients undergoing therapy for this disease.

MedNews/National Cancer Institute (NCI):
Esophageal Cancer ◉ ◉ ◉
http://www.meb.uni-bonn.de/cancernet/100089.html

Esophageal cancer information resources at this site include discussions of cellular classifications, stages of the disease, and treatment options. Typical treatment regimens for each stage of the disease and recurrent disease are also available. Information is technical and meant for health professionals. Users can also access a site through this address providing information on clinical trials for patients with esophageal cancer.

ThroatCancer.Com ⊙ ⊙ ⊙

http://www.throatcancer.com

This site contains numerous links to pages that provide diagnosis, prevention, treatment, drug facts, and laryngectomy information.

University of Kansas Medical Center:
Esophageal Cancer Links ⊙ ⊙

http://www2.kumc.edu/kci/cancerlinks/esophagus.htm

This address offers links to 15 other sites providing resources related to esophageal cancer. Most sites provide general information, therapy descriptions, support information, or practice guidelines.

Gastric Cancer

HealthAnswers.com: Gastric Cancer ⊙ ⊙

http://www.healthanswers.com/centers/body/
overview.asp?id=digestive+system&filename=000223.htm

Information on gastric cancer at this site includes a definition, causes, incidence, risk factors, symptoms, signs and diagnostic tests, treatment, support groups, prognosis, and complications. Information at the site is meant for nonprofessionals.

Helicobacter Foundation ⊙ ⊙ ⊙ (fee-based)

http://www.helico.com

This Foundation was started by an Australian physician in 1994 to provide the general public with information on Helicobacter Pylori and the effects of this infection on patient health. The site describes the organism in detail, its mechanism for survival in the stomach, typical treatment for the disease, conditions linked with infection, including gastric cancer, and answers frequently asked questions. Links to articles, a chat forum, and search engine are available for additional information.

National Cancer Institute (NCI): PDQ, Gastric Cancer ⊙ ⊙ ⊙

http://cancernet.nci.nih.gov/clinpdq/soa/Gastric_cancer_Physician.html

Gastric cancer information for health professionals is available at this site. Cellular classification and stages of the disease are described, including a discussion of treatments for each disease stage. Reference citations are listed, supporting information at the site.

National Institutes of Health (NIH): Rare Diseases
Clinical Trials Pertaining to Gastric Cancer ⚙ ⚙ ⚙

http://rarediseases.info.nih.gov/ord/wwwprot/menu/dx00025.html

Twenty-seven clinical trials investigating treatments for gastric cancer are listed at this site. Protocol information includes identification numbers, type, sponsorship, status, age range, projected accrual, objectives, outline, and entry criteria. Contact information for participating organizations/investigators is available.

OncoLink: Outline Summary of Stomach Cancer ⚙ ⚙ ⚙

http://oncolink.upenn.edu/disease/gastric/gastric_review.html

This document from the University of Pennsylvania Cancer Center provides statistics and epidemiology, risk factors, pathology, staging, and treatment information on gastric cancer. Outlines of clinical trial findings are provided for comparison and guidance when making treatment decisions. A table summarizing selected clinical trials and journal citations are available for further investigation.

Stomach Cancer Links ⚙ ⚙

http://www2.kumc.edu/kci/cancerlinks/stomach.htm

Eleven links are available at this address for specific resources on gastric cancer. Treatment information, patient resources, and images are offered through these links.

Liver Cancer

American Liver Foundation (ALF) ⚙ ⚙

http://gi.ucsf.edu/alf.html

The ALF site provides support, education, and research information. Also, information concerning various liver disorders, the Foundation, advocacy in legislation, news, and research work is offered to the user. A list of awards and grants, past winners, research news, and a calendar is provided.

Canadian Liver Foundation ⚙ ⚙

http://www.liver.ca

Readily available at this site is a physician-oriented newsletter, research information, organ donor materials, general information about cancer and other liver disorders, and offline and online contact details.

Children's Liver Alliance (CLA) ⚙

http://www.livertx.org

As a supportive and informational organization for patients and their families, the CLA provides services concerning all liver disease in children. Educational information about disease, support, transplantation, and seminars is provided along with links. A service is offered whereby the organization acts as a liaison between families and healthcare professionals.

Diseases of the Liver ◎ ◎

http://cpmcnet.columbia.edu/dept/gi/disliv.html

This reference site lists diseases and provides links to documents or information pages. There are also links to current papers in liver disease, books, and other sites. The disorders are in alphabetical order and are hyperlinked. Cancer topics include extra-hepatic bile duct carcinoma and hepatocellular carcinoma. The list is compiled by a staff member at Columbia University College of Physicians and Surgeons.

Liver Cancer Network ◎ ◎ ◎

http://www.livercancer.com

Presented by The Liver Program at Allegheny General Hospital, this site serves as a comprehensive resource and offers information about the disorder, treatments, the Program, contacts, news, and more. An easy to use fast-find feature lists specific information available at the site for patients and professionals.

Liver-Onc ◎ ◎

http://www.acor.org

A moderated online discussion for patients is provided by the Association of Cancer Online Resources (ACOR) at this site. Subscription information and instructions are provided.

University of Pittsburgh Cancer Institute: Liver Cancer Center ◎ ◎ ◎

http://www.upci.upmc.edu/Internet/Lcc/index.html

The Web site of the Cancer Center supplies information about the Center, its treatment facilities, and patient evaluation. In addition, treatment specifics and summaries of treatment results are listed along with reviews on hepatoma/HCC.

VAMC Pathology Service: Hepatocellular Carcinoma ◎ ◎ ◎

http://pathology.utmem.edu/seminars/hepato~1/page.htm

This page is supplied by the University of Tennessee and provides a detailed pathology guide for professionals. Topics covered are classifications, macroscopic details, cell types, patterns, metastasis, alpha-feto, E.M., HCC, HBV, and more. The site contains text descriptions with many images.

University of Iowa Virtual Hospital: Atlas of Liver Pathology ⊙ ⊙ ⊙

http://www.vh.org/Providers/Textbooks/LiverPathology/Text

The Virtual Hospital provides a number of texts and this one deals with all aspects of liver pathology. Chapter 11 deals specifically with tumors of the liver. In this chapter, benign, mesenchymal and epithelial tumors are discussed. Also provided are detailed text descriptions with links to images.

Pancreatic Cancer

European Registry of Hereditary Pancreatitis and Familial Pancreatic Cancer (EUROPAC) ⊙

http://www.liv.ac.uk/Surgery/europac.html

The goals of this registry are to establish incidence number, to analyze a possible gene mutation, and to develop screening techniques. Study information, contacts, and information about its mutation analysis and cell line service are provided.

Pancreas Cancer Home Page ⊙ ⊙ ⊙

http://www.path.jhu.edu/pancreas

Provided by The Johns Hopkins Medical Institution, this site is a comprehensive information resource for cancer of the pancreas. The site provides thorough information on facts, surgery, genetics research, cytogenetics, specific tumor types, information for clinicians/investigators, and much more.

Pancreatic Cancer ⊙ ⊙

http://www.cp-tel.net/pamnorth/panca.htm

This site, which includes statistics and information about pancreatic cancer, contains many links to information pages and research institutions. There is also a visual of the pancreas in a human anatomy atlas. Links to informational pages for other cancers are also provided.

Pancreatic Cancer Action Network (PANCAN) ⊙ ⊙

http://www.pancan.org

PANCAN is an advocacy, research funding, and educational organization for pancreatic cancer. Its site offers information about membership, fundraising events, future research support, and education. Quality links to related sites and informational pages are also provided.

Pancreatic Cancer Tumor Study Group ◎ ◎ ◎

http://www.mdanderson.org/DEPARTMENTS/pancreatic/default.htm

Provided by The University of Texas M. D. Anderson Cancer Center, this site provides a tremendous amount of information relating to pancreatic cancer in an easy-to-navigate Web site. The Center offers a multimodality program, and its site offers information about the program, its staff, and its treatments. In addition, there is an FAQ section, news, extensive clinical studies data, and diagnosis and treatment information. There is support and basic research information for patients as well.

Pancreatic Duct ◎ ◎ ◎

http://www.sterner.org/~dsterner/pancreas

This comprehensive information resource is geared mostly towards patients. It offers information and links to other sites and information pages that cover facts, therapy, emotional assistance, clinical trials, caregivers, and unconventional treatments.

Ronald S. Hirshberg
Pancreatic Cancer Research Center ◎ ◎

http://www.pancreatic.org

Facts related to pancreatic cancer, the Foundation, diagnosis and treatment methods, research, the Foundation's newsletter, and links are supplied here. Information about survival rates, tumor size, and disease progression is provided.

Small Intestine Cancer

HealthlinkUSA: Intestinal Diseases ◎ ◎

http://www.healthlinkusa.com/169.htm

This address contains links to information on all intestinal diseases, including cancer of the small intestine. Resources include answers to patient questions, fact sheets, information on diagnostic procedures, and news of ulcer cures when due to Helicobacter Pylori. Four pages of links are available from this site.

National Cancer Institute (NCI): PDQ, Small Intestine Cancer ◎ ◎ ◎

http://cancernet.nci.nih.gov/clinpdq/soa/Small_intestine_cancer_Physician.html

Resources for health professionals on small intestine cancer and its treatment are available at this site. Disease and survival rates are discussed, and visitors can also access cellular classification, staging, and treatment information. Standard treatments and treatments currently under evaluation are discussed for each stage of the disease. Information is supported with article citations.

**National Institutes of Health (NIH): Rare Diseases
Clinical Trials Pertaining to Small Intestine Cancer** ◎ ◎ ◎

http://rarediseases.info.nih.gov/ord/wwwprot/menu/dx01175.html

Seven clinical trials exploring treatments for small intestine cancer are listed at this site. Protocol information includes identification numbers, type, sponsorship, status, age range, projected accrual, objectives, outline, and entry criteria. Contact information for participating organizations/investigators is available.

9.8 **Gynecologic Cancers**

General Resources

Pathology Manual: Gynecologic Oncology Group ◎ ◎

http://www.vh.org/Providers/Textbooks/OBGYNOncology/PathologyManualHome.html

This site is provided by the University of Iowa's Virtual Hospital. Detailed pathology descriptions are offered for a variety of disorders related to gynecologic oncology. An appendix and sample synoptic reports are also supplied.

Society of Gynecologic Oncologists (SGO) ◎

http://www.sgo.org

The SGO site offers a tremendous amount of information to practitioners of Gynecologic Oncology. Consistent with the Society's philosophy of encouraging research and raising the standards of practice, the site offers up-to-date news from the SGO, upcoming symposia schedules, coding references, and abstracts.

Cervical Cancer

American Society for
Colposcopy and Cervical Pathology ◎ ◎

http://www.asccp.org

The Society's Web site provides information about symposia, disorders, educational materials, and a forum for discussion of educational topics. Membership and contact information is supplied. Forum registration is free.

Breast and Cervical Health Program (BCHP) in Washington State ❍ ❍

http://www.fhcrc.org/cipr/bchp

The BCHP program is a component of the Centers for Disease Control (CDC) program for breast and cervical cancer care. The site provides program information, contacts, and a publication listing. BCHP services such as clinical screening, mammography referral, and reimbursement are described. There are descriptions of mammography for physicians with referring provider information. Informative videos about the mammogram, questions to ask your doctor, the Pap test, results, and more are featured. Also, there is a document and slide clips library in the PDF format. Much of the site's information is provided in an audio text form for the visually impaired.

Cervical Screen ❍ ❍ ❍

http://cervicalscreen.rsc.com.au

This Australian site provides information for professionals that covers the physician's role in screening, taking a Pap smear, interpretation and management of results, epidemiology and pathology information, information to give patients, and common questions asked by patients. It also provides screening and educational information for patients.

Colposcopy Atlas ❍ ❍ ❍

http://lib-sh.lsumc.edu/fammed/Atlases/colpo.html

The site functions as a learning tool for colposcopists to help them better understand and perform the procedure. Supplied information includes introductions and overviews, step-by-step instruction, follow-up information, colposcopy news, and a glossary. There are discussions of Colposcopy in the Pregnant Patient and of Controversies and Decision-Making for Uterine Cervical Disease. Links for patient resources are also provided.

MDAdvice.com: Cervical Cancer ❍ ❍ ❍

http://www.mdadvice.com/topics/cervical_cancer/info/2.htm

Cancer of the cervix is described for patients and the general public at this site, including a description of the cervix and its location, the nature of cervical cancer, Pap smears, and different biopsies performed in the case of an abnormal Pap smear. Each stage of cervical cancer, treatment options, including different surgeries, radiation, and chemotherapy, are described, including a list of treatments commonly used at each stage of the disease. National Cancer Institute contact information is available for receiving additional information and educational booklets.

MedNews/National Cancer Institute (NCI): Cervical Cancer ⦿ ⦿ ⦿

http://www.meb.uni-bonn.de/cancernet/100103.html

Cervical cancer information at this site is technical and meant for health professionals. General information about the disease includes a discussion of recent treatment advances, statistics, staging and prognosis, and human papillomavirus infection. Cellular classifications, an overview of treatment options, and treatment discussions specific to each stage of the disease are also presented. All information is supported with references.

National Cervical Cancer Coalition (NCCC) ⦿ ⦿

http://www.nccc-online.org

The official Web site of the NCCC is geared mostly towards patients, and provides comprehensive information concerning their Pap test, DES, support, dealing with one's HMO, treatment options, books available, and clinical trials. For professionals, news, clinical trial information, and Clinical Laboratory Improvement Act guidelines are provided. There are also links to articles and to related sites.

National Institutes of Health (NIH): Consensus Development Statement, Cervical Cancer ⦿ ⦿ ⦿

http://text.nlm.nih.gov/nih/upload-v3/CDC_Statements/Cervical/cervical.html

The NIH provides Consensus Statements that are prepared by an independent panel of experts. These statements are reports from that panel based on presentations and open and closed discussions. They focus on cervical cancer and detail prevention, management of low and advanced stage cervical cancers, new directions for research, and panel information.

Reproductive Health Outlook: Cervical Cancer Research Topics ⦿ ⦿ ⦿

http://www.rho.org/html/cxca_restopics.htm

Summaries of current research related to cervical cancer control are presented at this site. Topics include epidemiology and natural history of cervical cancer, role of human papillomavirus tests and possible vaccine in cervical cancer control, primary prevention of cervical cancer, assessment of alternative screening approaches, evaluation of simple treatment approaches, and client perceptions of cervical cancer and prevention approaches. Each topic is presented with a summary of current research in that area, including references to supporting academic articles. All articles are listed with abstracts in a bibliography section.

Endometrial Cancer

Endometrial Cancer ◎ ◎
http://www.mef.hr/~mkopljar/ec/ec.htm

This site is geared towards students and the public and offers information and links. Topics covered are anatomy and physiology, etiology, pathogenesis, grading and staging, diagnostic process, complications, early symptoms, and differential diagnosis.

National Cancer Institute (NCI): Endometrial Cancer ◎ ◎ ◎
http://cancernet.nci.nih.gov/clinpdq/soa/Endometrial_cancer_Physician.html

Health professionals will find this site a useful source of information on endometrial cancer. Resources include a discussion of risk factors and statistics associated with the disease, patterns of metastasis, indicators of prognosis, cellular classification, and staging. An overview of treatment options is available, as well as a treatment discussion relevant to each stage of the disease and recurrent endometrial cancer.

ViaHealth: Endometrial Cancer ◎ ◎
http://www.viahealth.org/disease/gyn_oncology/endometr.htm

Endometrial cancer is described at this site, including risk factors, symptoms, causes, prevention, diagnosis, and treatment of the disease. Users can access other women's health resources from this site.

Ovarian Cancer

Corinne Boyer Fund ◎ ◎
http://www.corinneboyerfund.org

This organization provides research funds and support information for patients and their families. Information is available about the annual forum hosted by the organization, the organization's newsletter, educational forums, contacts, sponsored research, support groups, and ovarian cancer facts.

Early Detection of Ovarian Cancer ◎ ◎
http://www.fda.gov/opacom/catalog/ovarian.html

This page from the FDA Web site discusses methods of early detection, warning signs, and diagnostic procedures.

Gilda's Club

http://www.gildasclub.org

Gilda's Club provides support groups, work shops, lectures, and social events. The Web site is a forum for patients and their families to communicate and seek support. In addition, a program calendar, contact information, and membership details are provided.

National Ovarian Cancer Coalition (NOCC)

http://www.ovarian.org

A large collection of ovarian cancer information is available here. The site offers facts, opportunity for discussion, chapter locations, contact information, and news. The Resources section provides an opportunity to ask questions of experts in the field, supplies information about state resources, and allows for the search of a database, by state, that contains names of more than 600 gynecologic oncologists.

Ovarian Cancer Alliance Canada (OCAC)

http://www.ocac.ca

The OCAC site offers disease information for patients, a newsletter, support information, links, and downloadable pamphlets. A list of Canadian Gynecologic Oncologists with contact information is displayed. A special topics section offers some professionally written information documents.

Ovarian Cancer Research Notebook

http://www.slip.net/~mcdavis/ovarian.html

This comprehensive site provides a myriad of documents related to ovarian cancer. It provides detailed information for patients and oncologists and is organized in a manner such that each of the more that 2,500 documents available is summarized and grouped into categories to make location of information easy. Databases available include details about specific treatments in clinical or trial use, planned trials, human gene therapy protocols, biological approaches, anti-angiogenesis agents, and other presentations.

SHARE: Self Help for Women with Breast or Ovarian Cancer

http://www.sharecancersupport.org

This support organization for women, men, and children offers a listing of support groups, a calendar of programs, advocacy information, and information about its educational programs. Educational programs empower patients to make decisions about their treatment and to learn about research and nonconventional therapies. There is also extensive contact information available including hotline telephone numbers.

9.9 **Head and Neck**

General Resources

American Association of
Oral and Maxillofacial Surgeons (AAOMS) ◎ ◎

http://www.aaoms.org

The society consists of professionals who care for patients with disorders of the areas of mouth, teeth, jaw, and face including those with tumors and cysts. The site provides information about the AAOMS, news, continuing education programs, and conferences, residency, and contacts. A patient information section supplies details about the specialty and procedures.

Bobby R. Alford Department of Otorhinolanygology
and Communicative Sciences: Grand Round Archive ◎ ◎ ◎

http://www.bcm.tmc.edu/oto/grand/hnca.html

Provided by the Baylor College of Medicine, this site offers information about many neoplasms of the head and neck. There are 50 pages of articles, reviews, and information documents that cover a wide variety of topics such as Paranasal Sinus Carcinoma, Tracheal Tumors, Merkel Cell Carcinoma, Kaposi's Sarcoma, lip cancer, Cancer of the External Auditory Canal,and more.

Dysphagia Resource Center ◎ ◎ ◎

http://www.dysphagia.com

The Center offers a variety of links and information pages concerning swallowing and swallowing disorders of all types. Link topics are Vendors, American Speech-Language-Hearing Association (ASHA) Special Interest Division 13, Anatomy and Physiology, Research, Case Studies, Conference Announcements, Organizations, and more. A Tutorials and Articles section provides information about a variety of disorders including, larynx, oral, pharyngeal, stomach, and esophageal cancers. Information is provided for patients and professionals.

Eastman Dental Institute
for Oral Health Care Sciences ◎ ◎

http://www.eastman.ucl.ac.uk

This site provides information for all oral disorders. There are numerous abstracts, articles, reviews, research reports, pathology reports, and images that concern oral, lip, and tongue cancer. The site allows for a keyword search to group links to specific information pages.

ENT News Online ⊚ ⊚ ⊚ (fee-based)

http://www.ent-news.com

A review of current ENT and related fields, news, and access to past issues is available here. There are articles, conference reviews, calendars, award listings, and features in each installment. The site features a discussion forum and a bookstore. A free registration is required for site access.

Head and Neck Cancer Links ⊚ ⊚

http://www2.kumc.edu/kci/cancerlinks/head.htm

Twenty-five site links are listed at this address, providing resources related to thyroid cancer, head and neck cancers, laryngeal cancer, pharyngeal cancer, lip and oral cavity cancer, paranasal sinus, and nasal cavity cancer.

Lucas Project ⊚ ⊚ ⊚

http://www.odont.ku.dk/lucas

A cooperative effort among the dental schools of Copenhagen, Lund, and Sheffield, this site is an online teaching and information resource for odontogenic tumors. There are listings of various tumors that are linked to detailed descriptions and images that provide clinic, radiology, histology, diagnostic, therapy, and prognosis information.

M. D. Anderson Cancer Center: Head and Neck Center ⊚ ⊚

http://www.mdanderson.org/centers/headneck

The site for the Head and Neck Center provides patient guidelines and details of referrals, programs and services, staff, treatment options, and a patient-oriented FAQ.

Oral Cancer Information Center ⊚ ⊚ ⊚

http://www.oralcancer.org

This patient and professional information site provides details of oral cancer, educational programs, and other informational resources. Information is classified for patients or professionals and is online and offline. Access to parts of the site requires a free registration.

Support for People with Oral and Head and Neck Cancer, Inc. (SPOHNC) ⊚ ⊚

http://www.spohnc.org

A support organization that provides general information about head and neck cancers, SPOHNC offers a newsletter, support, and encouragement. Also available at the site is information about products available for patients, membership, books, and contacts. The newsletter has medical information that is relayed in terminology that patients can understand.

Adenoid Cystic Carcinoma

Aden-Cyst List ⊙ ⊙
http://www.outlookmagazine.com/resources/mailinglist/directory/aden-cyst.html

This site serves as a resource for professionals and patients for the discussion of treatment, support, research, clinical trials, and other information. The discussion is not moderated. There is a list of newsgroups.

Adenoid Cystic Carcinoma (ACC) Resource Center ⊙ ⊙ ⊙
http://www.paonline.com/knippd/acc

This personal site offers lists of ACC Medical Literature, Alternative Treatment and Nutrition details, a newsletter, a patient chat room, support information, and lists of treatment centers. The medical literature section provides links to professional documents and information pages at other sites.

Laryngeal Cancer

Cancer of the Larynx ⊙ ⊙
http://members.aol.com/fantumtwo/cancer1.htm

This site provides basic information about cancer of the larynx and links to related articles, PDQ files, informational pages, support groups, dealers of laryngectomy supplies and products, and links to otolaryngology centers and health providers.

International Association of Laryngectomies (IAL) ⊙ ⊙
http://www.larynxlink.com/ial/ial.htm

This nonprofit organization is made up of member clubs and seeks to provide patient information, support, and other services. The IAL Web site provides information concerning its Voice Institute, various clubs, speech instructors, events and products, and their distributors. An online information library offers health and laryngectomy articles. There is a newsletter and a section of links to other information sources.

Laryngeal and Hypopharyngeal Cancer Resource Site ⊙ ⊙
http://www3.cancer.org/cancerinfo/res_home.asp?ct=23

This site is provided by the American Cancer Society (ACS) and offers information about prevention and risk, detection and symptoms, treatment, survivorship, and publications. There are news, ACS materials, and resources sections at the site.

National Cancer Institute (NCI): Laryngeal Cancer ⊙ ⊙ ⊙

http://cancernet.nci.nih.gov/clinpdq/soa/Laryngeal_cancer_Physician.html

This resource for health professionals describes the morphology of the larynx, common presentations of laryngeal cancer, risk factors, and prognosis. Cellular classification and stages of the disease are defined, and users can read an overview of treatment options. The site also provides a discussion of treatment options for each stage of the disease and recurrent laryngeal cancer. All information is supported by academic article citations.

Voice Center at Eastern Virginia Medical School ⊙ ⊙ ⊙

http://www.voice-center.com

A professional reference site, this resource provides information concerning anatomy and function of the larynx, techniques for examining the larynx, topics in voice science, descriptions of most voice and laryngeal disorders, including cancer, and other details about otolaryngology. There are text descriptions with images and other learning tools.

Oral and Tongue Cancer

American Oral Cancer Clinic ⊙ ⊙

http://www.tonguecancer.com

This site offered by the Head and Neck Surgery Clinic of Houston provides information on lip cancer, oral cancer, voice box cancer, and tongue cancer. Visitors can read about the clinic and medical director, and access specific resources on each cancer.

British Dental Association: Oral Cancer Fact File ⊙ ⊙ ⊙

http://www.bda-dentistry.org.uk/factfile/fact17a.html

This fact file presents information on oral cancers, including causes, incidences (in table form), historical statistics on oral cancer cases and deaths, treatment, tumor locations, and recommendations on screening from the Association. Information is supported with article citations.

National Cancer Institute (NCI): PDQ, Lip and Oral Cavity Cancer ⊙ ⊙ ⊙

http://cancernet.nci.nih.gov/clinpdq/soa/Lip_and_oral_cavity_cancer_Physician.html

Health professionals can access this site for information on lip and oral cavity cancer, including a general discussion of the disease with morphology of the mouth and survival rates according to tumor location, cellular classifications, definitions of disease stages, and an overview of treatment options. Standard treatments and treatments under clinical evaluation are listed for each stage of the disease, including recurrent disease. Article citations are available, supporting information in the document.

National Library of Medicine (NLM): Guide to Clinical Preventive Services: Screening for Oral Cancer ⊙ ⊙ ⊙

http://text.nlm.nih.gov/cps/www/cps.22.html

This site explains issues related to mouth cancer screening, including the burden of suffering, accuracy of screening tests, effectiveness of early detection, and screening recommendations of other groups. A discussion of mouth cancer, current screening activities, and clinical intervention concludes this document. Reference citations are available for support and elaboration of information at the site.

Oral Cancer Awareness Initiative ⊙ ⊙ ⊙

http://www.oral-cancer.org

The Oral Cancer Awareness Initiative, comprised of professional dental schools and organizations, aims to alert the public to the importance of early detection and treatment of oral cancer. Resources on oral cancer at this site include a definition, incidence and mortality rates, annual costs, signs and symptoms, progression, risk factors, prevention, early detection and survival rates, and treatment and rehabilitation methods. General cancer resources and sites specific to oral cancer are found through links at this address.

PersonalMD.com: Cancer of the Tongue ⊙ ⊙

http://www.personalmd.com/healthtopics/crs/canctg.htm

This site provides patient resources on cancer of the tongue. A description of the disease, including morphology, causes, symptoms, diagnosis, and treatment is available. The site also answers common patient questions about duration of tongue cancer effects and how patients can administer proper self-care after diagnosis and treatment.

Salivary Glands/ Malignant Partoid Tumors

Diseases of the Salivary Glands ⊙ ⊙

http://www.roseway.demon.co.uk

Although a private professional site, this resource offers information about many salivary gland diseases including Malignant Partoid Tumors. The site offers basic information for patients and in-depth information for professionals. There are text descriptions with relevant figures that concern diagnosis, various glands, classification, and treatment. The site also offers links and publication information. Disorder information and links are organized by topic.

National Cancer Institute (NCI): PDQ, Salivary Gland Cancer ◉ ◉ ◉

http://cancernet.nci.nih.gov/clinpdq/soa/Salivary_gland_cancer_Physician.html

Professional resources on salivary gland cancer a this site include a general discussion of the disease and prognosis according to tumor site, cellular classification information, disease stage descriptions, and an overview of treatment options. Standard treatments and those currently under clinical evaluation are listed for each stage of the disease. Reference citations support information presented at the site.

9.10 Hematological Topics and Disorders

General Resources

Current Issues in Transfusion Medicine ◉ ◉ ◉

http://www.mdacc.tmc.edu/~citm

This Web site provides an online newsletter written by and intended for physicians. The newsletter is provided by the Section of Transfusion Medicine and Laboratory Immunology at The University of Texas M.D. Anderson Cancer Center. Topics discussed in the newsletter include screening, testing, complications, alternatives, and more.

Introduction to Blood ◉ ◉ ◉

http://cer.hs.washington.edu/John

This site is a reference tool that offers descriptions of blood banking and components. There are many microscopic and scanning electron images along with the descriptive text. Blood donation, typing, apheresis, and bone marrow transplantation are discussed.

Introduction to Blood Morphology ◉ ◉

http://healthlinks.washington.edu/courses/blood

This Web site provides data for the 19th edition of the *Cecil Text Book of Medicine* by James R. McArthur, M.D. It offers a large number of images of blood and marrow in a variety of conditions.

New York Blood Center ◉ ◉ ◉

http://www.nybloodcenter.org

A tremendous amount of information is available to professionals and patients at this site. Training and education, employment, donor, and publications information is provided for professionals. Major areas of research covered are virology, population genetics, and computer modeling, stem cell biology, plasma proteins, membrane biochemistry, molecular diagnostics, and transfusion transmitted disease, immunochemistry, immunogenetics, human genetics, hematopoietic stem cell processing, hematopoietic growth factors, epidemiology, cell biology, blood coagulation, biochemistry and molecular genetics, and biochemical virology. Research highlights, studies, staff, and publications in each area are provided. There is also a news area. Patient services and products are detailed. Transfusion, stem cell services, apheresis services, and donations are also discussed.

Aplastic Anemia

Aplastic Anemia (AA) Association of Canada ○ ○

http://www.aplastic.ualberta.ca

This site provides patient education and support information. Details of AA and Myelodysplasia, their causes, and treatments are provided along with a newsletter. Contact information for support, an FAQ section, and further details are provided.

Aplastic Anemia Foundation of America (AAFA) ○ ○

http://www.aplastic.org

This site provides newsletters and many information documents for professionals that concern Aplastic Anemia, Myelodysplastic Syndromes, and other bone marrow failure diseases. There are Annual Conference Listings, researcher awards listings, and links.

Fanconi Anemia Research Fund Home Page ○ ○ ○

http://www.fanconi.org

The site of this nonprofit organization offers details of the disorder, treatment, diagnosis, its relation to leukemia and other cancers, research, research grants available, family education, and support services and of upcoming events. The site has links to the organization's FA Family Newsletter and FA Science Letter. There is also a link to Fanconi Anemia: A Handbook for Families and Their Physicians, a guidebook with professional appendices.

HealthlinkUSA: Aplastic Anemia ○

http://www.healthlinkusa.com/23.htm

Site links are listed at this address providing patient information and support resources concerning aplastic anemia and related disorders. Most sites offer personal stories and experiences, and three full pages of links are available.

Medical Education Information Center (MedIC):
Aplastic Anemia: Introduction for the General Physician ◎ ◎ ◎

http://medic.uth.tmc.edu/ptnt/00001040.htm

The MedIC system, offered through the University of Texas, Houston, Department of Pathology and Laboratory Medicine, provides physician information on aplastic anemia at this site. A general description of the disease is followed by discussions of diagnosis, treatment, transfusions, natural history, and general prognosis for patients with this disease.

Desmoplastic Tumors

Desmoplastic Small Round Cell Tumor (DSRCT) ◎ ◎

http://www.dsrct.demon.co.uk

This patient-oriented site provides information about DSRCT, treatments, personal support stories, medical reports, histology slides, and links.

Hematopathology

Hematopathologic Phenotypes Made Mockingly Simple ◎ ◎ ◎

http://www.neosoft.com/~uthman/cdphobia/cdphobia.html

A physician at the University of Texas School of Medicine Department of Pathology and Laboratory Medicine is responsible for this site. The Web site offers charts that simplify antigen profiles and are used in diagnostic workup of lymphomas and leukemias. Links to reference information and relevant Web sites are also provided.

Hematopathology ◎ ◎ ◎

http://edcenter.med.cornell.edu/CUMC_PathNotes/Hematopathology/Hematopathology
.html

Provided by the Weill Medical College of Cornell University, this site offers a very detailed tutorial that covers the hematopoietic system, erythropoeisis, hypoproliferative anemias, leukopoeisis, and more. There is extensive text discussion with many figures, images and tables.

Hematopathology Laboratory ◎ ◎ ◎

http://www.depts.washington.edu/labweb/Division/Hematology/HP.Home.html

Provided by the University of Washington, this site offers an extensive collection of laboratory references including CD antigens useful for hematopathology, other antigens, ranges for peripheral blood lymphocyte populations, acute leukemia diagnosis, lymphoma classifications, and tables of lymphoid and myeloid differentiation. In addition, the site provides information about the testing conducted at the laboratory as well as information about specimen handling and about diagnostic tests and profiles.

Histiocytosis

Histiocytosis Association of America ⊙ ⊙
http://www.histio.org

The organization funds research and provides information to patients and professionals. The site offers conference and funding details and a number of discussion lounges. An information library provides news, research information, and links.

Histocompatibility

Histocompatibility ⊙ ⊙ ⊙
http://ntri.tamuk.edu/immunology/histocompatibility.html

This site offers a detailed reference document for professionals that discusses human and animal histocompatibility systems. There is significant discussion of the HLA complex in humans.

Histology Lessons ⊙ ⊙
http://www.mc.vanderbilt.edu/histo/blood/index.html

Based at Vanderbilt University, this page serves as a blood information reference for students. Included is an introduction and description of blood components, as well as discussions of polymorphonuclear leukocytes and mononuclear leukocytes.

Myelodysplastic Disorders

Myelodysplastic Syndromes and Sideroblastic Anemias ⊙ ⊙
http://mindspring.com/~sacremon/index.htm

This patient-oriented information and support site offers information about the disorders, blood, and patient conferences and events. There is also an extensive links section.

Myelodysplastic Syndromes (MDS) ⊙ ⊙ ⊙
http://www.leukemia.org/docs/pub_media/mds/fc_mds.html

The Leukemia Society of America provides a comprehensive site resource for MDS, giving an extensive overview of the disease, and brief descriptive profiles of symptoms, diagnosis, treatment, causes and risk factors, living with MDS, prognosis, emotional aspects, future expectations, a glossary, a further reading list, and other resources.

Myelodysplastic Syndromes (MDS) Foundation Home Page ⊚ ⊚ ⊚
http://www.mds-foundation.org

Founded by researchers and physicians, this organization seeks to facilitate the exchange of clinical, research, treatment, and other information relating to MDS. The site provides details of the foundation, pharmaceutical partners, press releases, symposia, membership, research, MDS centers, and continuing education. There are separate patient and professional discussion forums. A patient information section offers professionally written information documents about myelodysplastic syndromes.

Myeloproliferative Disorders

Myeloproliferative Disorders (MPD) Home Page ⊚ ⊚ ⊚
http://www.acor.org/diseases/hematology/MPD

An informational source for MPD, the Web site provides a newsletter, online support groups, an FAQ, reports from past MPD medical conferences, and many links to medical and other support information sources, citations, abstracts, and articles.

9.11 Hodgkin's Disease and Malignant Lymphoma

Hodgkin's Disease

Hodgkin's Disease Information ⊚ ⊚
http://www2.arnes.si/~uljfntfiz1/hodgkin/hodgkin.html

This address contains links to sites providing resources related to Hodgkin's disease. Categories include general information and resources, cancer and cancer treatment, Hodgkin's lymphoma, non-Hodgkin's lymphoma, support resources, and other general cancer resources. Sites are listed with short notes on target audience and available resources.

Hodgkin's Disease Resource Center ⊚
http://www3.cancer.org/cancerinfo/res_home.asp?ct=20

Provided by the American Cancer Society (ACS), this site provides medical information for patients, information about ACS materials, publications, and other resources dealing with Hodgkin's Disease.

Leukemia Society of America: Hodgkin's Disease and the Non-Hodgkin's Lymphomas ⊙ ⊙ ⊙

http://www.leukemia.org/docs/pub_media/hodgkins/whatitis.html

Information provided by this fact sheet includes a description of Hodgkin's disease and the non-Hodgkin's lymphomas, a description of the blood system with definitions of components, and a description of the lymph system. This general information is followed by more in-depth discussions of each disease, including symptoms, diagnosis, staging and associated tests, treatments and common complications of treatment, specific treatment options, bone marrow transplant, causes and risk factors, suggested sources for information and support, and current research and development in disease management. A useful glossary of terms is also available.

MedStudents: Hematology: Hodgkin's Disease ⊙ ⊙ ⊙

http://www.medstudents.com.br/hemat/hemat3.htm

This site offers information from a Brazilian physician on Hodgkin's disease for use by medical students. The article includes a definition of the disease and discussions of epidemiology, etiology and pathogenesis, pathology, clinical manifestations, and hematological abnormalities.

Non-Hodgkin's Lymphomas

AIDS Related Non-Hodgkin's Lymphoma ⊙ ⊙

http://www.thebody.com/treat/nhl.html

This page provides symposia proceedings, studies, and research articles. There are also links to information documents from other sites.

Introduction to Non-Hodgkin's Lymphomas ⊙ ⊙ ⊙

http://www.path.sunysb.edu/hemepath/tutorial/lymph_intro/lymph_intro.htm

This is an educational resource provided by the Department of Pathology, State University of New York at Stony Brook. There are easily navigable information pages that have images and hyperlinked text to term definition pages. In addition, there are discussions of immunophenotyping, epidemiology, and more.

Mantle Cell Lymphoma (MCL) ⊙ ⊙

http://eyesite.ucsd.edu/~mcl

The site provides informative statements from professionals concerning MCL and its treatment. There are also lists of relevant abstracts and links to useful sites.

National Cancer Institute (NCI):
PDQ, Childhood Non-Hodgkin's Lymphoma ☼ ☼ ☼

http://cancernet.nci.nih.gov/cancer_types/lymphoma.shtml

Professional resources are available at this site from the National Cancer Institute on childhood non-Hodgkin's lymphoma. General information, cellular classification details, definitions of disease stages, and an overview of treatment options are included. Specific treatment discussions relevant to each stage of the disease and recurrent disease are also available. All information is supported with appropriate article citations.

NHL Cyber Family ☼ ☼ ☼

http://www.wizard.com/NHL

A resource for patients and families that provides a wealth of information about education and support, the site provides clinical information, book reviews, case studies, links, newsgroups, inspirational information, and a newsletter. The links page is very extensive and has journal, research, informational, support, and conventional and alternative treatment links.

Non-Hodgkin's Lymphoma of Bone ☼ ☼

http://www.bonetumor.org/page96.html

This page from the bonetumor.org Web site provides a professionally oriented, detailed text description of Non-Hodgkin's Lymphoma of Bone, and a variety of images. A number of offline references are also provided.

Non-Hodgkin's Lymphoma Web Site ☼ ☼

http://www.westvirginia.net/~sigley/NHL_Web_Site.htm

A collection of information pages and resources that concern Non-Hodgkin's lymphoma and that are more patient oriented is housed at this site. There are support stories, references, and treatment and clinical trials information.

Non-Hodgkin's Lymphomas Tutorial ☼ ☼ ☼

http://www.medsch.wisc.edu/medsch12/indexNH.html

Provided by the University of Wisconsin Medical School, this tutorial is geared towards professionals. It is an educational slide presentation of facts, epidemiology, clinical features, and more. Slides are text, images, tables, and figures.

Lymphoma General Sites

Can.Survive ⊙ ⊙ ⊙
http://www.cansurvive.org.uk

This comprehensive site provides information about Hodgkin's disease, Non-Hodgkin's Lymphoma (NHL), and other cancers. There is also support, complimentary therapy, treatment, and news information. Treatment information concerns chemotherapy, radiotherapy, surgical oncology, BMT and stem cell transplant, clinical trials, and side effects. Support information comes in the form of nonprofit organizations, U.K. State benefits, patient stories, and psychological issues. Topics covered in the NHL and Hodgkin's sections are definitions, signs and symptoms, staging, predisposing factors, investigations, specific chemotherapy regimes, journal links, articles, and more. Information at this site is geared towards patients with some emphasis towards professionals.

Cure for Lymphoma Foundation ⊙ ⊙
http://www.cfl.org

This site provides news, lymphoma information, and resources. The nonprofit organization funds research and provides support for patients. Information about research grants, past awards, and the scientific advisory board is also provided. A grant application can be downloaded from this site.

Lymphoma Forum ⊙ ⊙ ⊙ (free registration)
http://www.lymphoma.org.uk

This forum is for the exchange of information and serves healthcare professionals, patients, and their families. The healthcare professionals section provides access to current topics, case studies, a resource library, notice board, and conference center. A free registration allows unlimited access to this section.

Lymphoma Information Network ⊙ ⊙ ⊙
http://www.lymphomainfo.net

A number of resources concerning Hodgkin's disease and Non-Hodgkin's lymphoma are located here. There is information about adult lymphomas, childhood lymphomas, and physician information. Detailed descriptions, diagnostic information, classification, resources, and support information are provided. Lymphoma in animals and links to resources geared towards children are also offered. The physician's section offers links to PDQ statements, book listings, treatment information, and many articles.

Lymphoma Research Foundation Canada (LRFC) ◎ ◎

http://www.lymphoma.ca

The foundation provides support and funds research with a focus on issues in Canada. Patient-oriented lymphoma information is provided along with descriptions of the LRFC funding guidelines, listings of Canadian conferences, news, and support and contact information. There is also a comprehensive listing of lymphoma research in Canada.

Lymphoma Research Foundation of America ◎ ◎ ◎

http://www.lymphoma.org/pages/index.html

This organization promotes research, offers educational and emotional support programs, conducts advocacy activities, and raises community awareness of lymphoma. The site provides information on patient and professional education programs, special events, research fellowship grants, support programs, lymphoma advocacy activities, an online bookstore, and message boards for Hodgkin's and non-Hodgkin's lymphoma.

Pathology of Lymph Nodes ◎ ◎ ◎

http://www.hitchcock.org/pages/path/levylecture/levylecture.html

This page, provided by the Dartmouth Hitchcock Medical Center, is a thorough informational page that covers many aspects of the lymph node and lymphopoiesis. There are overviews, anatomy diagrams, cytology discussions, images, pathology discussions, tables, and text linked to more information.

9.12 Leukemias

General Resources

Granny Barb and Art's Leukemia Links ◎ ◎ ◎

http://www.acor.org/leukemia/frame.html

This massive personal site provides a seemingly endless number of links to other sites and information pages concerning leukemia, bone marrow transplant, and cord blood transplant. Links are to government, personal, institutional, journal, and academic sites, and range from the most basic to intricate, professionally-oriented material. The links are organized by category and, in turn, are easy to find. Topics covered at the site are general facts, genetics, leukemia specific sites, resources for specific leukemias, causes, online journals, clinical trials, pathology, online support, and other organizations.

Leukemia Insights ⊚ ⊚ ⊚

http://www.mdanderson.org/leukemia/insights.html

The online newsletter of the University of Texas M.D. Anderson Cancer Center offers both patient and professional information. There is extensive case study, treatment, transplant, research, and clinical studies information. One is given access to the most recent as well as past newsletters. In addition, information about the center is provided.

Leukemia Online Support Group ⊚ ⊚

http://www.egroups.com/list/leukemia/info.html

This online support group for patients and caregivers allows the user to view previously posted messages or enter a new one. Instructions for use are provided.

Leukemia Research Foundation ⊚ ⊚

http://www.leukemia-research.org

The foundation funds research, provides financial aid to patients, provides support and promotes bone marrow registries. Its site contains contact information, application materials for research grants, links to relevant sites, and patient support information.

Leukemia Research Fund ⊚ ⊚

http://dspace.dial.pipex.com/lrf-

This U.K. organization is dedicated to raising funds to fight leukemia, Hodgkin's Disease and other lymphomas, myeloma, myelodysplasia, and aplastic anemia. Its site provides a handbook and guide to the investigation of clusters of diseases, a directory of research, access to publications, and symposia information. One can also view grant guidelines and download application materials. Links and many patient information materials are readily available.

Leukemia Research Fund Canada ⊚ ⊚

http://www.leukemia.ca

This Web site details the organization's goals to provide information and fund research in Canada. There is a listing of fellowships and operating grants as well as lists of past recipients. General information is offered concerning leukemia and related disorders along with news and links to relevant sites.

Leukemia Society of America ⊚ ⊚

http://www.leukemia.org

The society seeks to provide information, education, patient services, community services, and fund research dealing with leukemia, lymphoma, Hodgkin's disease, and myeloma. The society's site provides information about educational materials, publications, services offered, news, and events. The research link provides workshop information and applications, a professional education calendar, and grant information.

Macroscopic Patterns of
Leukemia Mortality in the United States ⊙ ⊙

http://www.inel.gov/resources/research/.research/.research_abstracts/.rb/index.html

A page from the Web site provided by the Idaho National Engineering and Environmental Laboratory (INEEL) provides an abstract that has many statistics and graphs that cover geographic distribution, distribution by sex, frequencies and more. In addition, there is a link to a table of state rates for leukemia.

Medicine Online: Leukemia Information Library ⊙ ⊙ ⊙

http://www.meds.com/leukemia/leukemia.html

This site offers professional information that concerns adult myelogenous leukemia. Topics covered include current issues, emerging trends in AML management, National Cancer Institute (NCI) documents, and key points. There is an atlas of acute leukemia that consists of detailed descriptions with many figures and tables. Patient information includes links, a terms glossary, and patient guides.

Newbury Leukemia Study Group (NLSG) ⊙ ⊙

http://www.newbury.net/nlsg

NLSG studies leukemia clusters to possibly determine causes of the disorder. The site provides an overview of the investigation with data collected, structure, and methods of operation information. The technical library offers a reports index, a critiques index, and a list of relevant Web sites.

Plain Talk about Leukemia ⊙ ⊙ ⊙

http://www.pt-able.com

This resource for patients provides facts, discussions of current news, information about Hodgkin's Disease, support information, patient profiles, and a newsletter. The topics section is quite extensive and has a large amount of information about acute leukemias, chronic leukemias, survival rates, and possible causes. There are many links to relevant Web sites and information pages.

University of Washington
Hematopathology Laboratory ⊙ ⊙

http://www.labmed.washington.edu/Division/Hematology/HP.home.html

The Laboratory provides useful information pertaining to lymphoma, leukemia and other diseases related to hematology. Tests are listed by disease category along with testing information. Reference information concerns useful CD antigens, acute leukemia diagnosis, peripheral blood lymphocyte population reference ranges, and myeloid and lymphoma differentiation.

Acute Lymphoid Leukemia

Acute Lymphoid Leukemia (ALL) ◎ ◎
http://www.tirgan.com/all.htm

This site focuses on signs, symptoms, diagnosis, classification, and treatment of Acute Lymphoid Leukemia (ALL), including information on the incidence of the disease in the population. Links provide further information on different treatment protocols.

Childhood Acute Lymphocytic Leukemia (ALL) ◎ ◎ ◎
http://cancernet.nci.nih.gov/Cancer_Types/Leukemia.shtml

This is a link to the National Cancer Institute, providing general information, cellular classification, treatment overviews, and articles on untreated childhood ALL, childhood ALL in remission, and recurrent ALL. There are bibliographic references for each descriptive profile.

Leukemia Society of America:
Acute Lymphocytic Leukemia ◎ ◎ ◎
http://www.leukemia.org/docs/pub_media/all/fc_all.html

This online booklet offers information on acute lymphocytic leukemia. Discussions provide details on normal blood and marrow, leukemia, acute lymphocytic leukemia, causes and risk factors, subtypes of the disease, symptoms and signs, diagnosis, treatment, chemotherapy, treatment side effects and their management, refractory leukemia and relapsed leukemia, social and emotional aspects of the disease, and follow-up care. The booklet concludes with information on current statistics on remission and survival, and future outlook based on research and trends. A glossary of terms and list of suggested readings are also available at the site.

Chronic Lymphoid Leukemias

Chronic Lymphoid Leukemias (CLL) ◎ ◎ ◎
http://www.tmc.tulane.edu/classware/pathology/krause/leukemias/cll/cll.html

The Department of Pathology at Tulane University Medical Center created this site which provides a description of CLL and accompanying magnified images of blood cells, bone marrow biopsy, and bone marrow core biopsy. The site has links to images for other forms of leukemia, including acute lymphoblastic leukemia, acute myeloblastic leukemia, chronic myeloid leukemia, hairy cell leukemia, and adult T-cell leukemia.

Acute Myeloid Leukemia

Adult Acute Myeloid Leukemia ⊙ ⊙ ⊙
http://cancernet.nci.nih.gov/Cancer_Types/Leukemia.shtml

CancerNet provides a detailed description of adult acute myeloid leukemia (click on "Acute Myeloid Leukemia, Adult" at the Leukemia site), including a general overview, cellular classification, stage information for untreated and "in remission" cancer, and a treatment option discussion. The material at this site is designed for health professionals rather than the general public.

Childhood Acute Myeloid Leukemia ⊙ ⊙ ⊙
http://cancernet.nci.nih.gov/Cancer_Types/Leukemia.shtml

Within CancerNet's Leukemia site, click on "Acute Myeloid, Childhood" to access this site, which provides healthcare professionals with a general introduction, cellular classification, histochemical evaluation, cytogenetic evaluation, stage information, and a treatment option overview.

Rare Disease Clinical Trials for Adult AML ⊙ ⊙ ⊙
http://rarediseases.info.nih.gov/ord/wwwprot/menu/dx01029.html

For the clinician, this site provides details on dozens of clinical trials for adult acute myeloid leukemia. There are both Phase I and Phase II studies relating to chemotherapy, bone marrow transplantation, and other therapies. This is not a site for the general public, as it is extremely technical.

Chronic Myeloid Leukemia

Chronic Myeloid Leukemia (CML) ⊙ ⊙
http://cait.columbia.edu:88/dept/medicine/bonemarrow/cml.html

Columbia Presbyterian Medical Center has provided a useful site serving as a general resource for CML. The information provided covers a summary of the nature of the disease, HLA typing, alternative donors, allogenic blood stem cell transplantation, conditioning regimens, irradiation, prognosis, relapse, and treatment. This is a technical site for physicians.

Hairy Cell Leukemia

Hairy Cell Leukemia Foundation ⊗
http://home.earthlink.net/~shanford/hcl.htm

The foundation provides support, information, and funds research. Its site provides basic information and contact information concerning its services.

Hairy Cell Leukemia (HCL) ⊗ ⊗
http://www.geocities.com/HotSprings/Spa/1350/index.html

Intended for those who have had or who currently have HCL, this site offers support information, a forum for patients to communicate with one another, archived and current reader's comments, and links to relevant sites. A section allows the user to ask questions, relay concerns, find help sources, and get more specific information.

Pediatric Resources

Childhood Leukemia Center ⊗ ⊗
http://www.patientcenters.com/leukemia

This Leukemia Center provides resources for parents and other family members. There are many articles, patient guides, an FAQ, and many links to information sources and support organizations. Article topics include diagnosis, working with your doctor, physician's rights, and coping with chemotherapy.

National Children's Leukemia Foundation ⊗ ⊗ ⊗
http://www.leukemiafoundation.org

This organization provides services, information, referrals, and support to patients and families. There is information about stem cell banking, a computerized donor search service, information about dream fulfillment, and access to a referral service. Online and offline contact information is provided.

9.13 **Lung Cancer**

General Resources

About.com: Lung Cancer ⊙ ⊙ ⊙
http://cancer.miningco.com/health/cancer/health/diseases/cancer/msublung.htm
This address lists links to sites providing detailed information related to lung cancer and chemotherapy, cost-effective combined treatments, costs of care for non-small-cell lung cancer, cigarette smoking, minority statistics, risks and prevention, lung carcinoid, and radiotherapy. A link offers an educational slide program on lung cancer, primarily for health professionals.

Alliance for Lung Cancer Advocacy, Support and Education (ALCASE) ⊙ ⊙ ⊙
http://www.teleport.com/~alcase
ALCASE is a patient education and support resource that provides extensive, professionally written information about the disorder, constipation, fatigue, anorexia, dyspnea, and PET imaging. There is a peer-to-peer telephone support program and a list of support groups around the U.S. There are links to other information, clinical trials, and support sites.

American Association for Respiratory Care (AARC) ⊙ ⊙ ⊙ (some features fee-based)
http://www.aarc.org
This professional and patient resource offers information about lung cancer and other respiratory disorders. There are a large number of AARC and industry articles and information about continuing education, government affairs, the AARC Fellowship Program, symposia, clinical practice guidelines, magazines and journals, and employment. A membership area has restricted access and details current professional news, AARC bylaws, resource documents and contact lists, an AARC helpline, and offers the current issue of *AARC Times*. Patients can find an FAQ section and a number of patient-oriented topical documents.

American Heart and Lung Institute ⊙ ⊙
http://www.best.com/~gek
This professionally managed site provides details on screening for cancer, small cell lung cancer, non-small cell lung cancer, diseases of the heart, diseases of the blood vessels, and cancer of the esophagus. Information about the organization divisions, institutes, and staff are provided.

Asbestos Update ◎ ◎ ◎

http://www.mesothel.com

A huge collection of medical articles, protocol lists, research findings and diagnosis, risk, and research information about Malignant Mesothelioma is housed at this site. There is a large database of non-medical information as well. All information is categorized and may be accessed independently from the main menu.

International Association for
the Study of Lung Cancer (IASLC) ◎ ◎ ◎

http://www.iaslc.org

Goals of the IASLC are to study etiology, epidemiology, prevention, treatment, and other aspects of the disorder and to present information to the public and professionals. Its site offers, past meetings, committees, upcoming events, IASLC publications, and news information. There is a link to the *Lung Cancer* journal and details of membership.

Lung Cancer ◎ ◎ ◎

http://rattler.cameron.edu/lungcancer

The Cameron University site is a gateway that offers a collection of organized links. Links are categorized under topics such as patient's introduction, newsgroups and listservers, clinical information, current news on lung cancer, disease information, and disease stages. Links are of use to the public as well as to professionals.

Lung Cancer ◎ ◎ ◎

http://www.meddean.luc.edu/lumen/MedEd/medicine/pulmonar/lungca/lungca.htm

An educational tool for students and professionals, this site provided by the Loyola University Medical Center discusses topics such as etiology, clinical manifestations, staging, solitary pulmonary nodule, pancoast tumor, superio vena cava syndrome, small cell carcinoma, and issues in patient management. Discussions cover topics such as calcification, radiological features, common diagnoses, symptoms, and cell types.

Lung Cancer Online ◎ ◎ ◎

http://www.lungcanceronline.org

Serving as a gateway to other sites, this professional and patient resource provides basic lung cancer information resources. Links to physicians, hospitals, clinical trials, support organizations, online support, patient stories, lung cancer information, diagnosis, testing, procedures, a pain management, database, journals, references, news, alternative medicine, research, professional and patient organizations, and therapy sites are provided. The links are easily accessed from the main page. Nearly every link includes introductory information about the link and topic.

Lung Tumors: A Multidisciplinary Database ◎ ◎ ◎

http://www.vh.org/Providers/Textbooks/LungTumors/TitlePage.html

This site from the University of Iowa's Virtual Hospital is an informational and educational resource for professionals. The site offers access to twenty-eight case studies. There are clinical presentations and diagnoses, staging, pathologic, treatment, and syndrome information for thoracic and pleural-based neoplasms.

National Familial Lung Cancer Registry ◎

http://www.path.jhu.edu/nfltr.html

The registry housed at the Johns Hopkins Medical Institutions aims to understand lung cancer causes and to provide information. Contact information for individual questions is provided.

Second Wind: A National Lung Transplant Patients Association ◎ ◎

http://www.2ndwind.org

This organization is for lung transplant recipients, lung surgery candidates, and the concerned public. It provides support, education, and advocacy. Information about the organization, transplantation, membership, activities, news, meetings, and disorders is listed.

9.14 Lymphedema

General Resources

Academy of Lymphatic Studies ◎ ◎

http://www.zutheracademy.com

The Academy offers general information about treatment with complete decongestive physiotherapy (CDP). There is information and registration material for CDP courses and contact listings.

Lymphedema Therapy ◎ ◎ ◎

http://www.lymphedema-therapy.com

This site is focused on information regarding complex lymphedema therapy (CLT). Reference articles and papers are offered along with multiple information pages. There is a photo gallery, contact information, and a section devoted to CLT and its use for lymphedema secondary to breast cancer.

Lymphoedema Association of Australia ⊙ ⊙
http://www.lymphoedema.org.au

Treatment, therapy, treatment results, newsletter, and membership information is available at this association's comprehensive site. Reviews of complex physical therapy and of compression instruments are supplied, as well as information about reference material.

Lymphoedema.Org ⊙ ⊙ ⊙ (some features fee-based)
http://www.lymphoedema.org

This well-designed site is divided into professional and public sections. The professional section has restricted access and offers papers, research information, and updates from worldwide lymphedema centers. The public section offers general information and links to the British Lymphology Society and the Lymphoedema Support Network. Both organizations are supported by this site. There is an information section for children and a link to *The Lymphnet*, an online publication.

Lymphovenous Canada ⊙ ⊙ ⊙
http://www.interlog.com/~mcpherc

The aim of this site is to link patients with local support groups and healthcare professionals and to provide research and treatment information. Sections of the site provide information about lymphovenous disorders, research developments, cancer lymphedema treatments, book reviews, and diuretics. There are listings of Internet chat and support groups for patients. There is also a section for parents of children with lymphovenous disorders.

National Lymphedema Network (NLN) ⊙ ⊙ ⊙
http://www.lymphnet.org

The NLN site provides education and information to patients and healthcare professionals. Included in this site are descriptions of lymphedema which include lists of many of the primary and secondary causes of lymphedema. Also provided is information regarding support groups, resources, guidelines, conferences, and the NLN newsletter. A database chronicles questions and answers from 1996 on.

Peninsula Medical ⊙ ⊙ ⊙
http://www.lymphedema.com

This site is an information resource for professionals and patients. A physician's section discusses topics such as sentinel node biopsy, surgical management, growth factors, and congestive heart failure. The site offers clinical data, news, links, and product information. For patients, there is an FAQ section, treatment information, a bulletin board, and an online discussion forum.

9.15 **Neuroblastoma**

General Resources

Causes of Neuroblastoma ⊙ ⊙ ⊙
http://www.chem-tox.com/neuroblastoma/index.htm

Topics presented within this neuroblastoma research index are chlordane, general information, case histories, immune systems, and proximity to agriculture. Journal articles and information pages are supplied at this site. There are also links to references.

National Cancer Institute (NCI): Neuroblastoma ⊙ ⊙ ⊙
http://cancernet.nci.nih.gov/Cancer_Types/Neuroblastoma.shtml

This site provides information for health professionals on neuroblastoma, obtained from the National Cancer Institute. General information includes an explanation of disease characteristics, common afflicted age groups, treatment, prognosis, survival statistics, screening experiments, and special biologic variables to consider during diagnosis and when making treatment decisions. Detailed information also relates to cellular classification, disease stages, and treatment options. Each stage of the disease is listed with a discussion of common or appropriate treatments, including treatment for recurrent disease. All information is supported with appropriate article citations.

Neuroblastoma Case Study ⊙ ⊙
http://everest.radiology.uiowa.edu/nlm/app/pedtumor/nblast/nblast.html

Provided by the Division of Physiologic Imaging, Department of Radiology at the University of Iowa, this study contains educational images including slice-by-slice computer images and movies.

Neuroblastoma Home Page ⊙ ⊙ ⊙
http://allserv.rug.ac.be/~fspelema/neubla/nb.htm

This home page is provided by the University Hospital Gent, Belgium. Images, details about the department and the disorder, links, and research information are offered. Some research protocols supplied involve molecular analysis of unbalanced translocation in neuroblastoma cell lines and primary tumors and mutation analysis of candidate tumor suppressor genes. Disorder information includes clinical aspects, genetics of neuroblastoma, and general information.

Neuroblastoma Online Researcher's Forum ❂ ❂ ❂
http://www.staff.ncl.ac.uk/s.j.cotterill/nbl-prof/index.htm

A discussion forum for researchers and physicians, this site provides the opportunity to discuss research, publications, and conference information. Registration information, links, and a linked list of relevant publications is provided.

Von Hippel-Lindau (VHL) Family Alliance ❂ ❂ ❂
http://www.vhl.org

This information and support site provides an FAQ, online chat, discussion groups, a newsletter, interviews, and meeting information. The site is available in multiple languages to accommodate international users. Information for professionals includes handbooks, links to informational pages, listings of DNA testing sources by area, conference schedules, and information about a VHL tissue bank. For professionals and patients, the site provides research information in the form of grant details, a collection of reports and articles, and access to a VHL research database.

Von Hippel-Lindau (VHL) Links Page ❂ ❂ ❂
http://neurosurgery.mgh.harvard.edu/NGlinks.htm#VHL

Provided by Massachusetts General Hospital and Harvard University, this is a central resource that has many links to documents, articles, and government pages that concern VHL.

Pediatric Neuroblastoma

Metastatic Neuroblastoma Case Study ❂ ❂
http://gamma.wustl.edu/mb002te143.html

A case study of a four-year-old boy with bone pain provides images and text descriptions with a full history, findings, ACR codes, references and more.

Neuroblastoma Children's Cancer Society (NCCS) ❂ ❂
http://www.graniteWebworks.com/nccs.htm

The NCCS provides advocacy, support, information, and research funding. Its site provides professionals and patients with PDQ information, a list of accomplishments, projects, and a list of resources. There is also a page for information exchange and contact data.

9.16 **Neurologic Tumors**

General Resources

American Neurological Association (ANA) ☉ ☉ ☉

http://www.aneuroa.org

ANA is a professional organization that serves those who deal with all disorders of the brain. Information available at the ANA Web site concerns brain tumors as well as other neurological disorders. Extensive ANA information is provided along with abstracts and listings, ANA archives, meeting information, member databases, links, and a newsletter.

Give Hope ☉ ☉

http://freespace.virgin.net/give.hope

Give Hope is a private site that serves as a resource for U.K. sites relating to brain tumors. Of greatest use is the resource section of the site that provides links to groups, U.K. research establishments, information sources, hospitals, education and equipment sources, and support groups.

International Paraneoplastic Association ☉ ☉ ☉

http://paraneoplastic.hypermart.net

Those suffering from neurological paraneoplastic syndromes can learn more about their condition and gain support here. Comprehensive information including notices, news, information about paraneoplastic cerebellar degeneration (PCD), medical contact information, coping and rehabilitation information, and journal access is easily accessible. A large number of links are provided for research information.

Making Headway Foundation Inc. ☉ ☉

http://www.makingheadway.org

The pediatric foundation for brain and spinal cord tumors and for other neurological illnesses focuses on providing services before, during, and after the hospital stay. Some services offered are the provision of psychologists, therapists and learning specialists, the donation of household items, and other assistance. The site offers a newsletter, a support group schedule, contact information, and complete information about services and programs offered.

Neuroanatomy and Pathology on the Internet ☉ ☉

http://www.neuropat.dote.hu

This comprehensive guide is intended as a resource for students, residents, and professionals. There are detailed images and descriptions in the anatomy section that are culled from worldwide resources. Similar sections exist for histology and pathology. There are also multiple choice quizzes, journals, and informative documents. Links to commercial software, shareware, and free software sites are also provided.

PET Brain Atlas ◎ ◎
http://www.crump.ucla.edu/PBA

This educational resource that presents over 100 patient cases where scans, reports, and other images are provided, includes teaching cases and tutorials that show model scans that can be presented in a quiz format. The user has many choices as to how the cases should be presented

Society for Neuro-Oncology ◎
http://www.soc-neuro-onc.org

The site of this multidisciplinary professional society offers a calendar of events, listings of employment and research opportunities, links, annual meeting information, a discussion forum, announcements, and a newsletter. There is a link to the *Neuro-Oncology* journal.

Whole Brain Atlas ◎ ◎ ◎
http://www.med.harvard.edu/AANLIB/home.html

From Harvard Medical School, this reference tool takes the user through a tour of the brain with images and text descriptions. Areas covered are neoplastic disease, the normal brain, cerebrovascular disease, degenerative disease, and inflammatory or infectious disease. In some cases, there are time lapse movies. There are 100 brain structures discussed.

Brain Stem Tumor

Brain Stem Tumor Links ◎ ◎ ◎
http://www.virtualtrials.com/btlinks/bookmark.cfm

This site offers a comprehensive series of topics and links specifically for brain stem glioma. Links take the user to information sites for patients and clinicians. There are explanations, case studies, articles, and reviews.

Brain Tumor

American Brain Tumor Association ◎ ◎

http://www.abta.org

The American Brain Tumor Association provides information to patients and health-care professionals and also funds and encourages research. Resources at the site for patients include links to brain tumor information, patient support resources, and to patient education tools.

Brain Tumor Center ◎ ◎ ◎

http://www.wfubmc.edu/surg-sci/ns/btc.html

This Web site, provided by the Wake Forest University School of Medicine, offers a tremendous amount of information concerning brain tumors and is a section of a larger entity that covers all aspects of neurosurgery. Much information is provided about the Center, its treatments and protocols, facilities, staff, and referrals process. In addition there are links and information pages devoted to primary and secondary metastatic brain tumors, pituitary tumor, meningioma, and acoustic neuroma. There is a link to the school's gamma knife center.

Brain Tumor Center at Duke Family Newsletter ◎ ◎

http://www.canctr.mc.duke.edu/btc/consult.htm

A large archive of family-oriented newsletters provides medical and support information. There are also links to other departments of the Center that describe neuro-oncology team members, specialists, program specifics, events, and other support sources. For professionals, there is information about clinical trials and laboratory investigations available at Duke.

Brain Tumor Foundation of Canada ◎ ◎

http://www.btfc.org

The foundation funds research and provides educational and support services to patients and their families. The foundation has helped to establish the Brain Tumor Tissue Bank, a depository of tissue samples that collects and distributes tissue samples to researchers. Current research deals with mechanisms for growth, chemo sensitivity, meningioma, and gap junctions.

Brain Tumor Information ◎ ◎ ◎

http://member.aol.com/lsdpout/brtmr.htm

As a collection of brain tumor links for patients and professionals, the site categorizes links under organizations, medical facilities, treatment types, medical information and resources, literature, chat rooms, personal stories, and support. There is also a link to an online support group.

Johns Hopkins Radiosurgery: Brain Tumor
Radiosurgery Association and Support: New Treatments ◎ ◎ ◎
http://www.med.jhu.edu/radiosurgery/nbtra/nbtra.html

This site offers general information on radiosurgery and resources related to the National Brain Tumor Radiosurgery Association. Contact details for the founder and president of the organization, a description of the Association, and membership details are available at the site. A link to Johns Hopkins information on brain tumor treatments and protocols leads to more detailed information on the treatment of brain tumors with radiosurgery.

Malignant Brain Tumors & Neuro-Oncology Resources ◎ ◎
http://neurosurgery.mgh.harvard.edu/nonc-hp.htm

This is a reference site provided by Massachusetts General Hospital and Harvard Medical School. There are discussions of many brain, spine, and peripheral tumors along with many links to documents and information pages related to malignant brain tumors.

Musella Foundation for Brain Tumor Research & Information ◎ ◎ ◎
http://www.virtualtrials.com/musella

This site provides information pertaining to various aspects of brain tumor trials. There is a database of brain tumor treatments that is a compilation of data collected from worldwide institutions. Here, one can browse listings by tumor type, by treatment type, or by a keyword search. In addition, there are descriptions of brain tumor treatments, live chats, a forum, and videos on trials and treatments. The site also has a link to a brain tumor virtual trial. This study is a database of treatment and outcome information that requires patient participation. Registration, update, and consent forms can be downloaded from the site.

New Approaches to Brain Tumor
Therapy (NABTT): A CNS Consortium ◎ ◎
http://www.nabtt.org

Funded by the National Cancer Institute, the consortium's goals are to ultimately improve therapies for the treatment of brain tumors and to participate in research for basic biology, pharmacology, and care. The site offers detailed information about the laboratory and other services offered, protocols, related institutions, and protocol status.

The Brain Tumor Society:
Brain Tumor Support Group Web Sites ◎ ◎

http://www.tbts.org/btsgws.htm

Support resources found through this address include links to online and traditional support groups, mailing lists, clinics and research groups, information sources, cancer centers, and foundations.

Wistar Institute's Albert R. Taxin
Brain Tumor Research Center ◎ ◎ ◎

http://www.wistar.upenn.edu

Information about the Center's employment and training programs, technology transfer, research, and public affairs is offered. The site also has a virtual library that gives the user access to the Center's reference collection, historical collection, archives, journal holdings, and museum. Major research occurs in the areas of tumor immunology, tumor biology, molecular genetics, structural biology, and gene therapy.

Pediatric Resources

Child-Neuro: Patient
Educational and Disease Oriented Resource Links ◎ ◎

http://www.waisman.wisc.edu/child-neuro/par-ed/Neurol-WWW/CNP-list.html

This computerized e-mail discussion group allows the sharing of information among patients, family members, and professionals. Information concerning subscription, digest format, archived messages, and sending messages is provided.

Childhood Brain Tumor Foundation (CBTF) ◎ ◎

http://www.monumental.com/cbtf

CBTF raises and provides funds for scientific research. It also raises public awareness of brain tumors. There are links to articles that are geared towards researchers and clinicians.

University of Newcastle upon Tyne:
Brain and Spinal Cord Tumors ◎ ◎ ◎

http://www.ncl.ac.uk/child-health/guides/clinks2a.htm

One hundred and sixty-one links are offered at this address cataloging Web resources on brain and central nervous system tumors. Organizations for patients and professionals, research centers, general resources, and information specific to childhood brain tumors, acoustic neuroma, and spinal cord tumors are found at this site. Resources are divided into those appropriate for both patients and healthcare professionals.

9.17 **Opthamological Cancers**

General Resources

American Academy of Ophthalmology (AAO) ◉ ◉ ◉

http://www.aao.org

The site of the professional organization provides a large number of resources for patients and professionals that concern all eye disorders. The professional area offers an academy overview, clinical education information, listings of meetings, member services details, practice services, and a products and publications listing. The patient area provides information about the AAO, about ophthalmology, eye health, anatomy, conditions and diseases, low vision resources, support groups, surgery, and news.

American Society of Ophthalmic
Plastic & Reconstructive Surgery ◉ ◉

http://www.asoprs.org

This Web site provides information about reconstructive surgery involving the eyelids, orbits, and lacrimal system. There is information about membership, fellowships, scientific meetings, journals, and contacts. A patient information section provides information about the field, procedures, eyelid skin cancers, tumors, and other conditions. There is a restricted section for members that provides professional information.

Association for Research in
Vision and Ophthalmology (ARVO) ◉ ◉

http://www.faseb.org/arvo

Information about ARVO, membership, abstracts, scientific programs, awards, and ARVO forms is supplied. There are links to investigative ophthalmology and visual science and to a guide to finding sources in eye and vision research.

Digital Journal of Ophthalmology ◉ ◉ ◉

http://www.djo.harvard.edu

This comprehensive, professional information site is provided by Massachusetts Eye and Ear Infirmary, a teaching affiliate of Harvard Medical School. It offers information about all eye disorders including cancers. There are many case studies, CD-ROM reviews, original articles, and quizzes. There is also information about CME and about publications. Patient information includes disorder, treatment, procedure and diagnosis details. The large links section is organized alphabetically and includes institutions, information sites, journals, professional organizations, and more.

Eye Care Foundation ◎ ◎
http://www.eyecarefoundation.com

The nonprofit organization's site provides information for patients and their families and professionals that concerns ocular oncology, macular degeneration, and other eye disorders. There are details of current treatment options, support programs, research, fellowship programs, and clinical trials.

EyeCancer Network ◎ ◎ ◎
http://www.eyecancer.com

This comprehensive information resource provides information about specific conditions, treatments, images, research, benign conditions, and metastasis. There are documents concerning radiation, enucleation, innovations, and studies. Patients can find information about second opinions and choosing a specialist. The site allows researchers to apply for research or clinical fellowships and provides an online bookstore. The site is available in English, Spanish, and German.

Ocular Oncology Service ◎ ◎
http://www.shieldsoncology.com

Provided by the Willis Eye Hospital and Thomas Jefferson University in Philadelphia, Pennsylvania, the site offers background, staff, patient care, and history details. There are descriptions of various eye tumor types, specific research papers, articles, fellowships available, and meetings.

Intraocular Melanoma

Collaborative Ocular Melanoma Study (COMS) ◎ ◎ ◎
http://www.med.jhu.edu/wctb/coms

COMS identifies treatments available for those afflicted with choroidal melanoma. Its site provides information about ocular melanoma, clinical trials, COMS design, clinical centers, and information about COMS. Also, there are detailed descriptions and examples of ophthalmic photography and ophthalmic echography.

National Cancer Institute (NCI): PDQ, Intraocular Melanoma ◎ ◎ ◎
http://cancernet.nci.nih.gov/clinpdq/soa/Intraocular_melanoma_Physician.html

Intraocular melanoma is discussed for health professionals at this site, including statistics on recurrence and prognosis. Specific resources, including cellular classification, stages of the disease, treatment options, and treatments for each stage of the disease or recurrent disease are also offered at the site. Article citations support all information at the site.

OncoLink: Intraocular Melanoma Articles ◉ ◉
http://cancer.med.upenn.edu/cancernet/99/jan/701170.html

Twelve article citations and abstracts describing recent research on intraocular melanoma, found through the National Cancer Institute's CancerLit system, are available at this site. Users can also access OncoLink resources on other cancer topics at this address.

Retinoblastoma

National Retinoblastoma
Research and Support Foundation (NRRSF) ◉ ◉
http://www.djo.harvard.edu/meei/PI/RB/NRRSF.html

The NRRSF provides information and support to families of patients. The site offers articles from the NRRSF newsletter, huge amounts of patient information dealing with many disorders of the eye, and links to other information sites.

Retinoblastoma.com ◉ ◉
http://www.retinoblastoma.com

This site provided by physicians presents a detailed guide of nine chapters for parents and a large number of offline references. Some chapter topics are genetic testing, classification, treatment, eye structure, and long term consequences.

Retinoblastoma International ◉ ◉
http://www.retinoblastoma.net

The nonprofit society provides support for education, research, and care for retinoblastoma. Its site primarily provides patient information for support and education.

9.18 Plasma Cell Dyscrasias

Amyloidosis

Amyloidosis Webforum ◉ ◉
http://neuro-www.mgh.harvard.edu/forum/AmyloidosisMenu.html

This forum is aimed towards professionals, although anyone can participate. New discussions can be started or archived discussions may be accessed.

Myeloma Amyloidosis
Monoclonal Gammopathy Group ◎ ◎ ◎

http://www.mayo.edu/mmgrg/rst/mmpage.htm

Provided by the Mayo Clinic, this resource is for patients, physicians, and scientists. A number of related disorders are covered in these pages. For professionals, there are listings of investigators and their work, employment, and education details and links. One can also access any of the numerous other sections of the Mayo Clinic Web site. Patients have access to diagnosis, treatment, and location information.

Specialist Services in Amyloidosis ◎ ◎

http://www.med.ic.ac.uk/dm/dmmh03/amyloidosis.html

Supplied by the Imperial College School of Medicine, London, this is an information page. Contact information, general descriptions, diagnostic imaging details, treatment information, and department services are provided.

Multiple Myeloma

Atlanta Area Multiple Myeloma Support Group ◎ ◎ ◎

http://www.mmsg.org/atlanta/default.asp

This group holds meetings in the Atlanta area, and provides information at its Web site for myeloma patients of all areas. Meeting information, news, a newsletter, survivor profiles, and discussion group details are provided at the site. In the discussion group section, one can view posted notes or post a new note.

International Myeloma Foundation (IMF) ◎ ◎ ◎

http://myeloma.org

This informative site details services provided by the IMF for patients and physicians. Basic and detailed information about myeloma is provided along with grant application materials, news items, links to other myeloma sites, patient seminar information, support group information, and publication and clinical meeting details. Reviews written about specific forms of myeloma and reviews concerning various aspects of myeloma are provided. The IMF has a 30-member international board of scientific advisors which provides counsel and support to the IMF in its education, treatment, and research goals. Contact information for each member of the board is available.

Multiple Myeloma ◎ ◎

http://www.cp-tel.net/pamnorth/bone.htm

Basic information and links to other sites are available here. There are details regarding plasma cell neoplasms, research organizations, and bone scans of myeloma.

Multiple Myeloma ⊙ ⊙ ⊙

http://www2.gasou.edu/facstaff/jariail/myeloma

This private site serves as an information resource for patients and professionals. It is very well organized, categorizing information under definitions, organizations, seminar reports, databases, articles, blood counts, medical centers, and clinical trials. Available links are to detailed information pages at other sites and pages.

Multiple Myeloma and Renal Disease ⊙ ⊙ ⊙

http://www.wramc.amedd.army.mil/departments/Medicine/nephro/Nephrology/lectures/myeloma/Sld001.htm

This site hosts a forty-six page slide presentation provided by the Walter Reed Army Medical Center. The site serves as an educational resource for professionals.

Multiple Myeloma Association ⊙ ⊙ ⊙

http://www.webspawner.com/users/myelomaexchange

Information for professionals and patients is provided. There is also an e-mail discussion group and information archives. Links are to transplant information sites, chat rooms, informative sites, PDQ statements, articles, programs, physicians, and research centers.

Multiple Myeloma Research Foundation (MMRF) ⊙ ⊙

http://www.multiplemyeloma.org

Goals of the MMRF are to fund research, raise awareness, and provide information. The site provides upcoming events, news, and contacts. Patient resources provided include fact sheets, articles, and links. Grant information and application materials are also supplied.

Multiple Myeloma Research Web Server ⊙ ⊙ ⊙

http://myeloma.med.cornell.edu

The Weill Medical College of Cornell University provides this useful database. The site offers information for patients, families, and professionals. Extensive information is provided concerning research, proceedings from recent relevant meetings, and multiple myeloma PDQ clinical trials. A lecture and case presentations section for second year medical students is offered. There is a myeloma chat room and a listing of newsgroups.

Myeloma Alphabet Soup Handbook ⊙ ⊙ ⊙

http://www.escapepod.com/myeloma

An information clearinghouse for patients, this site offers medical information that has been simplified into language suitable for the general public. There is information about research, pharmaceuticals, seminar notes, transplants, support groups, discussion groups, and more.

Myeloma Central ◎ ◎
http://members.home.net/vincentvr/myeloma.htm

A private physician's site that provides information to professionals and patients, Myeloma Central offers links, an FAQ, and select articles. In addition, there is an enormous listing of offline references for professionals.

Wheeless' Textbook of
Orthopedics: Multiple Myeloma ◎ ◎ ◎
http://www.medmedia.com/o6/129.htm

This detailed educational resource for professionals and students provides text descriptions with X-ray images. Topics of discussion include prognosis, clinical presentation, radiographic studies, lab studies, skeletal histology, survey, and treatment.

Waldenstrom's Macroglobulimnemia

International Waldenstrom's
Macroglobulinemia Foundation (IWMF) ◎ ◎
http://www.iwmf.com

This site provides medical information for the public and patients, a newsletter, and support information. There is also information about chapters of the IWMF and membership, and contact information. There are twelve national and two international chapters of the IWMF.

9.19 Urological Cancers

General Resources

American Foundation for Urologic Disease (AFUD) ◎ ◎
http://www.afud.org

The AFUD Web site offers information for a variety of urologic diseases including prostate cancer. The organization provides information for patients, the public, and professionals, and maintains health councils for each disorder area. Information concerning research, education, advocacy, membership, conditions, and the organization is available.

American Urological Association (AUA) ◎ ◎

http://www.auanet.org

This site of the AUA details information about the organization, publications, guidelines, events, managed care issues, education, member services, and the AUA annual meeting. The education section offers a residency program database and details of home study and other CME programs. A Web forum has restricted access for members. A section for the public offers disorder, general urology, and member information.

Johns Hopkins Medical Institutions:
Brady Urological Institute ◎ ◎ ◎

http://prostate.urol.jhu.edu

The institute provides patient care for all adult and pediatric urological disorders. Care is offered for prostate cancer, bladder cancer, renal cell carcinoma, testes cancer, reconstructive surgery, and other needs. Research is conducted in many areas of basic science, therapy, diagnostics, and heredity. The site offers information about services, programs, professional education programs, news, research programs, staff, and individual disorders. There is information about interstitial radiotherapy and cancer risk after prostate removal.

Patient Advocates for
Advanced Cancer Treatments, Inc. ◎ ◎

http://www.osz.com/paact

A nonprofit organization that provides support and advocacy for prostate cancer patients, this Web site offers a newsletter, contact information, links and information about detection, diagnosis, evaluation, and treatment of prostate cancer.

Urology Handouts ◎ ◎

http://www.ucihs.uci.edu/surgery/newpage22.htm

This page is from the University of California, Irvine Web site and offers a medical reference for professionals or students. Topics covered are scrotum cancer, penis cancer, kidney cancer, transitional cell cancer, and cancer of the testis. Details concerning diagnosis, evaluation, staging, treatment, and prognosis are offered.

UrologyChannel ◎ ◎ ◎

http://www.urologychannel.com

This site is a comprehensive resource site for urology disorders. Sections of the site are devoted to bladder cancer, kidney cancer, the prostate, upper tract tumors, uretheral/penile cancer, and testicular cancer. From this site, one can participate in a variety of live chats, learn of news and research, locate physicians, or ask questions directly to physicians. There are online educational videos, educational tools, and listings of patient associations, support groups, clinical trials, and events.

Uronet ⊙ ⊙ ⊙ (free registration)

http://www.uronet.org

A comprehensive prostate, bladder, and kidney cancer education, information, and discussion resource for professionals and patients, the site is provided by AstraZeneca Pharmaceuticals. It offers details of current controversies, research, publications, case studies, news, meeting reports and links in a pleasing and easy to navigate site. The URO Challenge section supplies questions and answers for professionals to test their urology/prostate cancer knowledge. A visual library provides sketches and other illustrations that are updated frequently. A free registration is required to access this service.

Uroweb ⊙ ⊙ ⊙

http://www.uroweb.org

The Uroweb service is for professionals and offers professionally screened information about all fields of urology. Topics such as urinary tract infections, benign prostatic hyperplasia, urological oncology, prostate cancer, bladder cancer, kidney and testis cancer, neurological urology, and pediatric urology are discussed. There is information about research, clinical trials, publications, and individual cancers. Some information is oriented towards the public. There is a specific link for oncology information.

Us Too International, Inc. ⊙ ⊙ ⊙

http://www.ustoo.com

A nonprofit group, Us Too seeks to raise awareness, supply political advocacy, provide education and support, and supply the latest information regarding trials and treatment. Information available at the Us Too site is updated frequently and is categorized under publications, treatment, clinical trials, advocacy, and links. Information about upcoming prostate cancer meetings and a calendar of upcoming events is provided along with contact information for support chapters located in nearly every state. This informative site is very easy to navigate and is linked to the Us Too Partners section wihch has support information for the partners of patients.

Bladder Cancer

Bladder Cancer WebCafe ⊙ ⊙ ⊙

http://webcafe.gi.nl

This is a resource site that provides information and links to sites about drug resistance tests, biomarkers, investigations, chemoprevention, gene therapy, superficial bladder cancer, and alternatives. There is an e-mail discussion list, extensive information for the newly diagnosed, and a list of references.

M. D. Anderson Cancer Center: Bladder Cancer ⊙ ⊙
http://www.mdanderson.org/~canprev/tlcf/tlchtml/bladder.html

Four links to resources on bladder cancer are available at this site. Visitors can find a patient's guide to bladder cancer from the Netherlands, general urology information, including anatomical illustrations, and information on bladder biopsy, bladder stones, and irritable bladder.

National Bladder Foundation (NBF) ⊙ ⊙
http://www.bladder.org

The NBF supports research and provides information for all bladder diseases. The site provides information concerning research, legislation, statistics, allied organizations, and the urology industry. There is a link to the *Digital Urology Journal*.

National Cancer Institute (NCI): PDQ, Bladder Cancer ⊙ ⊙ ⊙
http://cancernet.nci.nih.gov/clinpdq/soa/Bladder_cancer_Physician.html

Statistics on bladder cancer, most common presentations of the disease, and factors determining general prognosis are explained at this address. Detailed information relates to cellular classification, disease stages, and treatment options. Discussions of treatments specific to each disease stage, including recurrent bladder cancer, are also presented. Academic article citations supporting this information are found at the site.

University of Newcastle upon Tyne: Bladder Cancer ⊙ ⊙ ⊙
http://www.ncl.ac.uk/child-health/guides/clinks3d.htm

This Internet directory of bladder cancer resources includes 10 links for patients and the general public and 12 links for health professionals and researchers. Online patient education booklets, support groups, academic departments, genetic information, professional information sources, article citations and abstracts, and clinical trials resources are found at this address.

UrologyChannel: Bladder Cancer ⊙ ⊙ ⊙
http://www.urologychannel.com/bladdercancer/types.shtml

Detailed discussions of each type of bladder cancer are discussed at this site, including transitional cell carcinomas (papillary and carcinoma in situ), non-transitional cell carcinomas (squamous cell carcinoma and adenocarcinoma), and undifferentiated carcinoma. Visitors will also find information on the main causes of the disease, treatment, diagnosis, and disease staging.

Kidney Cancer

California Kidney Cancer Center (CKCC) ◎ ◎
http://www.ckcc.org

The CKCC is funded by a nonprofit associate agency, the California Kidney Cancer Foundation. The CKCC conducts research in the area of immunotherapy and information about research, treatment, and clinical protocols is available. For patients, there is basic information and listings of information pages at other sites.

Diagnostic and Interventional Radiology of Hepatocellular Carcinoma ◎ ◎ ◎
http://www.rad.unipi.it/works/hcc/presentation-hcc.html

The Department of Oncology at the University of Pisa in Italy is responsible for this research paper entitled "Diagnostic and Interventional Radiology of Hepatocellular Carcinoma." The table of contents which describes this paper includes an introduction, detection and characterization, staging workup, treatment strategy, follow-up of treated tumors, references, and authors. The entire document is accompanied by images and links to select areas that are discussed.

Kidney Cancer Association (KCA) ◎ ◎ ◎
http://www.nkca.org

The KCA is composed of and provides information for physicians, patients, family members and researchers. The site details membership, drug trials, research, public policy, disorders, patient meetings, and annual convention information. The site has online chat sessions and a mailing list. There is also information about current financial grants and past recipients.

Kidney Cancer Links ◎
http://www2.kumc.edu/kci/cancerlinks/kidney.htm

Nine links to Internet resources on kidney cancer are found at this site. Visitors will find a link to an introduction to the disease, fact sheets, treatment information, an online support group, and a foundation for research.

Prostate Cancer

American Prostate Society ◎ ◎ ◎
http://www.ameripros.org

This society provides patient and professional information for all diseases of the prostate including enlarged prostate, prostatitis, and cancer. There are sections regarding these disorders as well as conferences, the society mission, professional abstracts, and membership information. An online newsletter is also available.

Man to Man Prostate Cancer Education and Support Program ⊙ ⊙ ⊙

http://www.cancer.org/m2m/m2m.html

This program works in partnership, and shares some resources with the American Cancer Society (ACS). The Man to Man site has information on 155 group education and support programs, visitation and telephone support, and program goals and affiliations. Online patient education materials detail incontinence, other publications, and other sites. There are archived and current newsletters.

Prostate Cancer Answers ⊙ ⊙ ⊙

http://www.medsch.wisc.edu/pca

Provided by the University of Wisconsin Comprehensive Cancer Center, the site offers a wealth of information concerning prostate cancer research, prevention, detection, diagnosis, and treatment. There are links, listings of clinical trials, and an FAQ section.

Prostate Cancer InfoLink ⊙ ⊙ ⊙

http://www.comed.com/Prostate/index.html

A part of the CoMed Communications Internet Healthcare Forum, this site provides a medley of information concerning prostate cancer that includes recent news, clinical reviews, information surrounding treatment options, lists of clinical trials, and lists of U.S. clinics and cancer centers. There are also discussion sections where patients can ask questions and view question/answer sessions of others.

Prostate Cancer Research and Education Foundation (PC-REF) ⊙ ⊙ ⊙

http://www.prostatecancer.com

The organization that provides this site seeks to promote public education and to conduct research for prevention, therapy, and diagnosis. The site offers a discussion forum and information about prostate cancer, research, support resources, the organization, events, and links. Some areas of research are cryosurgery/immunology, prostate cancer vaccine, photodynamic laser therapy, and nutrition.

Prostate Pointers ⊙ ⊙ ⊙

http://www.prostatepointers.org/prostate

This site is a link and information resource for a variety of prostate cancer topics. The links are organized by category and are listed under topics such as abstracts, alternate ideas, biopsy, blood tests, clinical trials, cryosurgery, education, hormone therapy, and more.

PROSTATEinfo.com ◎ ◎ ◎

http://www.prostateinfo.com

The site offers extensive information for patients and professionals about the disease as well as news, products, educational information, and support. For professionals, the site offers treatment details, relevant associations listings, a prostate cancer management slide library, patient counseling information, and study data. Patients can find support group details and treatment, diagnosis, and disorder information. The site is sponsored by the AstraZeneca corporation.

University of Michigan Prostate Cancer Homepage ◎ ◎ ◎

http://www.cancer.med.umich.edu/prostcan/prostcan.html

The University of Michigan site serves as a comprehensive information and education resource for prostate cancer. There is content concerning diagnosis, staging, treatment options, specialists, current research, and clinical trials. There are articles, support group details, and descriptions of the University of Michigan Prostate Cancer Genetics Project.

Virgil's Prostate Online ◎ ◎

http://www.prostate-online.com

This centralized forum supplies links to other information sources, search engines, medical sites, support services, journals, medical societies, prostate cancer news sources, and more. Links are organized by topic with introductory information about each topic.

Testicular Cancer

National Cancer Institute (NCI): PDQ, Testicular Cancer ◎ ◎ ◎

http://cancernet.nci.nih.gov/clinpdq/soa/Testicular_cancer_Physician.html

Comprehensive professional resources on testicular cancer and its treatment are available at this address. A general discussion of the disease, diagnosis, treatment, and prognosis is followed by more specific resources. Cellular classification, disease stages, and treatment options are detailed. Treatments specific to each disease stage are also found at the site. Information is supported with academic article citations.

Testicular Cancer Resource Center ◎ ◎ ◎

http://www.acor.org/TCRC

A comprehensive resource, this site offers information about the disorder, self-exam, orchiectomy, radiation therapy, alternative treatments, laparoscopic techniques, extragonadal germ cell cancer, fertility, and more. The site offers excerpts from interviews with physicians, personal stories, support groups listings, and a virtual library. The library offers patient and physician information and a massive number of links. For professionals, there are specific sections for medical articles, case studies, tumor markers, extragonadal germ cell tumors, pictures, and urology.

Testis Cancer Tutorial   ⊙ ⊙ ⊙

http://www.uchsc.edu/sm/medonc/testorial/testis.html

The site provides a text and image-based tutorial for physicians that covers epidemiology, diagnosis, histology, tumor markers, staging, prognosis, therapy-stage A, therapy-advanced, and late complications.

Wilms' Tumor

National Cancer Institute (NCI): PDQ, Wilms' Tumor   ⊙ ⊙ ⊙

http://cancernet.nci.nih.gov/clinpdq/soa/Wilms'_tumor_Physician.html

The nature, causes, diagnosis, classification, prognosis, and treatment of Wilms' tumor, a rare renal carcinoma in children, are offered at this site. Resources include cellular classifications, disease stage definitions, and an overview of treatment options. Treatment discussions specific to each stage of the disease are available. All information is supported with research article citations.

National Wilms' Tumor Study Group (NWTSG)   ⊙ ⊙

http://www.nwtsg.org

NWTSG is a federally funded group that studies patients with Wilms' Tumor to better treat those with the disorder and to determine its causes. The study group is a collaboration of professionals of a variety of specialties from various institutions. The site offers information about the NWTSG and committee members as well as frequently-asked questions (FAQs).

PART TWO

GENERAL MEDICAL WEB RESOURCES

10. REFERENCE INFORMATION AND NEWS SOURCES

10.1 **Abstract, Citation, and Full-text Search Tools**

Doctor Felix's Free MEDLINE Page ◎ ◎
http://www.beaker.iupui.edu/drfelix/index.html

This site, a useful resource for those interested in performing MEDLINE searches for article citations, offers links to sites providing free MEDLINE access to visitors. More than thirty sites are profiled, with information on database coverage, frequency of updates, registration requirements, usage restrictions, document delivery information, and links to additional information on the site. Miscellaneous sources for full MED-LINE access trial periods are also listed.

Infomine: Scholarly Internet Resources ◎ ◎ ◎
http://infomine.ucr.edu/search/bioagsearch.phtml

Infomine offers searchable biological, agricultural, and medical resource collections. Web sites can be browsed by title of resource, subject and title, subject, and keyword. Recently added sites are stored in a separate section. The site also offers links to additional Internet medical resources.

Internet Grateful Med (IGM)
at the National Library of Medicine (NLM) ◎ ◎ ◎
http://igm.nlm.nih.gov

Internet Grateful Med (IGM) is one of the two NLM-sponsored free MEDLINE search systems. The default MEDLINE search includes articles published from 1966 to the present and includes PreMEDLINE. This version of IGM takes advantage of PubMed's ability to display related articles and links to the full text of participating online journals. Other searchable databases include AIDSLINE, AIDSDRUGS, AIDSTRIALS, BIOETHICSLINE, ChemID, DIRLINE, HealthSTAR, HISTLINE, HSRPROJ, OLDMEDLINE, POPLINE, SDILINE, SPACELINE, and TOXLINE. The site also offers a user's guide and specific information on new features of the site.

MEDLINE/PubMed at the National Library of Medicine (NLM) ◎ ◎ ◎
http://www.ncbi.nlm.nih.gov/PubMed

PubMed is a free MEDLINE search service providing access to 11 million citations with links to the full text of articles of participating journals. Probably the most heavily used and reputable free MEDLINE site, PubMed permits advanced searching by subject, author, journal title, and many other fields. It includes an easy-to-use "citation matcher" for completing and identifying references, and its PreMEDLINE database provides journal citations before they are indexed, making this version of MEDLINE more up-to-date than most.

10.2 Daily Medical News Sites

1st Headlines: Health ⊙ ⊙ ⊙

http://www.1stheadlines.com/health1.htm

This medical news information site offers a keyword search engine for access to nationwide health news derived from seventy-one daily publications and reputable broadcast and online networks, including USA Today's Health section, Reuters Health, MSNBC, and drKoop.com. News coverage includes treatment discoveries, pharmacological updates, the latest in managed care, product recalls, and hundreds of other breaking news bulletins.

Doctor's Guide to Medical and Other News ⊙ ⊙ ⊙

http://www.pslgroup.com/MEDNEWS.HTM

This site provides very current medical news and information for health professionals. Visitors can search the Doctor's Guide Medical News Database, and access medical news broadcast within the past week or the past month. News items organized by subject, firsthand conference communiqués, and journal club reviews are also available at this informative news site.

Health News from CNN ⊙ ⊙ ⊙

http://www.cnn.com/HEALTH

Health News from CNN is produced in association with WebMD. Specific articles are available in featured topics, ethics matters, research, and home remedies, and an allergy report is also provided. National and international health news is presented, and users can access specific articles on AIDS, aging, alternative medicine, cancer, children's health, diet and fitness, men's health, and women's health. Visitors can also access patient questions and answers of doctors, chat forums, and special community resources available through WebMD. Information and articles are also offered by Mayo Clinic and AccentHealth.com.

Medical Breakthroughs ⊙ ⊙ ⊙

http://www.ivanhoe.com/#reports

This site delivers daily News Flash Updates to your e-mail box. A fee of US$15 per quarter is required for receipt of bulletins on pending medical breakthroughs. Visitors can also search archived articles by keyword, read weekly general interest articles, find links to related sites, and watch videos related to current health issues. The site is sponsored by Ivanhoe Broadcast News, Inc., a medical news gathering organization providing stories to television stations nationwide.

Medical Tribune ⊙ ⊙ ⊙

http://www.medtrib.com

Daily medical news for health professionals is available at this site, and users can search archives for specific articles. The MD CyberGuide at the site describes and rates top medical Web sites, a valuable resource for physicians new to the Internet. Results of recent polls of physicians on many health topics and questions unrelated to health; clinical quizzes; a bulletin board; chat forums; and contact details are available at this informative site.

Reuters Health ⊙ ⊙ (some features fee-based)

http://www.reutershealth.com

Reuters provides an excellent site for breaking medical news, updated daily, as well as a subscription-based searchable database of the News Archives of Reuters News Service. Visitors can access MEDLINE from the site. Group subscribers have access to a database of drug information.

Science News Update ⊙ ⊙

http://www.ama-assn.org/sci-pubs/sci-news/1997/pres_rel.htm

This weekly online publication provides users with the Journal of the American Medical Association reports and a list of previous news releases. Visitors can also access site updates, search the site for specific articles, register for e-mail alerts of new issues, read classified advertisements, and find information on print subscriptions, reprints, and advertising rates.

This Week's Top Medical News Stories ⊙ ⊙ ⊙

http://www.newsfile.com/topcwh.htm

Conference coverage reports and summaries of recent research findings are available at this site from weekly online publications devoted to news such as HIV/AIDS, Alzheimer's disease, angiogenesis, blood products, cancer, gene therapy, genomics and genetics, CDC activities, hepatitis, immunotherapy, obesity, pain management, proteomics, transplants, tuberculosis and airborne diseases, vaccines, women's health, and world disease issues.

UniSci: Daily University Science News ⊙ ⊙

http://unisci.com

This site offers current articles related to all branches of science, including medicine. Many medical articles are available, and special archives offer additional medical resources. Users can access news from the past 10 days and perform searches for archived material.

USA Today: Health ☢ ☢ ☢

http://www.usatoday.com/life/health/archive.htm

USA Today's feature stories and headline archives are directly accessible at this Web site where visitors can view some of the best in nationwide medical news coverage. Interesting articles include the safety of online pharmacies, news on unconventional remedies, and genetic research and discoveries. Visitors will also find the latest in groundbreaking medical and pharmacotherapuetic research.

Yahoo! News: Health Headlines ☢ ☢ ☢

http://dailynews.yahoo.com/headlines/hl

Updated several times throughout the day, Health Headlines at Yahoo! offers full news coverage and Reuters News with top health headlines from around the globe. Earlier daily and archived stories may be accessed, and the site's powerful search engine allows viewers to browse, with full color, the latest in photographic coverage of news and events.

10.3 General Medical Supersites

American Medical Association (AMA) ☢ ☢ ☢

http://www.ama-assn.org

The AMA develops and promotes standards in medical practice, research, and education; acts as advocate on behalf of patients and physicians; and provides discourse on matters important to public health in America. General information is available at the site about the organization; journals and newsletters; policy, advocacy activities, and ethics; education; and accreditation services. AMA news and consumer health information are also found at the site. Resources for physicians include membership details, information on AMA CPT/RBRVS Electronic Medical Systems, Y2K information and preparation suggestions, AMA Alliance information (a national organization of physicians' spouses), descriptions of additional AMA products and services, a discussion of legal issues for physicians, and information on AMA's global activities. Links are provided to AMA member special interest groups for physicians and students. Information for consumers includes medical news; detailed information on a wide range of conditions; general health topic discussions; family health resources for children, adolescents, men, and women; interactive health calculators; healthy recipes; and general safety tips. Specific pages are devoted to comprehensive resources related to HIV/AIDS, asthma, migraines, and women's health. Healthcare providers and patients will find this site an excellent source for accurate and useful health information.

BioSites ⊙ ⊙ ⊙

http://www.library.ucsf.edu/biosites

BioSites is a comprehensive catalog of selected Internet resources in the Biomedical Sciences. The sites were selected as part of a project by staff members of Resource Libraries within the Pacific Southwest Region of the National Network of Libraries of Medicine. Sites are organized by medical topic or specialty field, and users can also search the site by keyword. Featured Web sites are listed by title, but detailed descriptions are not provided.

Centerwatch ⊙ ⊙ ⊙

http://www.centerwatch.com/main.htm

This clinical trials listing service offers patient resources, including a listing of clinical trials by disease category, links to current NIH trials, listings of new FDA drug therapy approvals, and current research headlines. Background information on clinical research is also available to patients unfamiliar with the clinical trials process. Industry professional resources include research center profiles, industry provider profiles, industry news, and career and educational opportunities. Links to related sites of interest to patients and professionals are available at the site.

Health On the Net (HON) Foundation ⊙ ⊙ ⊙

http://www.hon.ch

The Health On the Net Foundation is a nonprofit organization advancing the development and application of new information technologies, notably in the fields of health and medicine. This site offers an engine that searches the Internet as well as the Foundation's database for medical sites, hospitals, and support communities. A media gallery contains a searchable database of medical images and videos from various sources. The site also features a list of online journals, articles and abstracts, and papers from conferences and various other medical sources. The HON MeSH tool allows you to browse Medical Subject Headings (MeSH), a hierarchical structure of medical concepts from the National Library of Medicine (NLM). Users can select a target group (healthcare providers, medical professionals, or patients and other individuals) to receive more tailored search results.

HealthGate.com ⊙ ⊙ ⊙

http://www.healthgate.com

HealthGate offers information resources and health-related articles for healthcare professionals and the general public. Health professional resources include links to research tools, including online journals, drug information, and medical search engines, Continuing Medical Education (CME) resources, news, and patient education materials. Resources for the general public and patients include articles on current health issues and advances, drug and vitamin information, symptoms and medical tests information, and several Webzines devoted to specific topics, including alternative medicine, fitness, nutrition, mental well-being, parenting, travel health, and sexuality. A joint effort of two medical publishers allows site access to full-text journal articles. Search engines allow users to search the site, MEDLINE, or a medical dictionary for information. The site provides users with a good starting point for medical information.

Medical Matrix ⚙ ⚙ ⚙ (free registration)
http://www.medmatrix.org/reg/login.asp
Medical Matrix offers a list of directories categorized into specialties, diseases, clinical practice resources, literature, education, healthcare and professional resources, medical computing, Internet and technology, and marketplace resources containing classifieds and employment opportunities. Additional features include a site search engine, access to MEDLINE, clinical searches, and links to symposia on the Web, medical textbook resources, patient education materials, Continuing Medical Education information, news, and online journals. Free registration is necessary to access the site.

MedNets ⚙ ⚙ ⚙
http://www.internets.com/mednets
This site houses a collection of proprietary search engines, searching only medical databases. Users can access search engines by medical specialty or disease topic. Other resources include links to the home pages of associations, journals, hospitals, companies, research, government sites, clinical practice guidelines, medical news, and consumer and patient information. The site also includes a set of medical databases and links to search engines provided on the Internet by medical schools.

Medscape ⚙ ⚙ ⚙ (free registration)
http://www.medscape.com
Medscape offers a searchable directory of specialty Web sites that provide information on a wide range of medical specialties. Registration is free, and users can customize the site's home page from a particular computer by choosing a medical specialty. Information in a personalized home page includes news items, conference summaries and schedules, treatment updates, practice guidelines, and patient resources, all pertaining to the chosen field of specialization. The site also includes clinical feature articles and links to special clinical resources.

Megasite Project: A Metasite Comparing Health Information Megasites and Search Engines ⚙ ⚙ ⚙
http://www.lib.umich.edu/megasite/toc.html
The Megasite Project, created by librarians at Northwestern University, the University of Michigan, and Pennsylvania State University, evaluates and provides links to 26 Internet sites providing health information. Criteria for evaluation and comparison include administration and quality control, content, and design. Users can access

results of site evaluations, tips for successful site searches, lists of the best general and health information search engines reviewed, and site comparisons listed by evaluation criteria. A bibliography of articles on Web design and Internet resource evaluation is found at the address, as well as descriptions of other aspects of the project.

National Library of Medicine (NLM) ⚙ ⚙ ⚙
http://www.nlm.nih.gov

The National Library of Medicine, the world's largest medical library, collects materials in all areas of biomedicine and healthcare, and works on biomedical aspects of technology; the humanities; and the physical, life, and social sciences. This site contains links to government medical databases, including MEDLINE and MEDLINE plus (for consumers); information on funding opportunities at the NLM and other federal agencies; and details of services, training, and outreach programs offered by NLM. Users can access NLM's catalog of resources (LocatorPlus), as well as NLM publications, including fact sheets, published reports, and staff publications. Also available are NLM announcements, news, exhibit information, and staff directories. NLM research programs discussed at the site include topics in Computational Molecular Biology, Medical Informatics, and other related subjects.

The Web site features 15 searchable databases, covering journal searches via MEDLINE, AIDS information via AIDSLINE, AIDSDRUGS, and AIDSTRIALS, bioethics via BIOETHICSLINE, and numerous other important topics. The "master search engine," nicknamed Internet Grateful Med (IGM), searches MEDLINE using the retrieval engine called PubMed. It is very user-friendly. There are 9 million citations among MEDLINE, PreMEDLINE, and other related databases.

Additionally, the NLM provides sources of health statistics, serials programs, and services maintained through a system called SERHOLD; medical images; international medical resources; and a searchable NLM staff directory.

WebMD ⚙ ⚙ ⚙ (some features fee-based)
http://www.webmd.com

High-quality consumer health information and resources for healthcare professionals are available at this address. Consumer resources include information on conditions, treatments, and drugs; medical news and articles on specific topics; a medical encyclopedia; drug reference resources; a forum for asking health questions; online chat events with medical experts; transcripts of past chat events; message boards; and articles and expert advice on general health topics. Consumers can also join a "community" for more personalized information and forums. Physicians services are available for a fee of US$29.95 monthly (in a twelve-month contract), and includes access to medical news, online journals, and reference databases; online insurance verification and referrals; e-mail, voice mail, fax, and conference call capabilities; practice management tools; online trading; financial services; and other resources. The site includes a preview tour of the service for interested professionals.

10.4 **Government Information Databases**

CRISP: Computer Retrieval of Information on Scientific Projects ◎ ◎ ◎
http://www-commons.cit.nih.gov/crisp

CRISP is a searchable database of federally-funded biomedical research projects conducted at universities, hospitals, and other research institutions. Users, including the public, can use CRISP to search for scientific concepts, emerging trends and techniques, or to identify specific projects and/or investigators. This site provides a direct gateway into the searchable database. The NIH funds the operation of CRISP.

Government Information Locator Service ◎ ◎ ◎
http://www.access.gpo.gov/su_docs/gils/gils.html

Intended to pool access to government information through one search engine, this federal locator service enables a search by topic in which the search word or phrase is placed in quotation markets. Instructions for searching are located at the site.

Healthfinder ◎ ◎ ◎
http://healthfinder.gov/moretools/libraries.htm

Healthfinder provides links to national medical libraries, such as the National Library of Medicine and the National Institutes of Health Library, and other medical or health sciences libraries on the Internet. Directories of libraries are also available to find local facilities. Visitors can use a site search engine to find specific health Web resources.

MEDLINEplus: Health Information Database ◎ ◎ ◎
http://www.nlm.nih.gov/medlineplus/medlineplus.html

A comprehensive database of health and medical information, MEDLINEplus serves a different purpose from its sister service, MEDLINE, which is a bibliographic search engine to locate citations and abstracts in medical journals and reports. MEDLINEplus offers the ability to search by topic and obtain full information rather than citations. The search engine brings up extensive resources on every possible topic, giving complete information on all aspects of the topic. One can search body systems, disorders and diseases, treatments and therapies, diagnostic procedures, side effects, and numerous other important topics related to personal health and the field of medicine in general.

10.5 **Government Organizations**

Government Agencies and Offices

Administration for Children and Families (ACF) ⊙ ⊙ ⊙
http://www.acf.dhhs.gov

This site provides descriptions of, resources for, and links to ACF programs and services. These sites detail programs and services that relate to areas such as welfare and family assistance, child support, foster care and adoption, Head Start, and support for Native Americans, refugees, and the developmentally disabled. Updated news and information is provided as well.

Administration on Aging ⊙ ⊙ ⊙
http://www.aoa.dhhs.gov

This site provides resources for seniors, practitioners, and caregivers. Resources include news on aging, links to Web sites on aging, statistics about older people, consumer fact sheets, retirement and financial planning information, and help finding community assistance for seniors.

Agency for Toxic Substances and Disease Registry ⊙ ⊙ ⊙
http://www.atsdr.cdc.gov/atsdrhome.html

The mission of this agency is "to prevent exposure and adverse human health effects and diminished quality of life associated with exposure to hazardous substances from waste sites, unplanned releases, and other sources of pollution present in the environment." Toward this goal, the site posts national alerts and health advisories. It provides answers to frequently asked questions about hazardous substances and lists the minimal risk levels for each of them. The site has a HazDat database developed to provide access to information on the release of hazardous substances from Superfund sites or from emergency events and on the effects of hazardous substances on the health of human populations. A quarterly Hazardous Substances and Public Health Newsletter is available for viewing on the site, as are additional resources for kids, parents, and teachers.

Center for Nutrition Policy and Promotion (CNPP) ⊙ ⊙ ⊙
http://www.usda.gov/cnpp

The Center for Nutrition Policy and Promotion is "the focal point within USDA where scientific research is linked with the nutritional needs of the American public." It provides statistical information and resources for educators, and contains dietary guidelines for Americans, official USDA food plans, and means to request additional publications and information by mail or phone.

Department of Health and Human Services (HHS) Homepage ⊙ ⊙ ⊙

http://www.os.dhhs.gov

This site lists HHS agencies and provides links to the individual agency sites. It offers news, press releases, and information on accessing HHS records and contacting HHS officials. It also provides a search engine for all federal HHS agencies and access to HealthFinder.

Epidemiology Program Office ⊙ ⊙ ⊙

http://www.cdc.gov/epo/index.htm

Information and resources on public health surveillance is available here. Publications and software related to epidemiology are available for download. Updated news, events, and international bulletins are also featured at the site.

Federal Web Locator ⊙ ⊙ ⊙

http://www.infoctr.edu/fwl

This is a useful search engine for links to federal government sites and information on the World Wide Web. Users can search agency names and access a table of contents.

Food and Nutrition Service (FNS) ⊙ ⊙ ⊙

http://www.fns.usda.gov/fns

The Food and Nutrition Service (FNS) "reduces hunger and food insecurity in partnership with cooperating organizations by providing children and needy families access to food, a healthful diet and nutrition education in a manner that supports American agriculture and inspires public confidence." The site provides details of FNS nutrition assistance programs such as Food Stamps, WIC, and Child Nutrition. Research, in the form of published studies and reports, is also made available at the site.

Food and Drug Administration (FDA) ⊙ ⊙ ⊙

http://www.fda.gov

The FDA is one of the oldest consumer protection agencies in the United States, monitoring the manufacture, import, transport, storage, and sale of about $1 trillion worth of products each year. This comprehensive site provides information on the safety of foods, human and animal drugs, blood products, cosmetics, and medical devices. The site also contains details of field operations, current regulations, toxicology research, medical products reporting procedures, and answers to frequently asked questions. Users can search the site by keyword and find specific information targeted to consumers, industry, health professionals, patients, state and local officials, women, and children.

Food Safety and Inspection Service ◎ ◎ ◎

http://www.fsis.usda.gov

The Food Safety and Inspection Service (FSIS) is "the public health agency in the U.S. Department of Agriculture responsible for ensuring that the nation's commercial supply of meat, poultry, and egg products are safe, wholesome, and correctly labeled and packaged." This site offers a description of the FSIS and their activities, and provides news, consumer information, publications, and resources for educators.

Government Printing Office (GPO) Access ◎ ◎ ◎

http://www.access.gpo.gov/su_docs

Formed by the Government Printing Office to facilitate the transition of electronic documents, this site is the central location for accessing documents from all three branches of the federal government. It provides free access to the official government versions of some 140,000 titles in plain text or PDF format. GPO Access also contains links to governmental databases, including the Federal Register, the Code of Federal Regulations, and the Congressional Record.

Healthcare Financing Administration ◎ ◎ ◎

http://www.hcfa.gov

Information on Medicare, Medicaid, and Child Health insurance programs is provided here. Statistical data on enrollment in the various programs as well as analysis of recent trends in healthcare spending, employment, and pricing is also provided. The site offers consumer publications and program forms, which are available for download.

Indian Health Service (IHS) ◎ ◎

http://www.ihs.gov

Indian Health Service (IHS) is an agency "within the U. S. Department of Health and Human Services and is responsible for providing federal health services to American Indians and Alaska Natives." This site offers related news and press releases. It details management resources, medical programs, jobs, scholarships, office locations, and contact information.

National Bioethics Advisory Commission (NBAC) ◎ ◎

http://bioethics.gov/cgi-bin/bioeth_counter.pl

NBAC "provides advice and makes recommendations to the National Science and Technology Council and to other appropriate government entities regarding the appropriateness of departmental, agency, or other governmental programs, policies, assignments, missions, guidelines, and regulations as they relate to bioethical issues arising from research on human biology and behavior." It also advises on the applications, including the clinical applications, of that research. This site lists meeting dates, transcripts of meetings, reports, news, and links to related sites.

National Center for Chronic Disease Prevention and Health Promotion ☺ ☺ ☺

http://www.cdc.gov/nccdphp/nccdhome.htm

This site "defines chronic disease, lists major chronic diseases, and describes the cost burden of treating them as well as the cost-effectiveness of prevention." Risk behaviors that lead to chronic disease are discussed, and comprehensive and disease-specific approaches to prevention of chronic diseases are addressed. The site provides access to selected Center reports, newsletters, brochures, and CD-ROMs. Information on conferences, meetings, and news publications is provided along with links to related sites.

National Center for Environmental Health (NCEH) ☺ ☺ ☺

http://www.cdc.gov/nceh/ncehhome.htm

The NCEH "is working to prevent illness, disability, and death from interactions between people and the environment." Site links and information on programs and activities are provided, and access is available to publications and products including NCEH fact sheets, brochures, books, and articles. The site also offers current employment opportunities and information on training programs. Spanish and young adult versions of the NCEH site are also available.

National Center for Health Statistics (NCHS) ☺ ☺ ☺

http://www.cdc.gov/nchs/default.htm

The National Center for Health Statistics (NCHS) is the foremost federal government agency responsible for gathering, analyzing, and disseminating health statistics on the American population." To accomplish the mission of the Center, the NCHS Web site has a site-based search engine and collections of health related statistics organized alphabetically by topic. frequently asked questions are answered on various statistical topics. Useful resources at the site include contact information for obtaining copies of vital records, related catalogs, publications, and other information products.

National Center for Infectious Diseases ☺ ☺ ☺

http://www.cdc.gov/ncidod/ncid.htm

The mission of the National Center for Infectious Diseases "is to prevent illness, disability, and death caused by infectious diseases in the United States and around the world." The site contains an online bimonthly journal that tracks trends and analyzes new and reemerging infectious disease issues around the world. Resources include general information on infectious diseases, specific infectious disease discussions and descriptions, and links to organizations, associations, journals, newsletters, and other publications. One section of the site is devoted to resources related to travel health.

National Center for Toxicological Research (NCTR) ◎ ◎

http://www.fda.gov/nctr/index.html

The mission of NCTR "is to conduct peer-reviewed scientific research that supports and anticipates the FDA's current and future regulatory needs." This research is aimed at understanding critical biological events in the expression of toxicity and at developing methods to improve assessment of human exposure, susceptibility, and risk. The site details the accomplishments, current programs, and future goals of the NCTR.

National Guideline Clearinghouse (NGC) ◎ ◎ ◎

http://www.guidelines.gov/index.asp

The National Guideline Clearinghouse (NGC) is a database of evidence-based clinical practice guidelines and related documents produced by the Agency for Health Care Policy and Research (AHCPR), in partnership with the American Medical Association (AMA) and the American Association of Health Plans (AAHP). Users can search the database by keyword or browse by disease category.

National Institute for Occupational Safety and Health (NIOSH) ◎ ◎ ◎

http://www.cdc.gov/niosh/homepage.html

NIOSH "is part of the Centers for Disease Control and Prevention and is the only federal institute responsible for conducting research and making recommendations for the prevention of work-related illnesses and injuries." The site contains updated news, listings of special events and programs, and information on downloading or ordering related publications. It also provides access to databases such as a pocket guide to hazardous chemicals and a topic index of occupational safety and health information.

National Science Foundation, Directorate for Biological Sciences ◎ ◎ ◎

http://www.nsf.gov/bio/ibn/start.htm

The Division of Integrative Biology and Neuroscience (IBN) supports research aimed at understanding the living organism—plant, animal, microbe—as a unit of biological organization. Current scientific emphases include biotechnology, biomolecular materials, environmental biology, global change, biodiversity, molecular evolution, plant science, microbial biology, and computational biology (including modeling). Research projects generally include support for the education and training of future scientists.

IBN also supports doctoral dissertation research, research conferences, workshops, symposia, Undergraduate Mentoring in Environmental Biology (UMEB), and a variety of NSF-wide activities. This site describes in detail the activities and divisions of IBN, and offers a staff directory, award listings, and deadline dates for funding applications.

Office of National Drug Control Policy (ONDCP) ⊙ ⊙ ⊙

http://www.whitehousedrugpolicy.gov

This site states the missions and goals of the ONDCP. It has a clearinghouse of drug policy information with a staff that will respond to the needs of the general public, providing statistical data, topical fact sheets, information packets and more. There is information on related science, medicine, and technology. There are also resources on prevention, education, and treatment programs. Information on the enforcement of the policies is provided for the national, state, and local levels.

Office of Naval Research—Human Systems Department ⊙ ⊙

http://www.onr.navy.mil/sci_tech/personnel/default.htm#biological

This site details Medical Science and Technology, and the Cognitive and Neural Science and Technology programs of the Human Systems Department. Procedures for submitting proposals are also outlined at the site.

Public Health Service (PHS) ⊙ ⊙

http://phs.os.dhhs.gov/phs/phs.html

Links to public health service agencies and program offices, and Health and Human Services vacancy announcements are available at this site. The site is linked to the Office of the Surgeon General, providing transcripts of speeches and reports, a biography of the current Surgeon General, and a history and summary of duties associated with the position.

Substance Abuse and Mental Health Services Administration ⊙ ⊙ ⊙

http://www.samhsa.gov

The Substance Abuse and Mental Health Services Administration "is the federal agency charged with improving the quality and availability of prevention, treatment, and rehabilitation services in order to reduce illness, death, disability, and cost to society resulting from substance abuse and mental illnesses." The site provides substance abuse and mental health information, including details of programs for prevention and treatment in these areas, updated news and statistics, and notices of grant opportunities.

NIH Institutes and Centers

Center for Information Technology (CIT) ⊙ ⊙ ⊙

http://www.cit.nih.gov/home.asp

The Center for Information Technology incorporates the power of modern computers into the biomedical programs and administrative procedures of the NIH by conducting computational biosciences research, developing computer systems, and providing computer facilities. The site provides information on activities and the organization of the Center, contact information, resources for Macintosh users, and links to many useful Information Technology sites. Users can search the site or the CIT Help Desk Knowledgebase for specific information.

Center for Scientific Review (CSR) ◉ ◉ ◉
http://www.drg.nih.gov

The Center for Scientific Review is the focal point at NIH for the conduct of initial peer review, which is the foundation of the NIH grant and award process. The Center carries out a peer review of the majority of research and research training applications submitted to the NIH. The Center also serves as the central receipt point for all such Public Health Service applications and makes referrals to scientific review groups for scientific and technical merit review of applications and to funding components for potential award. To this end, the Center develops and implements innovative, flexible ways to conduct referral and review for all aspects of science. The site contains contact information, transcripts of public commentary panel discussions, news and events listings, grant applications, peer review notes, and links to additional biomedical and government sites.

Centers for Disease Control and Prevention (CDC) ◉ ◉ ◉
http://www.cdc.gov

The mission of the Centers for Disease Control and Prevention is to promote health and quality of life by preventing and controlling disease, injury, and disability. The site provides users with links to 11 associated Centers, Institutes, and Offices; a Web page devoted to travelers' health; publications; software; and other products, data, and statistics; training and employment opportunities; and subscription registration forms for online CDC publications. Highlighted publications include *Emerging Infectious Disease Journal* and *Morbidity and Mortality Weekly Report,* both of which can be e-mailed on a regular basis by registering on this site. Links are available to additional CDC resources, and state and local agencies concerned with public health issues. CDC offers a comprehensive, alphabetical list of general and specific health topics at the site. Visitors can also search the site by keyword, and read spotlights on current research and information presented by the Web site.

Computer Database for Scientific Topics ◉ ◉ ◉
http://www-commons.cit.nih.gov/crisp

CRISP (Computer Retrieval of Information on Scientific Projects) is a comprehensive compilation of abstracts describing the federally-funded research projects of academic, healthcare, and research institutions. The database, maintained by the Office of Extramural Research at the National Institutes of Health, includes projects funded by many of the major government agencies, such as the National Institutes of Health (NIH), the Food and Drug Administration (FDA), and the Centers for Disease Control and Prevention (CDCP). Visitors to the site can use the CRISP search interface to identify emerging research trends and techniques, or locate specific projects and/or investigators. General information about the CRISP database and answers to frequently asked questions about CRISP are also available.

Fogarty International Center (FIC) ◎ ◎ ◎

http://www.nih.gov/fic

The Fogarty International Center for Advanced Study in the Health Sciences leads NIH efforts to advance the health of the American public, and citizens of all nations, through international cooperation on global health threats. Resources at the site include Center publications, regional information on programs and contacts, research and training opportunities, a description of the Center's Multilateral Initiative on Malaria (MIM), details of the NIH Visiting Program for Foreign Scientists, and news and vacancy announcements.

Introduction to the National Institutes of Health (NIH) ◎ ◎ ◎

http://www.nih.gov

NIH is one of eight health agencies of the Public Health Service which, in turn, is part of the U.S. Department of Health and Human Services. The NIH mission is to uncover new knowledge that will lead to better health for everyone. NIH works toward that mission by conducting research in its own laboratories; supporting the research of non-federal scientists in universities, medical schools, hospitals, and research institutions throughout the country and abroad; helping in the training of research investigators; and fostering communication of biomedical information. The site provides a Director's message about the agency, e-mail and telephone directories, visitor information, employment and summer internship program information, science education program details, and a history of NIH. A site search engine and links to the home pages of all NIH Institutes and Centers are available.

National Cancer Institute (NCI) ◎ ◎ ◎

http://www.nci.nih.gov

The National Cancer Institute leads a national effort to reduce the burden of cancer morbidity and mortality, and ultimately to prevent the disease. Through basic and clinical biomedical research and training, the NCI conducts and supports programs to understand the causes of cancer; prevent, detect, diagnose, treat, and control cancer; and disseminate information to the practitioner, patient, and public. The site provides visitors with many informational resources related to cancer, including CancerTrials for clinical trials resources and CancerNet for information on cancer tailored to the needs of health professionals, patients, and the general public. Additional resources relate to funding opportunities, and events and research at NCI.

National Center for Biotechnology Information (NCBI) ⊙ ⊙ ⊙

http://www.ncbi.nlm.nih.gov

A comprehensive site that provides a wide array of biotechnology resources to the user, the NCBI includes sources such as a genetic sequence database (GenBank); links to related sites, a newsletter, site and genetic sequence search engines; information on programs, activities, and research projects; seminar and exhibit schedules; and database services. Databases available through this site include PubMed (for free MEDLINE searching) and OMIM (Online Mendelian Inheritance in Man) for an extensive catalog of human genes and genetic disorders.

National Center for Complementary and Alternative Medicine (NCCAM) ⊙ ⊙ ⊙

http://nccam.nih.gov

The National Center for Complementary and Alternative Medicine identifies and evaluates unconventional healthcare practices, supports, coordinates, and conducts research and research training on these practices, and disseminates information. The site describes specific program areas; answers common questions about alternative therapies; and offers news, research grants information, and a calendar of events. Information resources at the site include a citation index related to alternative medicine obtained from MEDLINE, a bibliography of publications; the NCCAM clearinghouse of information for the public, media, and healthcare professionals; and a link to the National Women's Health Information Center (NWHIC).

National Center for Research Resources (NCRR) ⊙ ⊙

http://www.ncrr.nih.gov

The National Center for Research Resources creates, develops, and provides a comprehensive range of human, animal, technological, and other resources to support biomedical research advances. The Center's areas of concentration are biomedical technology, clinical research, comparative medicine, and research infrastructure. The site offers more specific information on each of these research areas, grants information, news, current events, press releases, publications, research resources, and a search engine for locating information at the site.

National Eye Institute (NEI) ⊙ ⊙ ⊙

http://www.nei.nih.gov:80

The National Eye Institute conducts and supports research, training, health information dissemination, and other programs with respect to blinding eye diseases, visual disorders, mechanisms of visual function, preservation of sight, and the special health problems and requirements of the visually impaired. Information at the site is tailored to the needs of researchers, health professionals, the general public and patients, educators, and the media. Resources include a clinical trials database, intramural research information, funding, grants, contract information, news and events calendar, publications, visitor information, a site search engine, and an overview of the NEI offices, divisions, branches, and laboratories.

National Heart, Lung, and Blood Institute (NHLBI) ⊙ ⊙ ⊙

http://www.nhlbi.nih.gov

The National Heart, Lung, and Blood Institute provides leadership for a national research program in diseases of the heart, blood vessels, lungs, and blood, and in transfusion medicine through support of innovative basic, clinical, and population-based and health education research. The site provides health information, scientific resources, research funding information, news and press releases, details of committees, meetings and events, clinical guidelines, notices of studies seeking patient participation, links to laboratories at the NHLBI, and technology transfer resources. Highlights of the site include cholesterol, weight, and asthma management resources.

National Human Genome Research Institute (NHGRI) ⊙ ⊙ ⊙

http://www.nhgri.nih.gov

The National Human Genome Research Institute supports the NIH component of the Human Genome Project, a worldwide research effort designed to analyze the structure of human DNA and determine the location of the estimated 50,000–100,000 human genes. The NHGRI Intramural Research Program develops and implements technology for understanding, diagnosing, and treating genetic diseases. The site provides information about NHGRI, the Human Genome Project, grants, intramural research, policy and public affairs, workshops and conferences, and news items. Resources include links to the Institute's Ethical, Legal, and Social Implications Program and the Center for Inherited Disease Research, genomic and genetic resources for investigators, a glossary of genetic terms, and a site search engine.

National Institute of Allergy and Infectious Diseases (NIAID) ⊙ ⊙ ⊙

http://www.niaid.nih.gov

NIAID provides the major support for scientists conducting research aimed at developing better ways to diagnose, treat, and prevent the many infectious, immunologic, and allergic diseases that afflict people worldwide. This site provides NIAID news releases, contact information, calendar of events, links to related sites, a clinical trials database, grants and technology transfer information, and current research information (including meetings, publications, and research resources). Fact sheets for public use are available for different immunological disorders, allergies, asthma, and infectious diseases.

National Institute of
Arthritis and Musculoskeletal and Skin Diseases (NIAMS) ◉ ◉ ◉

http://www.nih.gov/niams

The NIAMS conducts and supports a broad spectrum of research on normal structure and function of bones, muscles, and skin, as well as the numerous and disparate diseases that affect these tissues. NIAMS also conducts research training and epidemiologic studies, and disseminates information. The site provides details of research programs at the Institute and offers personnel and employment listings, news, and an events calendar. Health information at the site is provided in the form of fact sheets, brochures, health statistics, and other resources, and contact details are available for ordering materials. Scientific resources include bibliographies of publications, consensus conference reports, grants and contracts applications, grant program announcements, and links to scientific research databases. Information on current clinical studies and transcripts of NIAMS advisory council, congressional, and conference reports are also available at the site.

National Institute of
Child Health and Human Development (NICHD) ◉ ◉ ◉

http://www.nichd.nih.gov

The NICHD conducts and supports laboratory, clinical, and epidemiological research on the reproductive, neurobiologic, developmental, and behavioral processes that determine and maintain the health of children, adults, families, and populations. Research in the areas of fertility, pregnancy, growth, development, and medical rehabilitation strives to ensure that every child is born healthy and wanted, and grows up free from disease and disability. The site provides general information about the Institute; funding and intramural research details; information about the Division of Epidemiology, Statistics, and Prevention Research; publications bibliography; fact sheets; reports; employment and fellowship listings; and research resources.

National Institute of Dental and Craniofacial Research (NIDCR) ◉ ◉ ◉

http://www.nidr.nih.gov

The National Institute of Dental and Craniofacial Research provides leadership for a national research program designed to understand, treat, and ultimately prevent the infectious and inherited craniofacial-oral-dental diseases and disorders that compromise millions of human lives. General information about the Institute, news and health information, details of research activities, and NIDCR employment opportunities are all found at the site. A site search engine and staff directory are also available.

National Institute of Diabetes and Digestive and Kidney Diseases (NIDDK) ◎ ◎ ◎

http://www.niddk.nih.gov

The National Institute of Diabetes and Digestive and Kidney Diseases conducts and supports basic and applied research, and provides leadership for a national program in diabetes, endocrinology, and metabolic diseases; digestive diseases and nutrition; and kidney, urologic, and hematologic diseases. NIDDK information at the site includes a mission statement, history, organization description, staff directory, and employment listing. Additional resources include news; a database for health information; clinical trials information, including a patient recruitment section; and information on extramural funding and intramural research at the Institute.

National Institute of Environmental Health Sciences (NIEHS) ◎ ◎ ◎

http://www.niehs.nih.gov

The National Institute of Environmental Health Sciences reduces the burden of human illness and dysfunction from environmental causes by defining how environmental exposures, genetic susceptibility, and age interact to affect an individual's health. News and Institute events, research information, grant and contract details, fact sheets, an Institute personnel directory, employment and training notices, teacher support, and an online resource for kids are all found at this site. Library resources include a book catalog, electronic journals, database searching, NIEHS publications, and reference resources. Visitors can use search engines at the site to find environmental health information and news, publications, available grants and contracts, and library resources.

National Institute of General Medical Sciences (NIGMS) ◎ ◎ ◎

http://www.nih.gov/nigms

The National Institute of General Medical supports basic biomedical research that is not targeted to specific diseases, but that increases the understanding of life processes, and lays the foundation for advances in disease diagnosis, treatment, and prevention. Among the most significant results of this research has been the development of recombinant DNA technology, which forms the basis for the biotechnology industry. The site provides information about NIGMS research and funding programs, information for visitors, news, publications list, reports, grant databases, a personnel and employment listing, and links to additional biomedical resources.

National Institute of Mental Health (NIMH) ◎ ◎ ◎

http://www.nimh.nih.gov

The National Institute of Mental Health provides national leadership dedicated to understanding, treating, and preventing mental illnesses through basic research on the brain and behavior, and through clinical, epidemiological, and services research. Resources available at the site include staff directories, information for visitors to the campus, employment opportunities, NIMH history, and publications from activities of the National Advisory Mental Health Council and Peer Review Committees. News, a calendar of events, information on clinical trials, funding opportunities, and intramural research are also provided. Pages tailored specifically for the public, health practitioners, or researchers contain mental disorder information, research fact sheets, statistics, science education materials, news, links to NIMH research sites, and patient education materials.

National Institute of Neurological Disorders and Stroke (NINDS) ⊗ ⊗ ⊗
http://www.ninds.nih.gov

The National Institute of Neurological Disorders and Stroke supports and conducts research and research training on the normal structure and function of the nervous system, and on the causes, prevention, diagnosis, and treatment of more than 600 nervous system disorders including stroke, epilepsy, multiple sclerosis, Parkinson's disease, head and spinal cord injury, Alzheimer's disease, and brain tumors. The site provides visitors with an organizational diagram, e-mail directory, links to advisory groups, the mission and history of NINDS, a site search engine, employment and training opportunities, and information on research at NINDS. Information is available for patients, clinicians, and scientists, including publications, details of current clinical trials, links to other health organizations, and research funding information.

National Institute of Nursing Research (NINR) ⊗ ⊗ ⊗
http://www.nih.gov/ninr

The National Institute of Nursing Research supports clinical and basic research to establish a scientific basis for the care of individuals across the life span, from management of patients during illness and recovery to the reduction of risks for disease and disability and the promotion of healthy lifestyles. NINR accomplishes its mission by supporting grants to universities and other research organizations as well as by conducting research intramurally at laboratories in Bethesda, Maryland. Visitors to this site can find the NINR mission statement and history, employment listings, news, conference details, publications, speech transcripts, answers to Frequently Asked Questions, information concerning legislative activities, research program and funding details, health information, highlights and outcomes of current nursing research, and links to additional Web resources.

National Institute on Aging (NIA) ⊗ ⊗ ⊗
http://www.nih.gov/nia

The National Institute on Aging leads a national program of research on the biomedical, social, and behavioral aspects of the aging process; the prevention of age-related diseases and disabilities; and the promotion of a better quality of life for all older Americans. The site presents recent announcements and upcoming events, employment opportunities, press releases, and media advisories of significant findings. Research resources include news from the National Advisory Council on Aging, links to extramural aging research conducted throughout the United States, and funding and training information. Health professionals and the general public can access publications on health and aging topics, or order materials online.

National Institute on Alcohol Abuse and Alcoholism (NIAAA) ◎ ◎ ◎
http://www.niaaa.nih.gov:80

The National Institute on Alcohol Abuse and Alcoholism conducts research focused on improving the treatment and prevention of alcoholism and alcohol-related problems to reduce the enormous health, social, and economic consequences of this disease. General resources at the site include an introduction to the Institute, extramural and intramural research information, an organizational flowchart, details of legislative activities, Advisory Council roster and minutes, information on scientific review groups associated with the Institute, a staff directory, and employment announcements. Institute publications, data tables, press releases, conferences and events calendars, answers to frequently asked questions on the subject of alcohol abuse and dependence, and links to related sites are also found at the site. The ETOH Database, an online bibliographic database containing over 100,000 records on alcohol abuse and alcoholism can be accessed from the site, as well as the National Library of Medicine's MEDLINE database.

National Institute on Deafness and Other Communication Disorders (NIDCD) ◎ ◎ ◎
http://www.nih.gov/nidcd

The National Institute on Deafness and Other Communication Disorders conducts and supports biomedical research and research training in the normal and disordered processes of hearing, balance, smell, taste, voice, speech, and language. The Institute also conducts and supports research and research training related to disease prevention and health promotion; addresses special biomedical and behavioral problems associated with people who have communication impairments or disorders; and supports efforts to create devices that substitute for lost and impaired sensory and communication function. The site provides visitors with many fact sheets and other information resources on hearing and balance; smell and taste; voice, speech, and language; hearing aids; otosclerosis; vocal abuse and misuse; and vocal cord paralysis. Other resources include a directory of organizations related to hearing, balance, smell, taste, voice, speech, and language, a glossary of terms, an online newsletter, information for kids and teachers, clinical trials details, and a site search engine. Information on research funding and intramural research activities, news and events calendar, and general information about NIDCD is also available at this site.

National Institute on Drug Abuse (NIDA) ◎ ◎ ◎

http://www.nida.nih.gov/NIDAHome1.html

The National Institute on Drug Abuse leads the nation in bringing the power of science to bear on drug abuse and addiction through support and conduct of research across a broad range of disciplines, and rapid and effective dissemination of results of that research to improve drug abuse and addiction prevention, treatment, and policy. The site contains fact sheets on common drugs of abuse and prevention strategies, Institute announcements, media advisories, congressional testimonies, speech transcripts, online newsletters, scientific meeting dates and summaries, funding, training, legislation information, and links to related sites. Recent research reports and news related to drug addiction are highlighted at the site.

National Library of Medicine (NLM) ◎ ◎ ◎

http://www.nlm.nih.gov

The National Library of Medicine, the world's largest medical library, collects materials in all areas of biomedicine and healthcare; and works on biomedical aspects of technology; the humanities; and the physical, life, and social sciences. This site contains links to government medical databases, including MEDLINE and MEDLINE plus (for consumers), information on funding opportunities at the National Library of Medicine and other federal agencies, and details of services, training, and outreach programs offered by NLM. Users can access NLM's catalog of resources (LocatorPlus), as well as NLM publications, including fact sheets, published reports, and staff publications. Also available are NLM announcements, news, exhibit information, and staff directories. NLM research programs discussed at the site include topics in Computational Molecular Biology, Medical Informatics, and other related subjects.

The Web site features 15 searchable databases, covering journal searches via MEDLINE, AIDS information via AIDSLINE, AIDSDRUGS, AIDSTRIALS, bioethics via BIOETHICSLINE, and numerous other important topics. The "master search engine," nicknamed Internet Grateful Med (IGM), searches MEDLINE using the retrieval engine called PubMed. It is very user-friendly. There are 9 million citations in MEDLINE and PreMEDLINE and the other related databases.

Additionally, the NLM provides sources of health statistics, serials programs, and services maintained through a system called SERHOLD, medical images, international medical resources, and a searchable NLM staff directory.

Warren Grant Magnuson Clinical Center ◎ ◎ ◎

http://www.cc.nih.gov:80

The Warren Grant Magnuson Clinical Center is the clinical research facility of the National Institutes of Health, supporting clinical investigations conducted by the Institutes. The Clinical Center was designed to bring patient-care facilities close to research labs, allowing findings of basic and clinical scientists to move quickly from labs to the treatment of patients. The site provides visitors with news, events, details of current clinical research studies, patient recruitment resources, links to departmental Web sites, and information resources for NIH staff, patients, physicians, and scientists. Topics discussed in the Center's Medicine for the Public Lecture Series and resources in medical and scientific education offered by the Center are included at the site.

10.6 Guides to Medical Journals on the Internet

Amedeo ○ ○ ○ (free registration)
http://www.amedeo.com

Amedeo is a free medical literature service, allowing users to select topics and journals of interest. The service sends a weekly e-mail with an overview of new articles reflecting the specifications indicated by the user, and creates a personal home page with abstracts of relevant articles. The site allows registered users to access a Network Center, which facilitates literature exchange among users with similar interests. This service is supported through educational grants by numerous pharmaceutical companies.

BioMedNet:
The Internet Community for Biological and Medical Researchers ○ ○ ○
http://www.biomednet.com/library

Owned by publishing giant Reed Elsevier, this site contains a full text library of over 170 biomedical journals, most of which are available for a fee ranging from US$1–$20. Other features include a shopping mall for books, software, and biological supplies; an evaluated Medline system; a list of biomedical site links; a job exchange; and a science news journal. Free BioMedNet membership provides access to many of the site's features. Some publications, such as the Current Biology journals, offer free access to editorials, short articles, and letters. Prices and special offers can be found on each journal's home page under "Prices/Subscriptions." All visitors to the site can search the journals library and view abstracts without incurring charges.

Blackwell Science ○ ○ ○
http://www.blackwell-science.com/uk/journals.htm

This site offers online access to information regarding well over 200 Blackwell Science Publications. Journals are sorted alphabetically by title and are available in all major fields of science and medicine. Blackwell Science provides a good general overview regarding the content and aim of each of its journals. Tables of contents are available for current and back issues of each title. Access to abstracts and articles requires a fee.

Elsevier Science ☺ ☺ ☺

http://www.elsevier.com

Covering the same Elsevier publications as Science Direct, this site's journal coverage is a bit more up-to-date, and it includes a table of contents search engine. The site also provides many links to journal-related information and subject categories for easy browsing of references in areas of interest. Information is also included on Elsevier's books, and an e-mail alerting service on subject-specific titles from Elsevier's books and journals is available free with registration.

EurekAlert ☺ ☺ ☺

http://www.eurekalert.org

This site allows professionals and consumers to search the archives for the latest articles, news items, events, awards, and grants in science and medicine, including psychiatry. Current news from the Howard Hughes Medical Institute and the National Institutes of Health, as well as numerous links to institutions, journals, and other online resources are available.

Hardin Library Electronic Journal Showcase ☺ ☺ ☺

http://www.lib.uiowa.edu/hardin/md/ej.html

The University of Iowa Hardin Library for the Health Sciences has compiled an index of free full-text journals on the Internet. Using this convenient listing, a user can go straight to a particular journal and retrieve the full text of an article, free-of-charge. Some journals are on a free-trial basis, and sample journal articles are provided for reference.

Highwire Press ☺ ☺ ☺

http://highwire.stanford.edu

One of the largest producers of online versions of biomedical journals, Highwire Press's Web page presents an organized list (by alphabet or subject) of its biomedical journals, including detailed information regarding what is available at no charge for each title. For each journal, there is a link to its page, where tables of contents and abstracts are available. Full text of entire journals or back issues are available for a good number of titles.

Instructions to Authors in the Health Sciences ☺ ☺ ☺

http://www.mco.edu:80/lib/instr/libinsta.html

Produced and maintained by the library staff of the Medical College of Ohio, this site contains a unique compilation of links to instructions for authors, for over 2,000 biomedical journals. All are links to the sites of the publishers who have editorial responsibilities for each title.

Karger ◎ ◎ ◎
http://www.karger.com

Karger provides online access to information on all of its publications. Journals are sorted by title and by subject area. Karger publishes hundreds of journals in an extensive variety of medical and related science fields. Table of contents and article abstracts are available free-of-charge. There is an extensive listing of back issues as well. A free sample issue of each publication is provided. However, a fee is assessed for access to articles.

MDConsult ◎ ◎ ◎ (fee-based)
http://www.mdconsult.com

MDConsult is a comprehensive online medical information service specifically designed for physicians. This is service is provided for a monthly fee of US$19.95, but a 10-day free trial is available. The service includes the ability to search 35 online medical reference books for information and 48 journals for full-text articles. Searches can also be performed for full text articles through MEDLINE and other databases. Members can also search patient education handouts, drug information, and practice guidelines. Additional resources include reviews of new developments from major journals, government agencies, and medical conferences, and a section devoted to what patients are reading in the popular press.

Medical Matrix ◎ ◎ ◎
http://www.medmatrix.org/reg/login.asp

Following a brief free registration, this site offers a wealth of information in all major medical fields, with continuous updating, rating, and annotating provided by an editorial board and contributors' group composed of physicians and librarians. Each link also includes a description of what can be accessed free-of-charge at that site. Most of the journal sites covered provide free access to table of contents and abstracts. However, some may assess a fee when accessing full text versions of journals. Links to other Web resources in a variety of specialty areas, diseases, and clinical practice subject are also provided, as well as a MEDLINE search engine, plus medical textbook and CME links.

MEDLINE Journal Links To Publishers ◎ ◎ ◎
http://www.ncbi.nlm.nih.gov/PubMed/fulltext.html

Through the National Library of Medicine, the MEDLINE service provides direct access to hundreds of medical journals in all fields, listed alphabetically by name, with direct links to their respective publishers. Upon accessing an individual publication, the reader can normally view the current issue table of contents and abstracts for the articles. In certain cases, the complete article texts are available without charge, but in other cases it is necessary to pay a fee and obtain an access password. Each page explains the available information and the conditions for access, since policies vary by publisher and journal.

PubList: Health and Medical Sciences ⊙ ⊙ ⊙

http://www.publist.com/indexes/health.html

This site contains an extensive list of links to medical journals, divided by subject areas. Useful information, such as frequency, publisher, and format is included for each publication, and a search engine can be used to identify titles of interest.

Science Direct ⊙ ⊙ ⊙

http://www.sciencedirect.com

A very useful site, Science Direct compiles an extensive list of links to online journal literature published by Elsevier Science in all major areas of scientific study, including clinical medicine. Access to full text is available by institutional subscription only; however, table of contents are provided free-of-charge for each journal. The site provides links to hundreds of journals categorized by subject and further subdivided by specialty. Journals are also listed alphabetically by title.

Springer-Verlag's LINK ⊙ ⊙ ⊙

http://link.springer.de

Covering the large list of journals published by Springer-Verlag, this site mostly contains abstracts, rather than full text. Full text is available for those titles for which individuals or institutions maintain print subscriptions. A bit slow to navigate, the site does cover a broad range of biomedical titles, all of which provide tables of contents from the most recent two to four years.

UnCover Web ⊙ ⊙ ⊙

http://uncweb.carl.org

This enormous database of medical and nonscientific journals' tables of contents permits searching by keyword, journal title, or author. Full articles can be faxed or e-mailed for a fee. For a modest price, the reveal service provides e-mailed tables of contents for specific journals as they are published and added to the database.

WebMedLit ⊙ ⊙ ⊙

http://webmedlit.silverplatter.com/index.html

WebMedLit provides access to the latest medical literature on the Web by indexing medical Web sites daily and presenting articles from each site organized by subject categories. All WebMedLit article links are from the original source document at the publisher's Web site, and most articles are available in full text.

Wiley Interscience ◎ ◎ ◎

http://www3.interscience.wiley.com/index.html

This site is maintained by John Wiley and Sons, Inc. and provides links to all Wiley publications. Hundreds of titles are available online via direct link from the publisher. Journals are available in business, law, and all areas of science, including life and medical science. The Journal Finder option allows the user to search journals by title and subject. Free registration allows access to table of contents and abstracts abstracts published within the last 12 months. Full text access is available via registration to both individual and institutional subscribers of the print counterparts of the Wiley online journals.

10.7 Health and Medical Hotlines

Toll-Free Numbers for Health Information ◎

http://nhic-nt.health.org/Scripts/Tollfree.cfm

A categorized list of toll-free health information hotlines is provided by this site. Each hotline provides educational materials for patients.

10.8 Hospital Resources

American Hospital Association ◎ ◎ ◎

http://www.aha.org

Everything pertaining to hospitals is either available at this site or at a link from this site, including advocacy, health insurance, extensive hospital information, research and education, health statistics, and valuable links to the National Information Center for Health Services Administration as well as other organizations and resources.

Hospital Directory ◎ ◎ ◎

http://www.doctordirectory.com/hospitals/directory

This useful site provides a listing of states and territories, each of which is a hot link to a further listing of cities in the state or territory. By clicking on a city, the database provides a listing of hospitals in that area, including name, address, and telephone numbers. The site offers other links for physicians pertaining to health plans, doctors, health news, insurance, and medical products.

HospitalWeb ◎ ◎ ◎

http://neuro-www2.mgh.harvard.edu/hospitalwebworld.html

This site is a guide to global hospitals on the World Wide Web (not including the United States). It lists over 50 countries. Under each country, the names of a number of hospitals in that country are listed. By clicking on the hospital name, the user is taken to the hospital's Web site which provides further information.

10.9 Internet Newsgroups

General Medical Topic Newsgroups
Internet newsgroups are places where individuals can post messages on a common site for others to read. Many newsgroups are devoted to medical topics, and these groups are listed below. To access these groups you can either use a newsreader program (often part of an e-mail program), or search and browse using a popular Web site, www.deja.com.

Since newsgroups are mostly unmoderated, there is no editorial process or restrictions on postings. The information at these groups is therefore neither authoritative nor based on any set of standards.

sci.med	sci.med.nutrition	sci.med.vision
sci.engr.biomed	sci.med.occupational	alt.image.medical
sci.med.aids	sci.med.orthopedics	alt.med
sci.med.cardiology	sci.med.pathology	alt.med.allergy
sci.med.dentistry	sci.med.pharmacy	alt.med.cfs
sci.med.diseases.cancer	sci.med.physics	alt.med.ems
sci.med.diseases.hepatitis	sci.med.prostate.bph	alt.med.equipment
sci.med.diseases.lyme	sci.med.prostate.cancer	alt.med.fibromyalgia
sci.med.diseases.viral	sci.med.prostate.prostatitis	alt.med.outpat.clinic
sci.med.immunology	sci.med.psychobiology	alt.med.phys-assts
sci.med.informatics	sci.med.radiology	alt.med.urum-outcomes
sci.med.laboratory	sci.med.telemedicine	alt.med.veterinary
sci.med.nursing	sci.med.transcription	alt.med.vision.improve

10.10 Locating a Physician

American Medical Association (AMA): Physician Select Online Doctor Finder ◉ ◉ ◉
http://www.ama-assn.org/aps/amahg.htm

The AMA is the primary "umbrella" professional association of physicians and medical students in the United States. The AMA Physician Select system provides information on virtually every licensed physician, including more than 650,000 physicians and doctors of osteopathy. According to the site, physician credentials have been certified for accuracy and authenticated by accrediting agencies, medical schools, residency programs, licensing and certifying boards, and other data sources. The user can search for physicians by name or by medical specialty.

HealthPages ☺ ☺ ☺
http://www.thehealthpages.com

This search tool allows visitors to locate doctors in their area by specialty and location. Over 500,000 physicians and 120,000 dentists are listed. Doctors may update their profiles free-of-charge. Local provider choices are displayed to consumers in a comparative format. They can access charts that compare the training, office services, and fees of local physicians; the provider networks and quality measures of area managed care plans; the size, services, and fees of local hospitals; and more. Patients can post ratings and comments about their doctors.

Physicians' Practice ☺ ☺
http://www.physicianpractice.com

This site allows the user to search for doctors in many specialty areas. Searches are performed by specialty and zip code. Physicians must pay a fee to be listed but enjoy other benefits such as referrals, Internet presence, and a newsletter.

10.11 Medical Abbreviations and Acronyms

Ask MedBot ☺ ☺ ☺
http://www.ncemi.org

The National Council for Emergency Medicine Informatics provides a searchable database for medical abbreviations and acronyms. Click on "Abbreviation Translator" and place the letters you wish to identify in the space and press "Enter." Single or multiple definitions will be printed on your screen.

Common Medical Abbreviations ☺ ☺
http://courses.smsu.edu/jas188f/690/medslpterm.html

Several hundred major medical abbreviations are defined in an alphabetical listing at this educational information site.

How to Read the Prescription ☺ ☺
http://www.ns.net/users/ryan/rxabrv.html

World Wide Pharmacy provides an alphabetical listing of abbreviations used in medical prescriptions.

10.12 **Medical and Health Sciences Libraries**

Medical Libraries at
Universities, Hospitals, Foundations, and Research Centers ◎ ◎ ◎
http://www.lib.uiowa.edu/hardin-www/hslibs.html

This site includes an up-to-date listing of libraries that can be easily accessed through links produced by staff of the Hardin Library at the University of Iowa. Libraries are listed state by state enabling easy access to hundreds of library Web sites. There are also numerous foreign medical library links. These sites can be easily accessed from the central site established by the Hardin Library at the University of Iowa.

National Institutes of Health (NIH): Library Online ◎ ◎ ◎
http://libwww.ncrr.nih.gov

This site presents information about the NIH Library including a staff listing, current exhibits, hours, materials available to NIH personnel and the general public, current job vacancies, maps for visitors, and answers to frequently asked questions about the Library. Users can search the Library's catalog of books, journals, and other periodicals, access public and academic medical databases, and find seminar and tutorial information, as well as links to related sites.

National Library of Medicine (NLM) ◎ ◎ ◎
http://www.nlm.nih.gov

The National Library of Medicine, the world's largest medical library, collects materials in all areas of biomedicine and healthcare, and works on biomedical aspects of technology; the humanities; and the physical, life, and social sciences. This site contains links to government medical databases, including MEDLINE and MEDLINE plus (for consumers); information on funding opportunities at the NLM and other federal agencies; and details of services, training, and outreach programs offered by NLM. Users can access NLM's catalog of resources (LocatorPlus), as well as NLM publications, including fact sheets, published reports, and staff publications. Also available are NLM announcements, news, exhibit information, and staff directories. NLM research programs discussed at the site include topics in Computational Molecular Biology, Medical Informatics, and other related subjects.

The Web site features 15 searchable databases, covering journal searches via MEDLINE, AIDS information via AIDSLINE, AIDSDRUGS, and AIDSTRIALS, bioethics via BIOETHICSLINE, and numerous other important topics. The "master search engine," nicknamed Internet Grateful Med (IGM), searches MEDLINE using the retrieval engine called PubMed. It is very user-friendly. There are 9 million citations in MEDLINE, PreMEDLINE, and other related databases.

Additionally, the NLM provides sources of health statistics, serials programs and services maintained through a system called SERHOLD, medical images, international medical resources, and a searchable NLM staff directory.

National Network of Libraries of Medicine (NN/LM) ◉ ◉ ◉

http://www.nnlm.nlm.nih.gov

Composed of 8 regional libraries, the NN/LM also provides access to numerous health science libraries in each region, located at universities, hospitals, and institutes. The Web site enables the user to link directly to each of the libraries in any regional of the United States. These libraries have access to the NLM's SERHOLD system database of machine-readable holdings for biomedical serial titles. There are approximately 89,000 serial titles that are accessible through SERHOLD-participating libraries.

10.13 Medical Conferences and Meetings

Cell Press Online: Meetings and Conferences ◉ ◉ ◉

http://jobs.cell.com/events

Focused on mostly research-oriented meetings, this is a comprehensive listing of forthcoming conferences, with searching capabilities, by research area, location, and keywords. A unique feature of this site is its e-mail alerting service.

Doctor's Guide to Medical Conferences and Meetings ◉ ◉ ◉

http://www.pslgroup.com/medconf.htm

This is a very extensive list of several hundred conferences and meetings, including Continuing Medical Education (CME) programs worldwide, organized by date, meeting site, and subject. Location and other details are provided.

Health On the Net (HON) Foundation ◉ ◉ ◉

http://www.hon.ch/cgi-bin/conferences

This site provides a limited listing of conferences and meetings in medical specialty areas, and they are not categorized or indexed by fields. Information is chronological by month.

Medical Conferences.com ◉ ◉ ◉

http://www.medicalconferences.com

This site covers a broad range of medical conference listings, including meetings related to many different areas of healthcare including pharmaceuticals and hospital supplies, as well as the clinical medical specialties. An easy-to-use search mechanism provides access to the numerous listings, each of which links to details concerning each conference. The site claims to be updated daily, providing details on over 7,000 forthcoming conferences.

MediConf Online ⊗ ⊗ ⊗ (some features fee-based)
http://www.mediconf.com/online.html

This well-organized site lists conferences by medical subject, chronology, and geographic location, mostly covering meetings to be held in the next month or two. The listings include research conferences, seminars, annual meetings of professional societies, medical technology trade shows, and opportunities for CME credits. What is provided free on the Internet is only a small percentage of the complete fee-based database, which includes more than 60,000 listings of meetings to be held through 2014, and is available through the information vendors, Ovid or Dialog.

MedMeetings ⊗ ⊗ ⊗
http://www.medmeetings.com

This site claims to be "an interactive guide to medical meetings worldwide." The site is a service of International Medical News Group (IMNG), which publishes six major independent newspapers for physicians. The database includes information on thousands of medical meetings and conventions. Searches can be performed by disease, specialty group, date, location, availability of CME credit, and other criteria.

Medscape: Conference Summaries & Schedules ⊗ ⊗ ⊗
http://www.medscape.com

This service enables members to attend important meetings, catch up on missed meetings, or review sessions later by way of "comprehensive next-day summaries by world-renowned faculty in the form of in-depth online coverage." Medscape also provides access to both free and fee-based continuing medical education courses online. Schedules for upcoming conferences in specialty areas are provided.

Physician's Guide to the Internet ⊗ ⊗ ⊗
http://www.physiciansguide.com/meetings.html

Dates and locations for major national medical meetings are listed alphabetically by association at this site. There are also some hyperlinks to association pages and contact persons.

Princeton Medicon: The Medical Conference Resource ⊗ ⊗ ⊗
http://www.medicon.com.au

This comprehensive site contains details regarding worldwide major medical conferences of interest to medical specialists and primary care professionals. It is also periodically published in printed form. Access to lists of meetings is provided through a useful search engine that permits searching by specialty, year, and geographic region.

10.14 **Medical Data and Statistics**

Centers for Disease Control and Prevention (CDC) National Institute for Occupational Safety and Health: Biostatistics/Statistics ⊙ ⊙ ⊙
http://www.cdc.gov/niosh/biostat.html

This address provides visitors with links to sources of national statistics. Resources include federal, county and city data, as well as statistics related to labor, current population, public health, economics, trade, and business. Sources for mathematics and software information are also found through this site.

Health Sciences Library System (HSLS): Health Statistics ⊙ ⊙ ⊙
http://www.hsls.pitt.edu/intres/guides/statcbw.html

The University of Pittsburgh's Falk Library of the Health Sciences developed this site to provide information on obtaining statistical health data from Internet and library sources. Resources include details on obtaining statistical data from United States population databases, government agencies collecting statistics, organizations and associations collecting statistics, and other Web sites providing statistical information. The site explains specific Internet and library tools for locating health statistics, and offers a glossary of terms used in statistics.

National Center for Health Statistics (NCHS) ⊙ ⊙ ⊙
http://www.cdc.gov/nchs/default.htm

The NCHS, located within the Centers for Disease Control and Prevention of the U.S. Department of Health and Human Services, provides an extensive array of health and medical statistics for the medical, research, and consumer communities. This site provides express links to numerous surveys and statistical sources at the NCHS.

University of Michigan Documents Center: Statistical Resources on the Web: Health ⊙ ⊙ ⊙
http://www.lib.umich.edu/libhome/Documents.center/sthealth.html

Online sources for health statistics are cataloged at this site, including comprehensive health statistics resources and sources for statistics by topic. Topics include abortion, accidents, births, deaths, disability, disease experimentation, hazardous substances, healthcare, health insurance, HMOs, hospitals, life tables, mental health, noise, nursing homes, nutrition, pregnancy, prescription drugs, risk behaviors, substance abuse, surgery, transplants, and vital statistics. Users can also access an alphabetical directory of sites in the database and a search engine for locating more specific resources.

World Health Organization (WHO)
Statistical Information System ☉ ☉ ☉

http://www.who.int/whosis

The Statistical Information System of WHO (WHOSIS) is intended to provide access to both statistical and epidemiological data and information from this international agency in electronic form. The site provides health statistics, disease information, mortality statistics, AIDS/HIV data, immunization coverage and incidence of communicable diseases, links to statistics from other countries, as well as links to the Centers for Disease Control and Prevention in the United States. This site is the premier resource for statistics on diseases worldwide. See also the WHO main site: http://www.who.int for some additional disease-related statistics.

10.15 Medical Dictionaries, Encyclopedias, and Glossaries

Bio Tech's Life Science Dictionary

http://biotech.icmb.utexas.edu/search/dict-search.html#H

This free online dictionary designed for the public and professionals contains terms that deal with biochemistry, biotechnology, botany, cell biology and genetics. The dictionary also contains some terms relating to ecology, limnology, pharmacology, toxicology and medicine. The search engine allows the user to search by a specific term or by a term contained within a definition.

Diagnostic Procedures Handbook ☉ ☉ ☉

http://www.bewell.com/dph/html/chapter/A.asp

This alphabetical listing of procedures, courtesy of Healthgate's supersite, provided an easy to access listing of diagnostic procedure information. Individual entries contain procedure synonyms, indications, contraindications, patient preparation, and special considerations and instructions. The techniques are fully described and related procedure links may be included.

Disease Finder from Healthanswers.com ☉ ☉ ☉

http://www.healthanswers.com/adam/index_new/index.asp?topic=Disease

A wide range of diseases are listed in this alphabetical directory of information for patients and consumers. Visitors can search by keyword or browse the directory for information. Details include alternative names, definitions, causes, incidences, risk factors, prevention, symptoms, signs and tests, treatment, prognosis, and complications. Any helpful diagrams or representative photographs related to the condition are also provided.

Diseases and Conditions from Yahoo! Health ⊙ ⊙ ⊙

http://health.yahoo.com/health/Diseases_and_Conditions/Disease_Feed_Data

Consumers will find an alphabetical list of health topics at this address. Each entry provides a definition or information on alternative names, causes, incidence, and risk factors, prevention, symptoms, signs and tests, treatment, and prognosis. Information is included on medical terms, diseases, medical conditions, vaccines, and other related topics.

Diseases and Conditions Index from MedicineNet.com ⊙ ⊙ ⊙

http://www.medicinenet.com/Script/Main/AlphaIdx.asp?li=MNI&d=51&p=A_DT

Medicinenet.com offers this comprehensive, user-friendly index to common and not so common diseases and conditions for reliable consumer information. Individual entries contain related terms as well as mini forums that offer concise encyclopedic articles on each disease, related news and updates, and ask the expert sections in which physicians answer common patient inquiries. Individual entries may also contain links to fact sheets on related topics of interest.

Glossary of Insurance—Related Terms at drkoop.com ⊙ ⊙

http://www.drkoop.com/hcr/insurance/glossary.asp

This site provides descriptions of both terms and phrases relating to health insurance. Terms are listed alphabetically.

HealthGate.com: Medical Tests ⊙ ⊙ ⊙

http://www.bewell.com/tests/index.asp

This page of the Healthgate supersite offers consumers information on over 400 diagnostic tests. Educational facts and descriptions are accessible by entering keywords or phrases or by scrolling through an alphabetical listing of topics. This complete guide to medical testing contains concise information for each test entry including category of test, material studied, estimated cost and time necessary for testing, predicted reliability rating, as well as purpose, risks, and required patient preparation.

HealthGate.com: Symptoms, Illness, and Surgery ⊙ ⊙ ⊙

http://www.bewell.com/sym/index.asp

As a service of Healthgate's supersite, this easy to use reference provides consumers with an excellent resource for a more complete understanding of disease diagnosis and treatment. By entering keywords or phrases or by browsing through an alphabetical listing of topics, visitors can obtain general information, signs and symptoms, causes, increased risk factors, and what to expect with respect to diagnostic and appropriate health care. Possible complications, prognosis, and general treatment measures are discussed for each entry listing.

Injury Finder from Healthanswers.com ◎ ◎ ◎

http://www.healthanswers.com/adam/index_new/index.asp?topic=Injury

Patients can access an alphabetical directory of common injuries at this address. Information available includes a definition and important considerations about the injury, causes, symptoms, prevention, and suggested first aid.

List and Glossary of Medical Terms ◎ ◎

http://allserv.rug.ac.be/%7Ervdstich/eugloss/welcome.html

This site offers a multilingual glossary of technical and popular medical terms.

MedDictionary.com ◎ ◎

http://www.meddictionary.com

MedDictionary.com is an online bookstore specializing in medical, nursing, and other health-related dictionaries. Additional products include software and terminology guides. Users can order all products online.

Medical Dictionary from MedicineNet.com ◎ ◎ ◎

http://www.medicinenet.com/Script/Main/AlphaIdx.asp?li=MNI&d=51&p=A_DICT

This valuable addition to the physician's electronic library contains all-inclusive entries that are revised on an ongoing basis for a considerable and ever-changing repertoire of classical and more modern medical terminology. The dictionary is unique in that it contains mini-encyclopedic entries for concise general information as well as definitions. With this easy to access reference tool, entries come complete with standard medical terms, related scientific terms, abbreviations, acronyms, jargon, institutions, projects, symptoms, syndromes, eponyms, and medical history.

Medical Spell-Check Offered by Spellex Development ◎ ◎ ◎

http://www.spellex.com/speller.htm

Spellex Medical and Spellex Pharmaceutical online spelling verification allows visitors to check the spelling of medical terms. The search returns possible correct spellings if the word entered was not found.

Merck Manual of Diagnosis and Therapy ◎ ◎ ◎

http://www.merck.com/pubs/mmanual

This online version of the 17th edition of the *Merck Manual* (1999) contains general medical text describing disorders and diseases that affect all organ systems. The site also provides links to the *Merck Manual of Geriatrics* and the *Merck Manual of Medical Information—Home Edition*. All manuals are searchable and use of the services is free-of-charge.

National Organization for Rare Disorders, Inc. (NORD) ◎ ◎ ◎ (some features fee-based)

http://www.rarediseases.org

The National Organization for Rare Disorders, Inc. (NORD) is a federation of more than 140 nonprofit organizations serving people with rare disorders and disabilities. The site provides access to current news items, conference details, an online newsletter, a rare disease database providing useful information for patients, an organizational database providing links to support and research organizations dedicated to rare disorders, and information specific to NORD. Users must pay a fee for full access to disease information.

Online Medical Dictionary from CancerWeb ◎ ◎ ◎

http://www.graylab.ac.uk/omd/index.html

This site offers a comprehensive medical dictionary online for clinical, medical student, and patient audiences, although a great many of the entries are very technical. It is a convenient source for a quick definition of an unfamiliar term.

Physical Fitness Encyclopedia ◎ ◎

http://www.phys.com/fitness/welcome/welcome2.html

This online encyclopedia includes exercise guides for working each part of the body. The encyclopedia also describes sports and activities, detailing the physical benefits, necessary equipment, related terms, and additional resources. It also provides tips for preparing, playing, and training for the activities.

Procedures and Tests Index from MedicineNet.com ◎ ◎ ◎

http://www.medicinenet.com/Script/Main/AlphaIdx.asp?li=MNI&d=51&f=685&p=A_PROC

MedicineNet.com offers this comprehensive, user-friendly index to common and not so common diagnostic tests and treatment procedures. Each diagnostic and treatment mini-forum contains a main article for general information, outlining the purpose and safety of the procedure, related diseases and treatments, articles written by physicians on related topics of interest, and interesting related consumer health facts.

Test Finder from Healthanswers.com ◎ ◎ ◎

http://www.healthanswers.com/adam/index_new/index.asp?topic=Test

Common medical tests are listed alphabetically at this address, providing patients and consumers with a definition of the test a descriptions of how the test is performed, patient preparation for the test, how the test will feel, risks, reasons the test is performed, normal values, the meaning of abnormal results, cost of the test, and special considerations.

Tests and Procedures, University of Michigan Health System ◎ ◎

http://www.med.umich.edu/1libr/tests/testa00.htm

An alphabetical directory of medical test and procedures is found at this address. Clear, non-technical explanations of each test are offered to interested consumers. Visitors will also find discussions of health topics and other UMHS resources through this site.

Vitamin Glossary A–Z ◎ ◎ ◎

http://www.intelihealth.com/IH/ihtIH/WSIHW000/408/408.html

The InteliHealth site provides a link to descriptions of vitamins and minerals. The glossary is divided into three main groups: fat soluble vitamins, water soluble vitamins, and minerals. Each description includes the following areas: Good to Know, Recommendations, Benefits, Food Sources, Day's Supply In, and Watch Out.

10.16 Medical Legislation

American Medical Association (AMA) ◎ ◎

http://www.ama-assn.org/ama/basic/category/0,1060,165,00.html

The purpose of this site is to encourage physicians around the country to get involved in the AMA's grassroots lobbying efforts. It covers information on legislation relevant to the medical profession, the AMA's Congressional agenda, and educational programs available through the AMA on political activism for physicians. The Web site is updated regularly with the latest news on medical issues in the government.

American Medical Group Association (AMGA) Public Policy and Political Affairs ◎ ◎

http://www.amga.org/gov/pos.htm

The AMGA Web site contains position papers concerning major issues in the medical profession currently debated in Congress, and information on ordering publications providing news, legal resources, and compliance information to healthcare professionals. One section is devoted to suggestions on communicating with Congressional representatives on policy issues.

American Medical Student Association (AMSA) Legislative Affairs ◎ ◎ ◎

http://www.amsa.org/lad/index.html

The AMSA is an organization that attempts to improve healthcare and medical education. Its Legislative Affairs section of the Web site contains news of legislation that affects medical education, educational information on how to be a health policy activist, information on internship and fellowship opportunities in the field of health policy, and legislative links.

American Medical Women's Association (AMWA) ⊙ ⊙
http://www.amwa-doc.org/index.html

The AMWA promotes issues related to women's health and professional development for female physicians. The site's advocacy and actions sections contain articles on news and legislation that is relevant to these issues and gives advice on how to get involved.

Hugnet Legislation ⊙ ⊙
http://www.hugnet.com

The Hugnet site has information on current legislation that concerns the medical community and those interested in healthcare. It encourages visitors to contact members of Congress to voice their opinions on this legislation.

Public Citizen ⊙ ⊙ ⊙
http://www.citizen.org

Public Citizen, a group founded by Ralph Nader, is an organization dedicated to political activism in issues concerning public health and safety. Within the site, there is information on legislation and activities related to the group's purpose of "protecting health, safety, and democracy." An extensive list of links to specific subjects include medically-related topics, such as "Healthcare Legislation," "HMO Accountability," and "Medical Malpractice Reform."

Thomas—U.S. Congress on the Internet ⊙ ⊙ ⊙
http://thomas.loc.gov

Within Thomas, one can find information on bills, laws, reports, or any current U.S. federal legislation. The site's engine can be used to find current congressional bills by keyword or bill number.

U.S. House of Representatives Internet Office of the Law Revision Counsel ⊙ ⊙ ⊙
http://law.house.gov/12.htm

The Office of the Law Revision Counsel of the U.S. House of Representatives prepares and publishes the United States Code pursuant to section 285b of title 2 of the Code. The Code is a consolidation and codification by subject matter of the general and permanent laws of the United States. U.S. Code can be searched by keyword or other classification criteria, and titles and chapters of the Code can be downloaded from the site. Classification tables listing sections of the U.S. Code affected by recently enacted laws are also available.

10.17 **Medical Search Engines and Directories**

Achoo Healthcare Online ⊙ ⊙ ⊙
http://www.achoo.com

This site offers a directory of Web sites in three main categories: Human Health and Disease, Business of Health, and Organizations and Sources. The site has extensive subcategories and short descriptions for each site. Daily health news of interest to patients, the public, or medical professionals is available at the site, as well as links to journals, databases, employment directories, and discussion groups.

All The Web ⊙ ⊙ ⊙
http://www.alltheweb.com

This comprehensive site provides a variety of search engines including Fast Search. Fast Search allows users to search the Internet in 25 language catalogs and covers over 200 million high quality Web pages in very high speed. Visitors can copy the code needed to add Fast Search to their Web sites. Additionally at this site are search engines to search pictures and sounds.

Argus Clearinghouse ⊙ ⊙ ⊙
http://www.clearinghouse.net

The Argus Clearinghouse provides a central access point for value-added topical guides which identify, describe and evaluate Internet-based information resources. Its mission is to facilitate intellectual access to information resources on the Internet. Users can search for Web resources at this site using a directory or search engine. Many general categories are available including "Health & Medicine" and "Science & Mathematics." Subcategories under "Health & Medicine" include disabilities, diseases and disorders, fitness and nutrition, general health, medical specialties, medicine and medical services and sexuality and reproduction. Information about each site includes the compiler name or organization, detailed ratings, related keywords and the date the site was last checked by Argus Clearinghouse.

BigHub ⊙ ⊙ ⊙
http://www.thebighub.com

Formerly known as iSleuth.com, the BigHub allows users to search multiple engines including Yahoo, AltaVista, Infoseek, Excite, WebCrawler, Lycos, HotBot and Goto, Web directories and news databases simultaneously, and receive one summary of results. The BigHub provides advanced search options in relevant specialty topics including Health, Science and Reference resources. Users can also access news, weather, financial information, and more.

CliniWeb International   ⊙ ⊙ ⊙

http://www.ohsu.edu/cliniweb

CliniWeb, a service of Oregon Health Sciences University, is a searchable index and table of contents to clinical resources available on the World Wide Web. Information found at the site is of particular interest to healthcare professional students and practitioners. Search terms can be entered in five different languages: English, German, French, Spanish, and Portuguese. The site offers links to sites for additional search resources, and is linked directly to MEDLINE.

Daily Diffs   ⊙ ⊙ ⊙

http://www.dailydiffs.com

This site catalogs and provides updates on useful sites in many categories, including Health and Medicine. This section provides current news items related to fitness and wellness, diseases and disorders, risks, prevention, current treatments, and many specific topics covered in detail. Users can also search for resources by keyword.

Direct Medical Knowledge   ⊙ ⊙ ⊙

http://www.dmk.org

By letting Direct Medical Knowledge do the research for you, valuable time and effort may be conserved. Medical professionals and consumers may choose to browse a list of articles on the chosen subject matter or view the Editor's Choice of article on the given topic. Articles of general interest, causes and origins of disease, and material specific to etiology, epidemiology, diagnosis, and prognosis are all included. Research on drug therapy, clinical trials, complementary therapies are available from a number of sources including related organizations, institutes, and research centers. Extra features include support group listings and emotional and economic issue discussions with many Web link support resources.

Doctor's Guide   ⊙ ⊙ ⊙

http://www.docguide.com

The Doctor's Guide to the Internet is provided by P\S\L Consulting Group, Inc. and its purpose is to provide a comfortable environment for physicians to search the Internet and World Wide Web. The site contains a professional edition for healthcare professionals and a section directed at patients. Information of medical and professional interest includes medical news and alerts, new drugs or indications, medical conferences, a Congress Resource Center, a medical bookstore, and Internet medical resources. Patient resources are organized by specific diseases or condition. Users can search the World Wide Web through Excite, InfoSeek, McKinley, and Alta Vista search engines or can search the Doctor's Guide Medical News and Conference database.

Dogpile ○ ○ ○

http://www.dogpile.com

Dogpile is a metasearch service that integrates several medium and large Web search and index guides into a single service. Visitors can complete a dogpile or geographic search (provides information about cities in the United States) or browse sites listed by categories such as "Health and Science" and their multiple subcategories. In addition this site offers yellow pages search, stock quotes, usenet articles, weather forecasts, job opportunities, shopping, and more.

drkoop.com ○ ○

http://www.drkoop.com

drkoop.com is an Internet-based consumer healthcare network. Included is a site search engine, reviews of Internet sites and multiple health-related topics and conditions to browse. In addition there are health-related news stories, a variety of resources such as information on drugs, books online, insurance, a physician locator, chat rooms, message boards, and much more.

Federal Web Locator ○ ○ ○

http://www.infoctr.edu/fwl

The Federal Web Locator is a service provided by the Center for Information Law and Policy and is intended to be the one stop shopping point for federal government information on the World Wide Web. Links to relevant sites are available in the following categories: legislative, judicial and executive branches, independent and quasi-official agencies, federal boards, commissions, committees and nongovernmental federally related sites. Additionally users can access a variety of search engines including Aliweb, Alpha Legal Directory, Alta Vista, Cyber411, EINET Galaxy, Excite, Google, Inference Find, InfoSeek, Law Crawler-Legal Search Information, Lycos, McKinley, Metacrawler, OpenText Index, SavvySearch, Snap, WebCrawler, World Access Inernet Navigator, and Yahoo.

Galaxy ○ ○ ○

http://galaxy.einet.net

This site houses a searchable directory of quality Web sites. Subcategories under medicine include diseases and disorders, health law, health occupations, history, human biology, medical informatics, operative surgery, philosophy, political issues, reference and therapeutics. There are also several site search options available.

Galen II ○ ○ ○

http://galen.library.ucsf.edu

Galen II is the digital library of the University of California San Francisco. The site includes UCSF and UC resources and services, links to the AMA Directory, Drug Info

Fulltext, Harrison's Online (requires a password), Merck Manual, Consumer Health, and a searchable database of additional resources and publications including electronic journals. Visitors can search the Galen II database or the World Wide Web using a variety of search engines.

Global Health Network ☉ ☉ ☉
http://www.pitt.edu/HOME/GHNet/GHNet.html

The Global Health Network offers national and international resources with information on agencies, organizations, academic programs, workshops, and conventions. The site maintains an online newsletter and offers links to related health networks. The site is also available in Japanese, Portuguese, Spanish, German, Chinese, Turkish, and Taiwanese.

Hardin Meta Directory of Internet Health Services ☉ ☉ ☉
http://www.lib.uiowa.edu/hardin/md/index.html

The purpose of the Hardin Meta Directory is to provide easy access to comprehensive resource lists in health-related subjects. It includes subject listings in large "one stop-shopping" sites such as MedWeb and Yahoo, and also independent discipline-specific lists. Sites are categorized by specific diseases and the number of links found at each site and only those that are well maintained are included. Additionally there is a list of free, full-text general medical journals available online.

Health A to Z ☉ ☉ ☉
http://www.healthatoz.com

This site offers visitors many useful resources for locating specific health information. A site search engine locates professionally reviewed health and medical information from other Internet resources including news headlines and updates, additional general health information, and a forum for asking questions of experts. Fact pages are dedicated to many specific health topics including diseases, alternative medicine, vaccines, nutrition, and fitness.

Health On the Net (HON) Foundation: MedHunt ☉ ☉
http://www.hon.ch/MedHunt

Health on the Net Foundation (HON) is a nonprofit organization and international initiative with a mission to help individuals and health care providers realize the potential benefits of the World Wide Web. This site provides several widely used medical search engines including MedHunt, Honselect, and Medline. Users can access databases containing information on newsgroups, LISTSERVs, medical images and movies, upcoming and past healthcare-related conferences, and daily news stories on health-related topics.

Health Sciences Information Service   ◎ ◎ ◎

http://www.lib.berkeley.edu/HSIS/other2.html

The Health Sciences Information Service at University of California, Berkeley offers links to Internet medical and health resources. Electronic journals, books, indexes, and databases on the Internet are cataloged. The Service offers links to sites providing general medical information, institutes, and organizations on the Web, current news related to health and medicine, clinical sites, and sites related to Medical Informatics.

Health Web   ◎ ◎ ◎

http://www.healthweb.org

HealthWeb provides links to specific, evaluated information resources on the World Wide Web, selected by librarians and information professionals at leading academic medical centers in the Midwest. Members, mainly universities or research centers, provide information that is sorted by alphabetical order and can be searched by keyword. Each member provides information on affiliated libraries as well as subject areas.

Indiana University Ruth Lilly Medical Library   ◎ ◎ ◎

http://www.medlib.iupui.edu

Although portions of this site are restricted, many WWW medical resources can be accessed through links, including other libraries, government libraries and information sources, national agencies, associations, and numerous other vital resources.

InfoMine   ◎ ◎

http://infomine.ucr.edu/search/bioagsearch.phtml

Provided by the University of California, InfoMine provides access to all types of Internet resources in the biological, agricultural, and medical sciences. Visitors can browse sites by subject, title, or keyword, or complete a search using InfoMine's search engine or a variety of Internet search and metasearch engines, virtual libraries and subject indexes, and mailing lists and newsgroups. Other features include access to BioAgMed and general references, online journals, the *Merck Manual* and educational resources.

MDchoice.com   ◎ ◎

http://www.mdchoice.com

MDchoice.com is a privately held company founded by academic physicians with the goal of making access to health and medical information on the Internet as efficient and reliable as possible. The site features an UltraWeb search with all content selected by board-certified physicians. In addition, users have access to MEDLINE, drug information, health news, and a variety of clinical calculators. Also offered are several interactive educational exercises, online journals and text books, and employment opportunities.

Med Engine ⊙ ⊙ ⊙

http://fastsearch.com/med/index.html

The Med Engine provides a general search engine called InferenceFind and several others including Microsoft's Multiple Search Engines, All-At-Once General Search, The Med Engine's I-Explorer, and Internet Sleuth. InferenceFind is unique in that it searches several search engines on the Internet, merges the results, removes redundancies and groups the results into understandable clusters. Additionally there are links to drug information, publications, physician directories, illnesses and diseases, educational sources, audio medicine, news, medical libraries and dictionaries, medical support, medical-legal issues, consumer information, associations and institutes, legislative action, hospital information, medical employment, government agencies, and more.

Med411.com ⊙ ⊙ ⊙

http://www.Med411.com

This medical search engine contains a collection of Web sites in the following categories: ancillary medical fields, associations, hospitals, import/export, insurance companies, journals/publications, medical equipment, medical legal, medical specialty, medical supplies, nursing, osteopathy, pharmaceuticals, and schools. Users can browse for sites by category or search for sites by keyword. A reference section titled "research" is available with links to medical associations, medical reference sites, medical libraries, medical dictionaries, sites that offer medical support, U.S. federal government sites and agencies and a search engine for the site of the Food and Drug Administration. Medical professionals may submit URLs of sites they are associated with to Med411.com online.

MedExplorer ⊙ ⊙ ⊙

http://www.medexplorer.com

MedExplorer is a comprehensive, searchable medical and health directory. Short descriptions of each site are provided. The site also lists related newsgroups and has information on conferences and employment.

MedFinder ⊙ ⊙ ⊙

http://www.netmedicine.com/medfinder.htm

MedFinder is an indexed database of WWW medical content. The database is searchable by type of Web page, with choices including information for patients, news articles, brief reviews, in-depth reviews or chapters, case presentations, simulations, practice guidelines, original research, and links directories. Searches can also be performed by topic, and specific criteria can be selected to further limit sites returned. Criteria can limit searches to pages containing peer-reviewed content, CME credits, audio or video resources, simulations, photos/animations, EKGs, radiographs, ultra-sound/echo, nuclear images, CT scans, MRIs, and other images.

Medical Matrix ⊙ ⊙
http://www.medmatrix.org/reg/login.asp

Medical Matrix offers peer-reviewed, annotated, updated clinical medicine resources, and assigns ranks to Internet resources based on their utility for point-of-care clinical application. Visitors can access several search engines including Medical Matrix, MEDLINE and others or access sites through categories such as medical specialties, diseases, clinical practice, literature, education, healthcare and professionals, medical computing and Internet and technology, and marketplace. Additional information available includes online journals and textbooks, news, CME, prescription assistance resources, symposia on the Web, and classifieds. Access to site requires free registration.

Medical World Search ⊙ ⊙ ⊙
http://www.mwsearch.com

This search engine indexes Web pages from selected medical Web sites. A directory of sites is not available. Users can chose to search indexed sites, selected general search engines, or MEDLINE. The search engine utilizes a medical thesaurus to increase the amount of returns from one query.

MedicineNet ⊙ ⊙ ⊙
http://medicinenet.com/Script/Main/hp.asp

MedicineNet is a network of doctors producing health information for public use. The site offers an alphabetically arranged directory that provides information about diseases, treatments, procedures, tests, and drugs. The site also provides a comprehensive medical dictionary with thousands of terms and disorders along with prefixes and association designations. Other features include news, treatment updates, and health facts.

Medmark ⊙ ⊙ ⊙
http://www.medmark.org

This comprehensive site provides users with a searchable directory of medical resources by specialty, free MEDLINE links, and other Internet resources. A search engine is available for locating additional medical and general sites.

Medscape ⊙ ⊙ ⊙
http://www.medscape.com

Medscape provides several databases from which users can search the Web. These include articles, news, information for patients, MEDLINE, AIDSline, Toxline, drug information, dictionary, book store, Dow Jones Library, and medical images. There is a wealth of additional information provided including articles, case reports, conference schedules and summaries, continuing medical education resources, job listings, journals, news, patient information, practice guidelines, treatment updates, links to medical specialty sites, and more. Requires free online registration.

MedSurf ⊙ ⊙ ⊙

http://www.medsurf.com/cgi-bin/OpenPage.cgi?Home.txt;Home

MedSurf offers links and a keyword search tool to find links to health and medical resources. The "Healthy Surfing" section provides news about the latest medical technologies and breakthroughs, while "Medicine Bag" guides physicians and health-care providers to news and in-depth information on new timesaving technologies, advanced treatment alternatives, aging research, and upcoming educational forums.

MedWeb ⊙ ⊙

http://www.medweb.emory.edu/Medweb

Offered by Emory University, this site provides a searchable database of Web sites providing medical and health information. Searching is possible by entering keywords or by browsing subject categories.

Metacrawler ⊙ ⊙

http://www.go2net.com/search.html

At the Metacrawler site users can search for Web resources through a directory or search engine. In addition, search engines are provided for newsgroups, audio, and shopping.

MMRL: Multimedia Medical Reference Library Medical Student Study Center ⊙ ⊙ ⊙

http://www.med-library.com/medlibrary

The Multimedia Medical Reference Library, developed by medical students and professionals at Tufts University School of Medicine, is a searchable database of reviewed medical Web sites. Visitors can find links to sites offering audio resources, clinical trials information, online journals, medical equipment auctions, medical reference libraries, medical services, software, products, and links to medical schools and professional organizations. Each site is listed with a short description.

NetMed.com ⊙ ⊙ ⊙

http://www.netmed.com/intro.html

NetMed.com provides users with links to useful sites grouped by medical condition. A relatively detailed description is given for most sites.

Online Medical Resources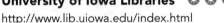

http://www.doctorbbs.com/searchall.htm

This site invites the user to search 20 different sites or online publications related to health and medicine. Links to MEDLINE and other general medical sites are also available.

Stanford MedWorld MedBot

http://www-med.stanford.edu/medworld/medbot

Offered by Stanford University, this site allows users to search medical and health resources on the Web using major general and medical search engines. More specific searches can be performed on index and reference, education and learning, news and information, and medical images, and multimedia resources topics. Users can specify engines to employ in the search.

University of Iowa Libraries

http://www.lib.uiowa.edu/index.html

This site includes links to OASIS, Healthnet, and other electronic resources available to University of Iowa students, faculty, and staff. Links are available to home pages for the Main Library and to each of the branch libraries.

Virtual Medical Center

http://www-sci.lib.uci.edu/~martindale/Medical.html

This site, hosted by the University of California and written by Jim Martindale, provides users with links to a wealth of useful information, including travel warnings and immunization details, reference resources on a wide range of scientific subjects, and pathology and virology educational resources. Co-contributors include the UCI Science Library, the Department of Defense, the National Institutes of Health, and the National Science Foundation.

Yahoo!

http://www.yahoo.com

Yahoo offers visitors the opportunity to search the Web and browse sites listed in multiple categories including health and science. Within each category are more specific subcategories that indicate the number of entries available. Most sites are suggested by users. Additionally Yahoo offers a wealth of services such as free e-mail, shopping, people search, news, travel, weather, stock reports, and more.

10.18 **Pharmaceutical Information**

Doctor's Guide: New Drugs and Indications ◎ ◎ ◎
http://www.pslgroup.com/NEWDRUGS.HTM

Doctor's Guide provides an ongoing source of new drug information, including FDA approvals and drug indications. Drug stories are presented in order of article datelines, with the most current stories listed first. Information for drug releases for the past 12 months is provided.

drkoop.com Drug Interactions Search ◎ ◎
http://www.drkoop.com/drugstore/pharmacy/interactions.asp

Users can enter several drug names into a search tool, checking for drug interactions.

Drug InfoNet ◎ ◎ ◎
http://www.druginfonet.com/phrminfo.htm

Information and links to areas on the Web concerning healthcare and pharmaceutical-related topics are available. The drug information is available by brand name, generic name, manufacturer, and therapeutic class. Visitors can ask questions of experts, and access disease information, pharmaceutical manufacturer information, healthcare news, and other resources.

Food and Drug Administration (FDA): Center for Drug Evaluation and Research ◎ ◎ ◎
http://www.fda.gov/cder/drug/default.htm

The Center for Drug Evaluation and Research broadcasts valuable information on prescription, consumer, and over-the-counter drugs at this address. Resources include alphabetical lists of new and generic drug approvals, new drugs approved for cancer indications, a searchable Orange Book listing all FDA approved prescription drugs, a National Drug Code directory, new over-the-counter labeling notices, patient information on over-the counter drugs, and alerts of new over-the-counter indications. Links are available to many resources related to drug safety and side effects, public health alerts and warnings, and pages offering information on major drugs. Reports and publications, special projects and programs, and cancer clinical trials information are also found through this address.

Food and Drug Administration (FDA) ◎ ◎ ◎
http://www.fda.gov

The FDA site provides extensive information on all aspects of drug research, regulations, approvals, trials, adverse reactions, enforcement, conferences, clinical alerts, reports, and drug news. The FDA Web Site Index is the first place to go to research a topic. There are several hundred subjects listed. One of these many sections covers

FDA-related acronyms and abbreviations, which itself is a very useful tool in understanding much of the material at this site. For many researchers and physicians, however, information about FDA drug approvals is of central concern. A separate service, not included within the FDA, offers a concise summary of such approvals by medical specialty and condition for each year up to the present. This information can be accessed at the following Web site: www.centerwatch.com/drugs/DRUGLIST.HTM.

Medications Index from MedicineNet.com ⊙ ⊙ ⊙

http://www.medicinenet.com/Script/Main/AlphaIdx.asp?li=MNI&d=51&p=A_PHARM

This all-inclusive pharmacological database from Medicinenet.com includes a mini forum for each prescription and nonprescription medication, containing a brief main article pertaining to the medication, related medications, related news and updates, diseases associated with the medication, and a listing of articles pertinent to the pharmacological agent's usage.

MedWatch—The FDA Medical Products Reporting Program ⊙ ⊙ ⊙

http://www.fda.gov/medwatch

The FDA Medical Products Reporting Program, MedWatch, is designed to educate health professionals about the importance of being aware of, monitoring for, and reporting adverse events and problems to the FDA and/or the manufacturer, and to disseminate new safety information rapidly within the medical community thereby improving patient care. To these ends, the site includes an adverse event reporting form and instructions, as well as safety information for health professionals, including "Dear Health Professional" letters and notifications related to drug safety. It also includes relevant, full-text continuing education articles and reports regarding drug and medical device safety issues.

Pharmaceutical Information Network ⊙ ⊙ ⊙

http://pharminfo.com

PharmInfoNet is a source of information on diseases, disorders, drug treatments, and research. In addition, there are links to more than one hundred pharmaceutical companies, both domestic and international. Organized by specialty areas, the site is a well-organized compilation of resources for physicians, researchers, medical students, and the public. The site is organized into information on disorders, archived articles, drugs used in the treatment of disorders, and other information sources, including newsgroups, e-mail lists, and related Web sites. An extensive Medical Sciences Bulletin Section and Pharmacotherapy Department provide articles on dozens of developments in research and drug therapies. Finally, the site provides a lengthy listing of drugs for treating disorders, with links to more extensive information sources.

Pharmaceutical Research and Manufacturers of America ⚙ ⚙ ⚙

http://www.phrma.org

This association Web site includes a "New Medicines in Development" database; a publications section containing reports relating to the pharmaceutical industry; various links for facts and figures on pharmaceutical research and innovation; and an issues and policies section covering many current topics of interest to pharmaceutical companies, such as genetics research and healthcare liability reform.

RxList—The Internet Drug Index ⚙ ⚙ ⚙

http://www.rxlist.com

This site allows users to search for drug information by name, imprint code, or keyword (action, interaction, etc.) The top 200 prescribed drugs for 1998, 1997, 1996, and 1995 are listed alphabetically or by rank. Patient monographs are available for a wide range of drugs, and one section is devoted to alternative medicine information and answers to frequently asked questions. The site also provides statistics related to site visits, and a forum for drug-specific discussions.

Virtual Library Pharmacy ⚙ ⚙ ⚙

http://www.pharmacy.org

This is truly a library of pharmacy information for professionals in all medical areas. The site provides information on pharmacy schools, companies, journals and books, Internet databases relating to pharmaceutical topics, conferences, hospital sites, government sites, pharmacy LISTSERVs, and news groups. Hundreds of site links are provided for the above areas.

World Standard Drug Database ⚙ ⚙

http://209.235.64.5:8888/cgi-bin/drugcgic.exe/START

Information on pharmaceutical products at this address includes ingredients, dosage, routes of administration, indications, contraindications, prescriber cautions, patient cautions, toxicity, side effects, liver disease cautions, renal failure procedures, pregnancy and lactation warnings, pharmacological actions, and diagnostic procedures. Visitors can search for relevant information by drug, ingredient, indications, contraindications, or side effects.

10.19 Physician Directories

Introduction

In order to obtain background information on practicing physicians in the United States, and to verify certification in various specialties, several important Web sites can be consulted, as listed below.

American Board of Medical Specialties (ABMS) ✪ ✪ ✪

http://www.certifieddoctor.com/verify.html

This is a very useful verification service containing all physicians certified by an ABMS member board. It permits the public to verify credentials and certification status of any physician free-of-charge, searching by name, city, state, and specialty within the 24 member board specialty areas. The user enters the name of the physician and information is immediately available.

Healthgrades.com ✪ ✪ ✪

http://www.healthgrades.com

This resource specializes in health care ratings, providing hospital ratings by procedure or diagnosis, physician ratings by specialty and geographic area, and ratings of health plans. Directories of hospitals, physicians, health plans, mammography facilities, and fertility clinics are also available. Visitors can access tips on choosing a hospital, physician, or health plan, as well as a glossary of terms and health news articles. Online health stores offer books, videos, magazines, greeting cards, flowers and gifts, pharmaceutical products, nutritional products, and insurance quotes. This service will soon include long-term care facilities, dentists, ambulatory surgery centers, and chiropractors in the ratings process.

Medi-Net Physician Background Information Service ✪ ✪ ✪

http://www.askmedi.com

Medi-Net describes itself as "an information delivery service that provides background information on every physician licensed to practice in the United States," providing name of medical school and year of graduation, residency training record, ABMS certifications, states where certified, and records of sanctions or disciplinary actions. There is a fee for reports.

11. PROFESSIONAL TOPICS AND CLINICAL PRACTICE

11.1 **Anatomy & Surgery**

Anatomy of the Human Body   ☺ ☺ ☺

http://rpisun1.mda.uth.tmc.edu/mmlearn/anatomy.html

This site offers images of the brain, elbow, arm, hand, knee, and foot. There are also sections that show slices of the ankle, foot, head, and neck in detail with nerves, muscles, and blood vessels identified.

Atlas of The Body   ☺ ☺ ☺

http://www.ama-assn.org/insight/gen_hlth/atlas/atlas.htm

The Atlas of the Body is a site offered by the American Medical Association that provides detailed information and labeled illustrations of the various systems and organs of the human body. The site also provides descriptions of disorders that affect these systems and organs.

Martindale's Health Science Guide,
The "Virtual" Medical Center—Anatomy and Histology Center   ☺ ☺

http://www-sci.lib.uci.edu/HSG/MedicalAnatomy.html

This site offers links to examinations, tutorials, and associations. It lists numerous atlases and sites with anatomical images, including some on embryology and developmental anatomy. Anatomy is just one of the many medical areas covered by the Virtual Medical Center, which also provides links to general medical dictionaries, glossaries, and encyclopedias, plus sites containing information on metabolic pathways and genetic maps.

Online Atlas Of Surgery   ☺ ☺ ☺

http://www.bgsm.edu/surg-sci/atlas/atlas.html

This site provides descriptions of specific surgical techniques, anatomy, instrumentation, positioning, room setup, and dissection. Also provided are indications leading to surgery and possible problems that may develop as a result of the surgery.

Online Surgery   ☺ ☺ ☺

http://www.onlinesurgery.com

Online Surgery gives the public an opportunity to view general and cosmetic surgical procedures online. Patients can fill out an application to finance an elective procedure and to be considered for a free procedure. Surgeries are viewed using RealPlayer.

Vesalius ○ ○ ○

http://www.vesalius.com

This site is a resource of medical illustrations with the purpose of providing educational material for surgeons and other medical professionals. Clinical Folios provide users with short educational narratives on surgical anatomy and procedures designed for online reference and study. There is an archive of images that demonstrate surgical techniques and other resources, including story boards, procedure descriptions using illustrations, photographs, x-rays, scans, animations and text, and short interactive programs or videos.

Virtual Body ○ ○ ○

http://www.medtropolis.com/vbody

This creative, informative site provides the viewer with labeled medical illustrations of various parts of the body. The human anatomy and body functions are presented in detail with interactive options that help the viewer learn the material.

Whole Brain Atlas ○ ○ ○

http://www.med.harvard.edu/AANLIB/home.html

This site, administered by the Harvard Medical School, shows imaging of the brain using magnetic resonance imaging (MRI), roentgen-ray computed tomography (CT), and nuclear medicine technologies. Structures within the images are labeled. Normal brain images are provided, as well as images of brains subjected to cerebrovascular disease, neoplastic disease, degenerative disease, and inflammatory or infectious disease. The entire atlas is available free-of-charge online or can be ordered on CD-ROM for a fee.

11.2 Biomedical Ethics

American Society of Bioethics and Humanities (ASBH) Home Page ○ ○ ○

http://www.asbh.org

The American Society of Bioethics and Humanities is an organization that promotes scholarship, research, teaching, policy development, and professional development in the field of bioethics. The site offers information on the Society, the annual meeting, position papers, awards, and links.

American Society of Law, Medicine, and Ethics (ASLME) ○ ○ ○

http://www.aslme.org

This site offers information on the American Society of Law, Medicine, and Ethics; *The Journal of Law Medicine and Ethics;* and *The American Journal of Law and Medi-*

cine. There is also information on research projects, a news section that gives information on recent developments in Law, Medicine, and Ethics, and information on future and past conferences held by the Society.

Bioethics Discussion Pages ☉ ☉ ☉
http://www-hsc.usc.edu/~mbernste/#Welcome

This page is a forum for people to discuss and share their views on selected topics in the field of biomedical ethics. There are also polls and articles on ethical issues.

Bioethics.net ☉ ☉ ☉
http://www.med.upenn.edu/bioethics/index.shtml

Produced by the Center for Bioethics of the University of Pennsylvania, Bioethics.net contains a host of resources relating to biomedical ethics. Included are sections on cloning and genetics, emergency room bioethics, surveys for pay, and assisted suicide. There is also a virtual library with links to Internet resources. A beginner's site (Bioethics for Beginners) contains material that is meant to educate the general public and people interested in the field about bioethics, its meaning, and its applications. At this beginner's site, there are resources for students and educators, and a list of different biomedical ethics associations.

Careers in Bioethics ☉ ☉
http://www.ethics.ubc.ca/brynw/jobs.html

This site has information on jobs that are being offered throughout the world in the field of Bioethics. Information on postdoctorals and fellowships is also available.

Center for Medical Ethics and Mediation ☉ ☉ ☉
http://www.wh.com/cmem

This site contains resources that help enable the Center to provide information on education, research, consultations, and mediations for healthcare professionals and organizations. These resources include information on workshops and seminars; requests for the Center to send a mediator to help with a dispute or conflict; profiles of the Center's mediators; and related links.

Hastings Center ☉ ☉ ☉
http://www.hastingscenter.org

The Hastings Center is a major center for the study of Biomedical Ethics. Their Web site provides information about the center as well as detailed explanations of current research activities. General listings of resources found at the Center, including an online library catalog, can also be accessed.

Health Priorities Group, Inc. ◎ ◎ ◎

http://www.bioethics-inc.com

The Health Priorities Group is made up of professionals in the field of Ethics, Medicine, Law, Nursing, and Theology. It offers training and support of corporate and hospital ethics committees, clinical case review, and help in health policy development for private and government institutions. The Web site has sections on services, publications, and reports on ethics issues.

Human Genome Project: Ethical, Legal, and Social Issues (ELSI) ◎ ◎

http://www.ornl.gov/TechResources/Human_Genome/resource/elsi.html

This site attempts to disseminate information on the Human Genome Project and the ethical, legal, and social issues surrounding the availability of genetic information. Available on this site are updates, publications, description of research in progress, and basic information on the Human Genome Project.

International Bioethics Committee ◎ ◎

http://www.unesco.org/ibc

Includes information on various ethical issues, including a section on the Human Genome Project. The site also has information on the International Bioethics Committee and its proceedings.

Medical Ethics—Where Do You Draw the Line? ◎ ◎

http://www.learner.org/exhibits/medicalethics

This site deals with issues by presenting real-life scenarios and letting the viewer take part in ethical decisions. There are also links to related resources and an ethics forum.

Midwest Bioethics Center ◎ ◎ ◎

http://www.midbio.org

This community-based Center is dedicated to the integration of ethical considerations in all health care decisions. Visitors to this address will find information about the organization, including a staff listing, membership details, and consortia information. Current events, publications, a discussion group, and advance directive pamphlets are also found at the site. Resources on community-state partnerships include policy, briefs, press releases, staff listings, a call for proposals, directories of grant seekers and recipients, and answers to questions. The Center's Compassion Sabbath program is also profiled at the site, offering information on conferences for clergy and other programs, lists of participants, answers to frequently asked questions, and links to related sites.

National Bioethics Advisory Commission (NBAC) ⊙ ⊙ ⊙
http://bioethics.gov/cgi-bin/bioeth_counter.pl

In addition to providing information on current research trends in the biotech industry, NBAC explores the ethical implications of technological advances. The site acts a forum for the ethical concerns of the public regarding a rapidly advancing technology. NBAC's policy is outlined at the site.

National Reference Center for Bioethics Literature ⊙ ⊙ ⊙
http://www.georgetown.edu/research/nrcbl

Linked to the Kennedy Institute of Ethics of Georgetown University, this Center holds the world's largest collections of literature on Biomedical Ethics. Serving as a resource for both the public and scholarly researchers, the library lists its resources on this Web site. The site also provides access to free searching of the world's literature in this area using BIOETHICSLINE or the Ethics and Human Genetics Database. Other relevant links are provided in the areas of Educational and Teaching Resources and other bibliographies and Internet links on bioethics.

Physicians Committee for Responsible Medicine (PCRM) ⊙ ⊙
http://www.pcrm.org

PCRM is dedicated to preventative medicine, higher ethical standards of research, and access to managed care. The organization provides extensive material on ethics and research as well as prevention and nutrition. The site also offers news and events about numerous PCRM activities, details on clinical research projects, and summaries of texts produced by the organization.

University of Buffalo
Center for Clinical Ethics and Humanities in Health Care ⊙ ⊙ ⊙
http://wings.buffalo.edu/faculty/research/bioethics/nav.html

Information about the Center, news and events notices, a library of bioethics and medical humanities documents, and the Ethics Committee Core Curriculum are available at this address. Links are presented to Internet resources on featured topics, including bioethics education, hospice and palliative care, advance directives, philosophy of mind, medical record privacy, genetics and ethics, and other relevant sites.

11.3 Biotechnology

Bio Online ⊙ ⊙ ⊙
http://www.bio.com

Bio Online is a comprehensive Web site for the life sciences and the biotechnology industry. This site provides general information, current news, an industry guide, academic and government links, and an extensive career center. It is an excellent resource for seeking information on the biotech industry and related sciences.

Biofind.com ☺ ☺ ☺

http://www.biofind.com

Biofind.com provides insight into the biotechnology industry and is a resource for general information, news, and developments in emerging technologies. The site also contains a job search database, chat room, the "Biotech Rumor Mill" for anonymous public discussion of current events in the field, and links to other biotech Web sites. A subscription service is also available for a fee, which provides daily e-mail updates on jobs, candidates, business opportunities, innovations, press releases, or company "rumors" posted at the site.

Bioresearch Online ☺ ☺ ☺

http://www.bioresearchonline.com/content/homepage

Bioresearch Online is a virtual community, forum, and marketplace for biotechnology professionals. Users have access to the latest headlines, product information, new and industry analyses, as well as career information. There are also specific pages devoted to pharmaceutical research and laboratory science.

Biotechnology: An Information Resource ☺ ☺ ☺

http://www.nal.usda.gov/bic

Dedicated to providing current information in all areas of biotechnology, this site is a subsidiary of the National Agricultural Library and the U.S. Department of Agriculture. The site catalogs press releases and offers an exhaustive listing of links to other Web-based resources from around the world, and is an excellent source for information, especially in the area of Agricultural Biotechnology.

Biotechnology Industry Organization ☺ ☺ ☺

http://www.bio.org/welcome.html

This industry-sponsored Web site provides weekly news updates on developing technology and world news. The site also offers general information, links to corporate Web sites, an online library, and a number of other educational resources. Although corporate sponsored, the site does not focus solely on product promotion, but has a genuine educational quality. Those seeking to learn more about this growing industry will find this site to be a valuable resources.

BioWorld Online ⊙ ⊙ ⊙

http://www.bioworld.com

BioWorld Online tracks the growth of the biotechnology market. In addition to providing stock and financial information, the site provides access to current industry headlines, job search resources, forums, and news worldwide.

CorpTech Database ⊙ ⊙ ⊙

http://www.corptech.com

This comprehensive database provides details on companies involved in high-tech industries, including biotechnology and pharmaceutical companies. Basic information such as each company's description, address, annual sales, and CEO name is available free; however, more in-depth financial and business data is only accessible to fee-paying subscribers. Searches for products or names of company officers are also available, again with some amount of information provided at no cost.

Enzyme Nomenclature Database ⊙ ⊙

http://www.expasy.ch/enzyme

Enzyme information of a very specific nature is available at this site devoted exclusively to this important medical subject. The database at this Web site provides access to enzyme information by EC (Enzyme Commission) number, enzyme class, description, chemical compound, and cofactor. There is an accompanying user manual for the enzyme database as well.

Infobiotech ⊙ ⊙ ⊙

http://www.cisti.nrc.ca/ibc/home.html

Infobiotech is a collaboration of government, academic, and private sector resources. This Canadian-based site provides general information, resources, and links to both Canadian and non-Canadian sites. In addition, it offers a large list of related sites providing current information on advances in the biotech industry.

International Food Information Council ⊙ ⊙ ⊙

http://ificinfo.health.org

The International Food Information Council collects and disseminates scientific information on food safety, nutrition, and health by working with experts to help translate research findings into understandable and useful information for opinion leaders and consumers. This site provides information and news on emerging technologies in the food industry. Resources available through this site include publications, recent news articles, government guidelines and regulations, and links to other resources on the Internet.

MedWebPlus: Biotechnology ⊙ ⊙ ⊙

http://www.medwebplus.com/subject/Biotechnology.html

MedWebPlus contains an extensive guide to online resources in biotechnology and a wide variety of other fields. The site catalogs hundreds of Internet resources containing many forms of information on the biotech industry. In addition, links are provided to journals, online publications, and recent articles of interest. Vast amounts of information are provided at this site, and links are kept current.

National Center for Biotechnology Information (NCBI) ⊙ ⊙ ⊙

http://www.ncbi.nlm.nih.gov

A collaborative effort produced by the National Library of Medicine and the National Institutes of Health, NCBI is a national resource for molecular biology information. The Center creates public databases, conducts research in computational biology, develops software tools for analyzing genome data, and disseminates biomedical information in an effort to improve the understanding of molecular processes affecting human health and disease. In addition to conducting and cataloging its own research, NCBI tracks the progress of important research projects worldwide. The site provides access to public molecular databases containing genetic sequences, structures, and taxonomy; literature databases; catalogs of whole genomes; tools for mining genetic data; teaching resources and online tutorials; and data and software available to download. Research performed at NCBI is also discussed at the site.

Recombinant Capital ⊙ ⊙ ⊙

http://www.recap.com

This online magazine provides analysis of the biotechnology industry. This is a good resource for those seeking to invest in companies on the forefront of the rapidly growing biotech industry. Although much of the information presented here is from a financial perspective, the site gives a good overview of the entire industry and provides daily news updates. The progress of developing technology can be closely monitored via this site.

World Wide Web Virtual Library: Biotechnology ⊙ ⊙ ⊙

http://www.cato.com/biotech

This is an excellent directory of sites in the field of Biotechnology. This site catalogs hundreds of reviewed links, including publications, educational resources, general information, and government links. There is also a rating system used by the editor of the site to point out links of specific importance.

11.4 **Chronic Pain Management**

American Academy of Pain Management (AAPM) ⊙ ⊙ ⊙
http://www.aapainmanage.org

The American Academy of Pain Management is the largest multidisciplinary pain society and largest physician-based pain society in the United States, providing credentials to practitioners in the area of pain management. This site provides information about AAPM and its activities, resources for finding a professional program in pain management, accreditation and Continuing Medical Education (CME) resources, and a membership directory for locating a pain management professional. It also provides good general information on pain management and a listing of relevant links. Access to the National Pain Data Bank is available at the site, containing statistics on various pain management therapies based on an outcomes measurement system. The site is divided into two sections with information tailored to the needs of patients and healthcare professionals.

Back and Body Care ⊙ ⊙
http://www.backandbodycare.com

Produced by physical therapists, this site is a good starting point for consumers seeking an overview of the causes and treatments chronic pain. It provides general information in the areas of back, neck, arm, and wrist pain. The site lists possible causes of chronic problems, treatments and exercises, and preventive measures. A search engine for locating a local, qualified physical therapist is featured at the site.

Pain.com ⊙ ⊙ ⊙
http://www.pain.com/index.cfm

This site is an excellent resource for seeking information on pain and pain management, and contains a great deal of information for the specific needs and interests of health professionals and patients. It offers an online pain journal, articles about recent advances and news in pain management, medical forums and chat rooms, and an extensive list of other Web-based resources.

Pain Net, Inc. ⊙ ⊙
http://www.painnet.com

Pain Net, Inc. provides visitors with useful information and links on pain control and prevention. Patients can find information on new treatments as well as a listing of pain management practitioners categorized by state. Doctors can search a database of important links and organizations, and can list their practice in the public information directory.

11.5 Clinical Practice Management

Cut to the Chase ⊙ ⊙ ⊙ (free registration)

http://www.cuttothechase.com

Healthcare management information for physicians is available at this site, including articles about practice management issues, career development resources, publications and software sources, information about other products and services related to healthcare management, and links to sites offering additional healthcare management resources. Free site registration is required for access to these resources.

Guide to Clinical Preventive Services ⊙ ⊙ ⊙

http://158.72.20.10/pubs/guidecps

This guide is a comprehensive online reference source covering recommendations for clinical practice on 169 preventive interventions, including screening tests, counseling interventions, immunizations, chemoprophylactic regimens, and other preventive medical tools. Sixty (60) target conditions are discussed in the report.

Health Services/Technology Assessment Text (HSTAT) ⊙ ⊙ ⊙

http://text.nlm.nih.gov

This electronic resource for physicians provides access to consumer brochures, evidence reports, reference guides for clinicians, clinical practice guidelines, and other full-text documents useful in making healthcare decisions. Users can download documents from the site, access general information about the system, and browse links to additional sources for information. Searches can be comprehensive or limited to specific databases within the HSTAT system, and users can also search by keyword.

InfoMedical.com v3.0—The Medical Business Search Engine ⊙ ⊙ ⊙

http://www.InfoMedical.com

This engine allows users to search for companies, news, and press releases from submitted sites in the following categories: companies, distributors, products, organizations, services, and World Wide Web resources.

Martindale's Health Science Guide ⊙ ⊙ ⊙

http://www-sci.lib.uci.edu/~martindale/HSGuide.html

An all-encompassing site for physician resources, including clinical practice and research information, this Web service offers access to teaching files, medical cases, multimedia courses and textbooks, tutorials, and other databases. There is information on different medical disciplines including Bioscience, Chemistry, Nursing, Dental Medicine, Pharmacology, Public Health, and Biotechnology.

MDGateway ⊙ ⊙

http://www.mdgateway.com

Described as an Internet "onramp for physicians busy in clinical practice," this site offers health news articles and information on clinical, professional, and personal resources. Clinical resources include links to clinical applications, medications information, practice guidelines, and patient education literature. Professional links are available with respect to coding and billing information, resources for creating and maintaining a medical practice, medical societies, and sources for medical meetings/Continuing Medical Education information. Personal finance information is also found at the site.

MedConnect ⊙ ⊙ ⊙

http://www.medconnect.com

Important medical resources at MedConnect include literature reviews, cases of the month, featured articles, journal clubs, Board reviews, free MEDLINE access, and teaching files discussing ECGs, x-rays, and CAT scans. This information is presented in separate journals of emergency medicine, pediatrics, managed care, and primary care.

MedPlanet ⊙ ⊙ ⊙

http://www.medplanet.com

Visitors to this site can search medical product classified advertisements, including surgical, anesthesia, monitoring, critical care, imaging, and laboratory equipment. The site also provides links to medical equipment manufacturers, dealers, and financing agencies. Users can add their own classified ads and include links to Web sites of equipment and product suppliers.

Medsite.com ⊙ ⊙ ⊙

http://www.medsite.com

This site describes itself as an e-services portal for the medical community. Services provided include books, medical software, and supplies at discounted prices; financial resources; a scheduling tool geared for medical professionals; and free e-mail accounts. The service requires free registration.

National Guideline Clearinghouse (NGC) ⊙ ⊙ ⊙

http://www.guideline.gov/index.asp

Four hundred and seventy-nine evidence-based clinical practice guidelines are offered at this indispensable site. Visitors can browse for guidelines by disease or condition or search for guidelines by keyword. Topical categories include immunologic, viral, endocrine, musculoskeletal, respiratory tract, urologic and male genital, nutritional and metabolic, otorhinolaryngologic, occupational, neonatal, eye, parasitic, nervous system, obstetric and gynecologic, skin and connective tissue, hemic and lymphatic, digestive system, and cardiovascular diseases, bacterial infections and mycoses, injuries, poisonings, and neoplasms.

Online Clinical Calculator ☼ ☼ ☼
http://www.intmed.mcw.edu/clincalc.html

Directed at clinical practitioners, this site offers useful analytical tools and clinical formulas for a variety of medical purposes, including body surface calculations, heart disease risk, ingested substance blood level, pregnancy due date, weights and measures, and other subjects.

Online Directory of Medical Software ☼ ☼
http://www.healthcarecomputing.com/onlindir.html

This directory provides the names, addresses, telephone numbers, and e-mail or Web site information for each of the state medical boards. Physicians can contact a board for information on licensing in that state or for other information regarding medical regulation or standards.

PDR.net ☼ ☼ ☼ (some features fee-based)
http://www.PDR.net

PDR.net is a medical and healthcare Web site created by the Medical Economics Company, publisher of healthcare magazines and directories including the PDR (Physicians' Desk Reference). The site has specific areas and content for physicians, pharmacists, physician assistants, nurses, and consumers. Access to the full-text reference book is free for U.S.-based MDs, DOs and PAs in full-time practice. There is a fee for other users of this service, but most of the site's features are free.

Physician's Guide to the Internet ☼ ☼ ☼
http://www.physiciansguide.com

This site contains a directory of Web sites for physicians. Features include physician lifestyle resources, such as sites offering suggestions on stress relief; news items; clinical practice resources, including access to medical databases and patient education resources; and postgraduate education and new physician resources. Other resources include links to sites selling medical books, products, and services for physicians; links to Internet search tools; and Internet tutorials.

Practice Management Information Corporation ☼ ☼
http://medicalbookstore.com/arm.htm

This site provides an opportunity for physicians to order books that offer information on topics that relate to the management of a private medical practice. Books on medical coding and reimbursement are also available.

State Medical Boards Directory ◎ ◎

http://www.fsmb.org/members.htm

This directory provides the names, addresses, telephone numbers, and e-mail or Web site information for each of the state medical boards. Physicians can contact a Board for information on licensing in that state or for other information regarding medical regulation or standards.

11.6 **Genetics**

Frontiers in Clinical Genetics ◎ ◎ ◎

http://www.frontiersingenetics.com/main.htm

Presented by The George Washington University Medical Center, this site offers lectures on various genetics topics presented on the Web via Real Audio. Directed at physicians requiring CME credit, the lectures assume a good deal of prior knowledge of genetics. There is also a listing of links to related sites. Lectures are archived for a period of two years to permit future study and reference.

GeneClinics ◎ ◎ ◎

http://www.geneclinics.org

GeneClinics is a knowledge base of expert-authored, up-to-date information relating genetic testing to the diagnosis, management, and counseling of individuals and families with inherited disorders. Indexed articles are of a specific and technical nature intended for use by healthcare professionals. The site also includes an extensive listing of disease profiles that is continuously updated.

Genetics Revolution at Time.com ◎ ◎

http://www.pathfinder.com/time/daily/special/genetics/index.html

This article from Time.com tracks the progress of the rapid advances in genetic technology. The site gathers a great deal of up-to-date information and offers links to a number of additional related Web-based resources.

Genetics Virtual Library ◎ ◎ ◎

http://www.ornl.gov/TechResources/Human_Genome/genetics.html

This site contains a comprehensive listing of links to major Web sites on specific topics in genetics. Links are subdivided by organism, providing genetics information on many animals, from transgenic mice to humans. Brief descriptions are provided for many links.

Institute for Genomic Research (TIGR) ⚙ ⚙ ⚙

http://www.tigr.org

The Institute for Genomic Research is a not-for-profit research institute with interests in structural, functional, and comparative analysis of genomes and gene products in viruses, eubacteria, archaea, and eukaryotes. Information on recent advances in genetics and continuing research projects in the area of human genomics, an extensive searchable database of previous research, and links to other genome centers worldwide are available at this site.

Kyoto Encyclopedia of Genomes and Genetics (KEGG) ⚙ ⚙ ⚙

http://www.genome.ad.jp/kegg

The Kyoto Encyclopedia of Genes and Genomes (KEGG) attempts to computerize current knowledge of molecular and cellular biology in terms of information pathways consisting of interacting molecules or genes, and also provides links to gene catalogs produced by genome sequencing projects. Information indexed at this site ranges from basic genetic information to extremely technical descriptions of molecular pathways. Also provided is a listing of links to other major Internet sites containing information relevant to genetic research.

Molecular Genetics Jump Station ⚙ ⚙ ⚙

http://www.horizonpress.com/gateway/genetics.html

This site provides a comprehensive listing of Web-based resources for geneticists. Sites indexed here are technical in nature and intended for investigators. Resources include links to molecular biology, microbiology, and genetics jump sites (containing catalogs of links); sites containing protocols on laboratory techniques; journals and other online publications, news groups, and mail lists; institutes and organizations; conferences and meetings announcements; commercial sites; and sources for ordering technical books. The site is sponsored by Beckman, Horizon Scientific Press, *Journal of Molecular Microbiology and Biotechnology,* and MWG-Biotech.

National Center for Biotechnology Information (NCBI): Online Mendelian Inheritance in Man (OMIM) ⚙ ⚙ ⚙

http://www.ncbi.nlm.nih.gov/Omim

Dr. Victor A. McKusick, a researcher at Johns Hopkins, and his colleagues have authored this database of human genes and genetic disorders. The database was developed for the World Wide Web by the National Center for Biotechnology Information. Reference information, texts, and images are found through the site, as well as links to the Entrez database of MEDLINE articles and sequence information. Visitors can search the OMIM Database, OMIM Gene Map, and OMIM Morbid Map (a catalog of cytogenetic map locations organized by disease) from the site. Information on the OMIM numbering system, details on creating links to OMIM, site updates, OMIM statistics, information on citing OMIM in literature, and the OMIM gene list are all found at the site. Links are available to allied resources, and the complete text of OMIM and gene maps can be downloaded from the site.

National Human Genome Research Institute (NHGRI) ⊙ ⊙ ⊙

http://www.nhgri.nih.gov

The National Human Genome Research Institute supports the NIH component of the Human Genome Project, a worldwide research effort designed to analyze the structure of human DNA and determine the location of the estimated 50,000–100,000 human genes. The NHGRI Intramural Research Program develops and implements technology for understanding, diagnosing, and treating genetic diseases. The site provides information about NHGRI, the Human Genome Project, grants, intramural research, policy and public affairs, workshops and conferences, and news items. Resources include links to the Institute's Ethical, Legal, and Social Implications Program, and the Center for Inherited Disease Research. The site also provides genetic resources for investigators, a glossary of genetic terms, and a site search engine.

Office of Genetics and Disease Prevention ⊙ ⊙ ⊙

http://www.cdc.gov/genetics

Created by the Centers for Disease Control and Prevention, this site offers access to current information on the impact of human genetic research and the Human Genome Project on public health and disease prevention. The site provides general information, indexes recent articles, lists events and training opportunities, and offers an extensive listing of links to other resources. Users can search the site by keyword and access the Human Genome Epidemiology Network (HuGENet), a global collaboration of individuals and organizations committed to the development and dissemination of population-based epidemiologic information on the human genome.

Primer on Molecular Genetics ⊙ ⊙ ⊙

http://www.ornl.gov/hgmis/publicat/primer/intro.html

The United States Department of Energy presents an excellent resource for those seeking basic background information on genetics and genetic research at this site. Discussions at the site include an introduction to genetics, DNA, genes, chromosomes, and the process of mapping the human genome. Mapping strategies, genetic linkage maps, and various physical maps are available, as well as links to mapping and sequence databases and a glossary of terms. The site also summarizes the predicted impact of the Human Genome Project on medical practice and biological research.

University of Kansas Medical Center: Genetics Education Center ⊙ ⊙ ⊙

http://www.kumc.edu/gec

Links are available at this address to Internet resources for educators interested in human genetics and the Human Genome Project. Sites are listed by topic, including the Human Genome Project, education resources, networking, genetic conditions, booklets and brochures, genetics programs and other resources, and glossaries. Lesson plans are offered both by the University of Kansas and other sources at the site. A description of different careers in genetics are also available. This site is an excellent tool for finding useful genetics Internet resources for nonprofessionals and educators.

11.7 **Geriatrics**

Administration on Aging: Resource Directory for Older People ☺ ☺ ☺
http://www.aoa.dhhs.gov/aoa/dir/intro.html

The National Institute on Aging and the Administration on Aging has compiled this directory of resources, serving older people and their families, health and legal professionals, social service providers, librarians, researchers, and others interested in the field of aging. The directory includes names of organizations, addresses, telephone numbers (including toll-free numbers), and links to Internet sites, when available. Visitors can search the directory by keyword or view the entire table of contents from this address.

American Geriatrics Society (AGS) ☺ ☺ ☺ (some features fee-based)
http://www.americangeriatrics.org/index.html

A national nonprofit association of geriatrics health professionals, research scientists, and other concerned individuals, the American Geriatrics Society is dedicated to "improving the health, independence, and quality of life for all older people." The site offers a description of the Society, adult immunization information, AGS news, conference and other events notices, legislation news, career opportunities, directories of geriatrics health care services in managed care, position statements, educational, and practice guidelines, awards information, and other professional education resources. Patient education resources, a selected bibliography in geriatrics, links to related organizations and government sites, surveys, and a site search tool are also found at this address.

11.8 **Grants and Award Guides**

Foundation Center ☺ ☺ ☺
http://fdncenter.org

The Foundation Center provides direct, hot links to thousands of grant-making organizations, including foundations, corporations, and public charities, along with a search engine to enable the user to locate sources of funding in specific fields. In addition, the site provides listings of the largest private foundations, corporate grant makers, and community foundations. There is also information on funding trends, a newsletter, and grant-seeker orientation material. More than 900 grant-making organizations are accessible through this useful site.

National Institutes of Health (NIH): Funding Opportunities ⊙ ⊙ ⊙
http://grants.nih.gov/grants

Funding opportunities for research, scholarship, and training are extensive within the federal government. At this site for the National Institutes of Health, there is a Grants Page with information about NIH grants and fellowship programs, information on Research Contracts containing information on Requests for Proposals (RFPs), Research Training Opportunities in biomedical areas, and an NIH Guide for Grants and Contracts. The latter is the official document for announcing the availability of NIH funds for biomedical and behavioral research and research training policies. Links are provided to major divisions of NIH that have additional information on specialized grant opportunities.

National Science Foundation (NSF) Grants & Awards ⊙ ⊙ ⊙
http://www.nsf.gov/home/grants.htm

Because approximately 20% of the federal support to academic institutions for basic research comes from the National Science Foundation, this site is an important source of information for award opportunities, programs, application procedures, and other vital information. Forms and agreements may be downloaded as well, and regulations and policy guidelines are set forth clearly.

Polaris Grants Central ⊙ ⊙
http://polarisgrantscentral.net

For the grant seeker, this site provides resources that are available from numerous organizations pertaining to grant identification and application. There are books and publications on grant sources, descriptions of grant information providers, clearing-houses for grant information, federal contacts, grant training materials, and resources on disk or CD-ROM. Within the site, useful sections provide "Tips and Hints" on writing grant proposals, "Grants News" from different government agencies and other organizations, "Scholarships or Grants to Individuals," and information on grant workshops.

Society of Research Administrators (SRA) GrantsWeb ⊙ ⊙ ⊙
http://sra.rams.com/cws/sra/resource.htm

The Society of Research Administrators has created an extremely useful grant information site, with extensive links to government resources, general resources, private funding, and policy/regulation sites. The site section devoted to U.S., Canadian, and other international resources provides links to government agency funding sources, the commerce business daily, the Catalog of Federal Domestic Assistance, scientific agencies, research councils, and resources in individual fields, such as health, education, and business. Grant-application procedures, regulations, and guidelines are provided throughout the site, and extensive legal information is provided through links to patent, intellectual property, and copyright offices. Associations providing funding and grant information are also listed, with direct links.

11.9 Imaging and Pathology

Center For Biomedical Imaging Technology ⊙ ⊙ ⊙

http://panda.uchc.edu/htbit/indiv/research.html

Current research performed by the Center for Biomedical Imaging Technology is presented at this site in the form of medical imaging examples accomplished by the Center. A short tutorial on the classification of MR images, videos, and abstracts on light microscopy of living cells, and the structure and function of the endoplasmic reticulum are available through links at the site.

Center For Human Simulation ⊙ ⊙ ⊙

http://www.uchsc.edu/sm/chs

This site provides a browser to view cross sections from any part of the bodies from the Visible Human Project. Also included are images, animations, videos, and 3-D polygonal models of various parts of the human anatomy that were created using new imaging technology.

CT Is Us ⊙ ⊙ ⊙

http://www.ctisus.org

The CT (computed tomography) site offers information on medical imaging with a specific focus on spiral CT and 3D imaging. Images of the body and various medical conditions are organized by region, and information on Continuing Medical Education (CME) courses, teaching files, medical illustrations, and a 3D vascular atlas are all available at the site.

Digital Imaging Center ⊙ ⊙ ⊙

http://info.med.yale.edu/library/imaging

This Web site, provided by Cushing/Whitney Medical Library of Yale University, serves as a starting point for help on the various resources available through the Digital Imaging Center, including a digital camera, computer resource lab, color printers, scanners, and digital video editing capabilities. Resources at this site are most useful to visitors with access to the Cushing/Whitney Medical Library Digital Imaging Center.

Dr. Morimoto's Image Library of Radiology ⊙ ⊙ ⊙

http://www.osaka-med.ac.jp/omc-lib/noh.html

This site provides users with access to images and videos collected by Dr. Morimoto, Department of Radiology, Osaka National Hospital. Images were scanned and stored with JPEG, GIF format, and movies with QuickTime format. Visitors can download the images freely but need permission for redistribution. Ultrasonographic anatomy images related to the liver, pancreas, and bile duct include an illustration of portal anatomy, normal bile duct, tumor of liver hilum, bile duct cancer, pancreatic cancer, esophageal varix, and obstructive jaundice. Heart and major vessels images include a normal heart, major vessels of the body, and abdominal aortic aneurysm. Head images include a surface image of human head and an image of an arachnoid cyst. Images related to the kidney and urinary tract include that of a renal cell carcinoma.

Health On the Net (HON) Foundation ⊙ ⊙ ⊙

http://www.hon.ch/Media/anatomy.html

This site provides links to radiological and surgical images on the Internet. Images are available of the abdomen, ankle, arm, full body, brain, elbow, eye, foot, hand, head, heart, hilum, hip, kidney, knee, leg, liver, lung, muscle, neck, pancreas, pelvis, shoulder, skin, skull, teeth, thorax, trachea, blood vessels, and wrist.

Integrated Medical
Curriculum Human Anatomy ⊙ ⊙ ⊙ (free registration)

http://www.imc.gsm.com

An extensive database of images can be easily accessed for educational purposes. The site covers Human Anatomy, Microscopic Anatomy, Radiologic Anatomy, Cross-Sectional Anatomy, as well as essentials of Human Physiology, essentials of Immunology, and Clinical Pharmacology. A simple, free registration is required.

Medical i-Way ⊙ ⊙ ⊙

http://www.largnet.on.ca/oldlargnet

Medical i-Way demonstrates pathology through the use of medical imaging. A separate section is devoted to each anatomical group, with a list of specific pathologies available for view. Details of each image include case history, diagnosis, image findings, and descriptions of similar cases. Users can also find images through a keyword index.

Medical Images on the Web ⊙ ⊙ ⊙

http://www.unmc.edu/library/medimag.html

Eleven links are available at this address to Internet sources for medical images. All links are accompanied by short descriptions of resources at the site.

Mudi-Muse Biomedical Imaging and Processing ⊙ ⊙ ⊙
http://www.expasy.ch/LFMI

The MultiDimensional-MultiSensor/MultiModality Biomedical Imaging and Processing Web site provides examples and applications of different techniques used in biomedical imaging. Multidimensional, multimodality, and multi-sensor applications are described in detail with specific examples of medical applications, and discussions of new developments in this growing field are available.

National Library of Medicine (NLM) New Visible Human Project ⊙ ⊙ ⊙
http://www.nlm.nih.gov/research/visible/visible_human.html

The Visible Human Project, devoted to the creation of complete, anatomically detailed, three-dimensional representations of the normal male and female human bodies, is an outgrowth of the National Library of Medicine's 1986 Long Range Plan. The Project has recently completed acquisition of transverse CT, MR, and cryosection images of representative male and female cadavers. The site describes the Visible Human Data Set and how to obtain data, and provides links to primary contractors for the Project, a sampler of images and animations from the project, and links to articles and other press releases discussing the Project. Applications and tools for viewing images are discussed, and links to sources of images and animations are provided. This site is also available in Spanish.

Neurosciences on the Internet: Images ⊙ ⊙ ⊙
http://www.neuroguide.com/neuroimg.html

Internet sites are found through this address offering resources relating to human neuroanatomy and neuropathology, neuroscience images and methods, medical imaging centers, medical illustration, medical imaging indexes, and neuroanatomy atlases of animals.

Normal Radiologic Anatomy ⊙ ⊙
http://www.vh.org/Providers/TeachingFiles/NormalRadAnatomy/Text/RadM1title.html

This site provides visitors with X-Ray, CT, MR, and ultrasound images of the head and neck, thorax, abdomen, pelvis, upper extremity, and lower extremity. Images are labeled to identify normal anatomic structures.

PERLjam Online/Medical Images, Including Neuroanatomy ⊙ ⊙ ⊙
http://erl.pathology.iupui.edu

This site is an online version of the PERLjam CD-ROM of pathology, histology, and laboratory medicine resources distributed to Indiana University School of Medicine students. The Indiana University School of Medicine Pathology Educational Resources Laboratory provides general and systemic pathology, histology, laboratory medicine, and dermatology images at this site. Images are categorized by organ system.

Three-Dimensional Medical Reconstruction ◎ ◎ ◎

http://www.crd.ge.com/esl/cgsp/projects/medical

Three-dimensional (3-D) reconstruction technology and medical imaging was employed to make short videos showing various sections of the human anatomy at this site. Information on the Visible Human Project and several short videos on this topic, surgical planning, and virtual endoscopy are also available.

University of Illinois College of Medicine
at Urbana-Champaign-The Urbana Atlas of Pathology ◎ ◎ ◎

http://www.med.uiuc.edu/PathAtlasf/framer2/path3.html

The site provides an extremely comprehensive collection of images sectioned into general, cardiovascular, endocrine, pulmonary, and renal pathology. The general pathology section includes images of the kidney, heart, spleen, thyroid, testis, cervix, small intestine, lung, artery, pancreas, liver, lymph nodes, brain, colon, skin, mesentery, joints, uterus, and peritoneal cavity.

University of Iowa College Of Medicine—
Division of Physiological Imaging Department Of Radiology ◎ ◎ ◎

http://everest.radiology.uiowa.edu

This site describes work done by the Division of Physiological Imaging of the University of Iowa College of Medicine. This group is dedicated to the research and advancement of medical imaging technology. Within the Web site are examples of medical imaging, selected papers on the field, descriptions of new technology and projects, and a list of links to related sites.

Visible Human Slice and Surface Server ◎ ◎ ◎

http://visiblehuman.epfl.ch

This site provides a viewer that enables the user to see images of planar and curved surfaces from the bodies of the Visible Human Project.

11.10 Medical Informatics

American Medical Association (AMA):
Electronic Medical Systems & Coding ◎ ◎ ◎

http://www.ama-assn.org/med-sci/cpt/oems.htm

The American Medical Association plays a key role in the field of medical informatics. This site provides information on coding and medical information systems relative to the transmission of computerized patient and claims information. There are also links for electronic medical records, telemedicine, electronic data exchange, national uniform claim standards, and administrative simplification legislation.

American Medical Association (AMA): Coding and Medical Information Systems ◉ ◉ ◉

http://www.ama-assn.org/med-sci/cpt/cpt.htm

This site provides information on the AMA's new current procedural terminology (CPT) information services, the resource-based relative value scale, and electronic medical systems, including systems for storing electronic medical records, telemedicine resources, and electronic data interchange. Information is also available on the National Uniform Claim Committee and Administrative Simplification Legislation.

American Medical Informatics Association (AMIA) ◉ ◉ ◉

http://www.amia.org

With the proliferation of medical information, the growth of medical research, the development of medical information systems, and the creation of management systems for computerized patient data, the medical informatics field has grown substantially. This leading association provides its own organization, meeting, policy, and information access features, and also provides links to other organizations in the informatics field. Major themes of the AMIA are privacy and confidentiality of medical records, public policy development for legislation in the field, conferences of medical informatics professionals, and the issuance of papers and publications covering various aspects of the medical information field.

Medical Informatics Resources from Health Network ◉ ◉

http://www.healthwave.com

A dozen U.S. and international centers and medical departments dealing with Medical Informatics can be accessed from this central listing (click on Professional Medicine, Medical Informatics), including centers at Oregon Health Sciences University, Stanford, Columbia, and at European institutions. There are also articles, directories, and discussion group links for further resources on Medical Informatics.

11.11 Patent Searches

Introduction

The following sites provide easy access to patent information for medical researchers and healthcare professionals interested in learning about the latest techniques, therapies, products, and drugs.

Intellectual Property Network ◉ ◉ ◉

http://www.patents.ibm.com

Ideal for physicians and researchers with an interest in patents, this IBM service offers a searchable database of patent information, titles and abstracts, and inventors and companies. The database brings up patents on any topic by typing in the subject, along with inventor information, dates of filing, application numbers, and an abstract of the patent.

U.S. Patent and Trademark Office ⊙ ⊙ ⊙
http://www.uspto.gov/patft/index.html

Access to the database of the U.S. Patent and Trademark Office is available through this site, for detailed searching of patents by number, inventor, and topic. There are both a full-text database and a bibliographic database.

12. STUDENT RESOURCES

12.1 **Fellowships and Residencies**

Accreditation Council for Graduate Medical Education (ACGME) ◉ ◉ ◉

http://www.acgme.org

The ACGME reviews and accredits residency programs, establishes standards of performance, and provides a process to consider complaints and possible investigations by the Council. The site offers information about ACGME, meetings, workshops, institutional reviews, contact details, links to residency review committees, and a listing of accredited programs.

American Medical Association (AMA): Fellowship and Residency Electronic Interactive Database Access (FREIDA) Online System ◉ ◉ ◉

http://www.ama-assn.org/physdata/datacoll/datacoll.htm

Operated as a service of the American Medical Association (AMA), the FREIDA System provides online access to a comprehensive database of information on approximately 7,500 graduate medical educational programs accredited by the Accreditation Council for Graduate Medical Education (ACGME). FREIDA enables the user to search this comprehensive database and offers other services, including label printing for mailing purposes.

Educational Commission for Foreign Medical Graduates (ECFMG) ◉ ◉ ◉

http://www.ecfmg.org

The Educational Commission for Foreign Medical Graduates, through its certification program, "assesses the readiness of graduates of foreign medical schools to enter residency or fellowship programs in the United States that are accredited by the Accreditation Council for Graduate Medical Education (ACGME)." The site is a very useful source of information for foreign students to learn about testing and examination dates, clinical skills required, and available publications to review requirements for applications.

Electronic Residency Application Service ◉ ◉ ◉

http://www.aamc.org

The Association of American Medical Colleges (AAMC) provides this application service for students. It transmits residency applications, recommendation letters, Dean's letters, transcripts, and other supporting credentials from medical schools to residency program directors via the Internet. At present, the service covers Obstetrics and Gynecology, Pediatrics, Surgery, and Psychiatry. The system allows tracking of an application 24 hours a day via a special document tracking system.

National Residency Matching Program (NRMP) ◎ ◎ ◎

http://nrmp.aamc.org/nrmp

The NRMP is a mechanism for the matching of applicants to programs according to the preferences expressed by both parties. This is an extremely useful site and service, which last year placed over 20,000 applicants for postgraduate medical training positions into 3,500 residency programs at 700 teaching hospitals in the United States. The applicants and residency programs evaluate and rank each other, producing a computerized pairing of applicants to programs, in ranked order. This process provides applicants and program directors with a uniform date of appointment to positions in March, eliminating decision pressure when options are unknown. The site offers information about the service, contact details, publications, and forms for registration. Prospective residents can register with the service for a fee and access the directory of programs.

Residency Page ◎ ◎ ◎

http://www.Webcom.com/~wooming/residenc.html

The Residency Page Web site provides an online listing of medical residencies organized by specialty. Program directors can access resumes of residency applicants, and prospective residents can review documents related to residency matching programs and publications offering advice on obtaining a position.

12.2 Medical School Web Sites

American Universities ◎ ◎ ◎

http://www.clas.ufl.edu/CLAS/american-universities.html

All American university home pages are listed at this site.

Gradschools.com ◎ ◎ ◎

http://www.gradschools.com/noformsearch.html

Sponsored by several universities and other teaching institutions, Gradschools.com offers a listing of graduate programs nationwide. Programs are found by indicating a specific area of study. A directory of distance learning programs is also available.

Medical Education ◎ ◎ ◎

http://www.meducation.com/schools.html

Accredited medical schools are listed, with links, at this site.

Medical Schools ⊙ ⊙ ⊙

http://www.scomm.net/~greg/med-ed/schools.html

This medical site provides direct links to all of the medical schools of U.S. and Canada accredited by the AAMC. These include hundreds of medical school Web sites in the United States and elsewhere.

12.3 Medical Student Resources

American Medical Women's Association (AMWA) ⊙ ⊙ ⊙

http://www.amwa-doc.org

A national association, the AMWA provides information and services to women physicians and women medical students, and promotes women's health and the professional development of women physicians. Resources include news, discussions of current issues, events, conferences, online publications, fellowship and residency information accessed through FREIDA, general information and developments from AMA staff members, advocacy activities, a listing of AMWA continuing education programs, and links to sites of interest. A variety of topics related to women's health are discussed at the site.

Association of American Medical Colleges (AAMC) ⊙ ⊙ ⊙

http://www.aamc.org

This nonprofit Association committed to the advancement of academic medicine consists of American and Canadian medical schools, teaching hospitals and health systems, academic and professional societies, and medical students and residents. News, membership details, publications and other information resources, meeting and conference calendars, medical education Internet resources, research findings, and discussions related to health care are all found at the site. Employment opportunities at the AAMC are also listed.

IMpact: The Internal Medicine Newsletter for Medical Students ⊙ ⊙ ⊙

http://www.acponline.org/journals/impact/impmenu.htm

This online newsletter focuses on different medical specialties with each issue, and includes full-text articles of interest to physicians and medical students. The newsletter is produced by the American College of Physicians—American Society of Internal Medicine (ACP-ASIM). Students can apply for free membership in the ACP-ASIM if they are currently enrolled in medical school.

Medical Books at Amazon.com ☺ ☺ ☺

http://www.abcba.com/books/medical.htm

This site allows users to search by medical topic or keyword for medical textbooks. Dictionaries, encyclopedias, and Physician's Desk References on different subjects may be ordered through the site.

Medical Student Section of the AMA ☺ ☺ ☺

http://www.ama-assn.org/ama/pub/category/0,1120,14,FF.html

The Medical Student Section of the American Medical Association (AMA) is dedicated to representing medical students, improving medical education, developing leadership, and promoting activism for the health of America. The site offers information about the section, current issues and advocacy activities, business issues of the section, chapter information, and leadership news. Special interest groups within the section include those for residents, young physicians, organized staff, students, international medical graduates, and senior physicians.

Medical Student Web Site ☺ ☺ ☺

http://www.medicalstudent.com

This is an excellent, current site for medical students, describing itself as "a digital library of authoritative medical information for all students of medicine." It contains an extensive medical textbook section organized by discipline, patient simulations, consumer health information, access to MEDLINE and medical journals online, continuing education sources, board exam information, medical organizations, and Internet medical directories.

Stanford MedWorld ☺ ☺ ☺

http://www-med.stanford.edu/medworld/home

MedWorld, sponsored by the Stanford Medical Alumni Association, offers information for students, patients, physicians, and the healthcare community. Resources include case reports and global rounds, links to quality medical sites and MEDLINE, doctor diaries and medical news, and newsgroups and discussion forums. Visitors can access Stanford's medical search engine, MEDBOT, to simultaneously utilize many Internet medical search engines.

Student Doctor Network:
The Interactive Medical Student Lounge ☺ ☺ ☺

http://www.medstudents.net

This is an excellent site for medical students with interests in all medical specialties as well as all aspects of the medical community. The site provides information on applying to medical school, financial aid, internships and residencies, medical chat rooms, databases, discussions of educational issues, links to online journals, news, updates, and broadcasts. In addition, the site provides access to discounts on medical equipment and books, the purchase and sale of used medical texts, medical software and medical CD-ROMs. Students can also access medical reference material, medical school sites, medical search engines, student groups, externships, foreign residencies, and medical missions abroad.

13. PATIENT EDUCATION AND PLANNING

13.1 **Patient Resources**

Introduction

Patient information regarding various medical conditions and health issues can be obtained at any of the general medical search engines that are included. Below are listings of health Web sites accessible through the well-known search engines, as well as other sites that cover wide-ranging topics of interest to patients.

Allexperts.com ⊙ ⊙

http://www.allexperts.com/medical

Allexperts.com is a free online question and answer service. A message board and many frequently asked questions are present. Available medical topics are listed alphabetically, and users can choose a specific "volunteer expert" to contact after reading short biographies and descriptions of specialty areas.

allHealth.com ⊙ ⊙ ⊙

http://www.allhealth.com

Resources at this site include a site search engine; a drug database; information on specific conditions; weight management information; and special information centers devoted to seniors', women's, and men's health, pediatrics, mental health, sexual health, alternative medicine, asthma, headaches, smoking cessation, HIV/AIDS, heartburn, and family health. Physician directories for home and when traveling, elder care directories, interactive health calculators, an online newsletter, research information, chat forums, and news articles are also provided.

America Online (AOL) ⊙ ⊙

http://www.aol.com/timesavers/health.html

Sponsored by America Online, this site is a useful medical information source for the general public. The user can search for a disease; use a symptom analyzer; learn about rare illnesses; obtain advice; find support groups; and research topics on health, medicine, and wellness.

American Academy of
Family Physicians Health Information Page ⊙ ⊙ ⊙

http://familydoctor.org

This site allows visitors to search information by keyword or category, and is written and reviewed by the physicians and patient education professionals at the Academy of Family Physicians.

American Medical Association (AMA): Health Insight ⚙ ⚙ ⚙
http://www.ama-assn.org/consumer.htm

Information for consumers at this site includes medical news; detailed information on a wide range of conditions; general health topic discussions; family health resources for children, adolescents, men, and women; interactive health calculators; healthy recipes; and general safety tips. Specific pages are devoted to comprehensive resources related to HIV/AIDS, asthma, migraines, and women's health. Patients will find this site an excellent source for accurate, useful health information. American Medical Association information at this site includes a directory of advisory board members and contact information for the Association.

BestDoctors.com ⚙ ⚙ (free registration)
http://www.bestdoctors.com

Best Doctors' Inc. provides information and searching services for superior medical care to major insurers, managed care companies, self-insured corporations, foreign governments, and individuals. The site provides visitors with news, feature articles from a participating doctor, drug information, general information, and suggested sites relating to over 40 health topics. Contact information, employment details, a directory of the company's medical advisory board, rating information on medical Web sites, news and events information, contact information for a physician referral service, and answers relating to recent Internet health-related rumors are all found at the site. Registered users can ask health questions, participate in chat forums, and gain access to medical newsletters.

Boston University Medical Center— Community Outreach Health Information System ⚙ ⚙ ⚙
http://www.bu.edu/cohis

This site provides the general public with an excellent resource for health information. A wide range of health topics are discussed at the site, including AIDS/HIV, infectious diseases, sexually transmitted diseases, cancer, blood and heart diseases, nutrition, smoking cessation, domestic violence, teen pregnancy, and alcohol and substance abuse. More specific topics are also listed. Visitors can submit health questions and access a physician directory.

Columbia University College of Physicians and Surgeons Complete Home Medical Guide ⚙ ⚙ ⚙
http://cpmcnet.columbia.edu/texts/guide

Patients will consider this site an excellent resource for healthcare information. Topics include receiving proper medical care, the correct use of medications, first aid and safety, preventative medicine, and good nutrition. Chapters containing more specific information on health concerns for men, women, and children; disorders; infectious diseases; mental and emotional health; and substance abuse are also available.

Combined Health Information Database (CHID) ◉ ◉ ◉

http://chid.nih.gov

The Combined Health Information Database (CHID) is produced by several agencies of the federal government offering a searchable file of health promotion publications, education materials, and program descriptions. The site offers simple and detailed search options, and users can also indicate specific search criteria, including date and language of the publication. Availability and ordering information is provided for the resources included. Site updates are performed quarterly.

DiscoveryHealth.com ◉ ◉ ◉

http://www.discoveryhealth.com/DH/ihtIH?t=20707&st=20707&r=WSDSC000

In association with InteliHealth, this site from the makers of the Discovery Channel offers consumer health resources. News items, feature articles and reports, a site search engine, links to health reference materials, chat forums, a forum for asking health questions, and descriptions of recent research advances are all found at this site. Visitors can learn interesting health facts and access information specific to men, women, senior citizens, children, mental health, and health in the workplace. Nutrition, fitness, and weight management tools are also available at this site.

DoctorDirectory: HealthNews Directory ◉ ◉

http://www.doctordirectory.com/HealthNews/Directory/Default.asp

In addition to daily news and a national directory of doctors listed by state, this site contains links to resources related to various health topics, including AIDS, allergies/asthma, alternative medicine, cancer, children's health, clinical trials, cosmetic surgery, dentistry, diabetes, women's health, geriatrics, healthcare companies, insurance, and other subjects.

drkoop.com ◉ ◉ ◉

http://www.drkoop.com

This site provides patients and the general public with an excellent source for current health information. Free registration and e-mail newsletters, site search engines, health news, chat topics, general information about clinical trials, and a drug interaction search tool are some of the most useful features. Please note that some sections of the site offering specific information are sponsored by pharmaceutical products, i.e., a company producing a smoking cessation medication sponsors a section designed to help users quit.

Family Village—
A Global Community of Disability-Related Resources ⚙ ⚙ ⚙

http://www.familyvillage.wisc.edu/index.htmlx

This site provides the general public with cataloged information about a wide range of disorders and disabilities. Chat room links and other networking resources, support and medical resources, technology/products links, recreation programs, research programs, publications, and educational resources for children are all found at this comprehensive patient support site.

Health-Center.com ⚙ ⚙

http://site.health-center.com/default.htm

This site contains a variety of links to fact sheets on family issues, senior citizen related topics, general wellness topics, mental health information, and medications. There are also links to professional resources, including postings of online continuing education resources.

HealthAnswers.com ⚙ ⚙ ⚙

http://www.healthanswers.com

This site provides the general public with informational resources on a wide range of health topics, including senior health, pregnancy, alternative medicine, diseases, and healthy lifestyle tips. Partners include the American Academy of Pediatrics, the Center for Pharmacy, the National Health Council, the National Transplant Society, Reuters Health News, and other national groups and information resources.

HealthCentral.com ⚙ ⚙ ⚙

http://www.healthcentral.com/home/home.cfm

News items, feature columns, quizzes and polls, a doctor's column, drug and herb information, health profiles and assessment tools, online shopping, and medical reference materials are all available at this useful site. Information centers offer specific resources on "hot topics," alternative medicine, fitness, life issues, wellness, consumer health, health improvement, such as weight loss and smoking cessation, and medical conditions.

HealthlinkUSA ⚙ ⚙ ⚙

http://www.healthlinkusa.com

At this site, links to many general health sites are listed in alphabetical order by topic or disorder. Interested persons can access links to specific health issues or browse for sites by medical category.

HealthWorld Online ☼ ☼ ☼

http://www.healthy.net

A subject map appears at the beginning of this site indicating the many aspects of the health and medical world covered by numerous links. There is a topical site search engine, access to publications through MEDLINE at the National Library of Medicine, information on specific diseases and alternative therapies, a referral network, a global calendar, and information on wellness, fitness, and nutrition.

InteliHealth: Home to Johns Hopkins Health Information ☼ ☼ ☼

http://www.intelihealth.com/IH/ihtIH?t=408&st=408&r=WSIHW000

This comprehensive site offers consumers tips on healthy living, information, and other resources on specific conditions, a site search engine for specific information, health news by topic, special reports, an online newsletter, pharmaceutical drug information, and an online store offering health items for the home. Conditions and health topics discussed at the site include allergy, arthritis, asthma, babies, cancer, caregivers, childhood, diabetes, digestive, fitness, headache, heart, mental health, pregnancy, vitamin and nutrition, and weight management. Links are available to other sites offering consumer health resources.

Johns Hopkins Medical Institutions ☼ ☼ ☼

http://infonet.welch.jhu.edu/advocacy.html

A database of patient advocacy groups is housed at this site. Telephone contact information and links to an associated Web site is offered for most organizations. A search tool is available to find groups for specific disorders.

KidsHealth.org ☼ ☼ ☼

http://kidshealth.org/index2.html

This site, created by the Nemours Foundation Center for Children's Health Media, provides expert health information about children from before birth through adolescence. Specific sections target kids, teens, and parents, with age-appropriate information and language.

Mayo Health ☼ ☼ ☼

http://www.mayohealth.org/index.htm

Visitors to this informative site will find answers to patient questions, news and articles on featured topics, registration details for e-mail alerts of site updates, and site search engines for health information and prescription drug information. Specific information centers are devoted to allergy and asthma, Alzheimer's disease, cancer, children's health, digestive health, heart health, general medicine, men's and women's health, and nutrition. A library of answers to health questions, a glossary of medical terms, and a forum for asking specific questions are also available at the site.

MDAdvice.com ⚙ ⚙
http://www.mdadvice.com

In addition to containing links to informative fact sheets on a variety of health topics (arranged alphabetically), this site provides detailed information on pharmaceuticals, medicine in the news, information on health centers, expert advice, and chat rooms.

Med Help International ⚙ ⚙ ⚙
http://www.medhelp.org

This all-encompassing site describes itself as "the largest online consumer health information resource with tens of thousands of entries." It includes a medical search engine, library access and doctor forums, medical and health news, and support groups.

MedicineNet ⚙ ⚙ ⚙
http://www.medicinenet.com

An efficient and thorough source of information on hundreds of diseases and medical conditions, MedicineNet enables the user to click on subjects in an alphabetical list. The site's medical content is produced by Board certified physicians and allied health professionals. Topics include diseases and treatments, procedures and tests, a pharmacy section, a medical dictionary, first aid information, and a list of poison control centers.

Mediconsult.com, Inc. ⚙ ⚙ ⚙
http://www.mediconsult.com

Mediconsult provides medical news and information on a variety of topics, including cancer, chronic pain, eating disorders, and migraines. The information at the site is drawn from journals, research centers, and other sources, and is subject to a rigorous clinical review process. Specific sections are devoted to health issues relevant to women, men, seniors, children, and caregivers. Additional resources include a medical directory of disease information, drug information, fitness and nutrition discussions, a question and answer forum, and live chat events.

MEDLINEplus ⚙ ⚙ ⚙
http://www.nlm.nih.gov/medlineplus

This site is a source for information on various diseases and health topics for the public, featuring a directory of links divided into categories such as health topics, dictionaries, other directories, organizations, and publications. The site links to MEDLINE, either through PubMed or the Internet Grateful Med.

National Women's Health Information Center (NWHIC) ◎ ◎ ◎
http://www.4woman.org

This searchable site offers lists of publications and organizations for information on a wide range of women's health topics. There are also links to resources for special groups, journals, FAQs, news items and affiliated organizations, as well as information about the NWHIC itself.

NetWellness ◎ ◎ ◎ (some features fee-based)
http://www.netwellness.org

NetWellness is a Web-based consumer health information service with one of the largest groups of medical and health experts who answer consumer questions on the Web. Developed by the University of Cincinnati Medical Center, The Ohio State University, and Case Western Reserve University, over 200 health faculty answer questions on over 40 topics. Responses are usually provided within two to three days. Users can also search archives of articles.

New York Online Access to Health (NOAH) ◎ ◎ ◎ (some features fee-based)
http://www.noah.cuny.edu

This site is offered as a public resource by many providers, including hospitals, institutes, foundations, research centers, and city and state agencies. Users can access information concerning a wide range of health topics, including diseases, mental health, nutrition, and links to patient resources. A site-based search engine is available. A health information database containing abstracts and articles from selected health-related periodicals is only available to users accessing the site from specific institutions, including the New York Public Library branches.

OnHealth.com ◎ ◎ ◎
http://www.onhealth.com/ch1/index.asp

Visitors to this site can search for health information by keyword or condition, access news and reports, ask health questions, and find many useful information resources related to specific topics, such as smoking cessation, pharmaceutical drugs, alternative medicine, vitamins and minerals, and first aid. Chat forums, information on live chat events, physician and medical center directories, online shopping opportunities, and interactive health assessment tools are all found at this site.

Prevention Magazine Online ◎ ◎ ◎
http://www.healthyideas.com

Prevention Magazine offers resources for healthier living at this site. Health tools include a calorie calculator, exercise and weight loss information, recipes, vitamin and herb information, and tips on skin care. Online newsletters and stores, chat forums, and subscription details for the magazine are available, as well as resource centers offering specific information on health conditions, men's and women's health, and pediatrics. Links are also found to women.com for specific women's resources.

Psci-com ☼ ☼ ☼
http://www.psci-com.org.uk

Psci-com is described as "a gateway to public understanding of science and science communication information on the Internet." The site offers a searchable catalog of Internet resources selected and cataloged by the Wellcome Trust for the benefit of the UK public.

Quackwatch ☼ ☼ ☼
http://www.quackwatch.com

Quackwatch is a nonprofit corporation combating "health-related frauds, myths, fads, and fallacies." The group investigates questionable health claims, answers consumer inquiries, distributes publications, reports illegal marketing, generates consumer-protection lawsuits, works to improve the quality of health information on the Internet, and attacks misleading Internet advertising. Operation costs are generated solely from the sales of publications and individual donations. Sister sites, Chirobase and MLM Watch, offer a consumer's guide to chiropractors and a skeptical guide to multilevel marketing. Information for cancer patients includes alerts of questionable alternative health treatments, a discussion of how questionable practices may harm cancer patients, and other related discussions. Cancer prevention information alerts are also posted. Visitors to the site can purchase publications, read general information about questionable medical practices, and read information about specific questionable products and services. Links to government agencies and other sites providing information about health fraud are available at this important site.

Thrive ☼ ☼ ☼
http://www.thriveonline.com

Thrive Online offers information resources in the areas of general medicine, fitness, sexuality, nutrition, serenity and mental wellness, and weight. Users can find information by choosing from a list of medical conditions, or employ search capabilities by keyword or in question form.

University of California (UC), Davis Medical Center Patient Care ☼ ☼ ☼
http://www.pcs.ucdmc.ucdavis.edu

This site contains information about patient care services at UC Davis Medical Center as well as a list of health resources on the Internet. Specific resources include topics in patient care, education, and epidemiology and infection control.

University of Iowa Virtual Hospital ◎ ◎ ◎ (some features fee-based)
http://www.vh.org

The Virtual Hospital is a service of the University of Iowa, providing patients and healthcare professionals with a digital library of health information. The library contains hundreds of books and brochures on health related issues, and also provides physicians with Continuing Medical Education resources. The site provides information about the departments at the University of Iowa hospitals, a link to the Virtual Children's Hospital, Continuing Medical Education information, and resource sections for patients and healthcare providers. Two sections are restricted to University of Iowa students, faculty, and affiliates.

Yahoo! ◎ ◎ ◎
http://www.yahoo.com

A reliable source of information in most fields, Yahoo offers a Health Section covering diseases, medical topics, patient information, fitness, and other health topics. It is a good place to start for a patient seeking general information.

13.2 Support Groups

Ask NOAH About: Support Groups ◎ ◎ ◎
http://www.noah.cuny.edu:8080/support1.html

This directory of Web sites and other resources includes links to other directories, general health sites, toll-free telephone numbers, face-to-face support groups, support organizations, newsgroups, mailing lists, chat forums, and other online support resources. Visitors can browse listings by type of resource or by specific medical conditions.

Support-Group.com ◎ ◎ ◎
http://www.support-group.com

Support-Group.com allows people with health, personal, and relationship issues to share their experiences through bulletin boards and online chats, and provides plenty of links to support-related information on the Internet. The A to Z listing offers hundreds of connections to disease-related support, bereavement assistance, marriage and family issue groups, and women's/men's issues, to name a few. The Bulletin Board Tracker lists the most recent messages and provides a complete cross-reference of topics. By visiting the Support-Group.com Chat Schedule page, dates, times, and group facilitators for upcoming chat events can be viewed. Users have the option of participating in real time Chat Groups via Internet Relay Chat or JavaChat using a Java-capable Web browser. Complete instructions are available at the Web site.

13.3 **Medical Planning**

Blood Bank Information

America's Blood Centers   ⊙ ⊙

http://www.americasblood.org

America's Blood Centers are found in 46 states and collect approximately 47% of the U.S. blood supply. This site provides contact information for each of this organization's centers.

American Association of Blood Banks   ⊙ ⊙ ⊙

http://www.aabb.org

This site provides a contact list for each state on locating and arranging blood donation, including information on storing blood for an anticipated surgery or emergency (autologous blood transfusion). It also answers general questions about blood and blood transfusion.

Caregiver Resources

Caregiver Network   ⊙ ⊙ ⊙

http://www.caregiver.on.ca/content_main.html

This resource center, based in Canada, offers support, advice, seminars, and information for caregivers of the elderly and chronically ill. Text excerpts from an educational video program are available, and visitors can order the video series online. A caregiver resource guide offers telephone numbers and other contact information for government agencies, organizations, service providers, support agencies, publications, and periodicals. Suggested book and video lists and links to related Internet resources are available.

Caregiver Survival Resources   ⊙ ⊙

http://www.caregiver911.com

Maintained by professionals in the field of caregiving, this site offers bulletin boards, forums for questions, telephone numbers for related organizations, and links to government agencies and other sites for additional information searches. Visitors can access a list of suggested publications, read book excerpts, and books online from the site.

National Family Caregivers Association (NFCA)

http://www.nfcacares.org

The NFCA is national organization offering education, information, support, public awareness campaigns, and advocacy to American caregivers. The address discusses caregiving and provides statistics, a survey report, news, an informational pamphlet, a reading list, caregiving tips, and contact details. Caregivers will find this site a source of support, encouragement, and information.

Chronic and Terminal Care Planning

American Association for Retired Persons (AARP): Basic Facts about Reverse Mortgages

http://www.aarp.org/hecc/basicfct.html

This fact sheet within the AARP Web site describes reverse mortgages, including eligibility requirements, how reverse mortgages work, what a borrower receives from the mortgage, typical payments, and contact details for information on other programs or services not involving a loan against the home.

Chronic Pain Solutions

http://www.chronicpainsolutions.com

Chronic Pain Solutions is a quarterly guide for chronic pain sufferers linking traditional and natural medical care. The site contains the online newsletter, contact and home subscription details, an online store for ordering therapeutic products, and biographies of contributing writers.

Consumer Guide to Viatical Settlements

http://www.nvrnvr.com/guide.html

This online booklet, *Every Question You Need To Ask Before Selling Your Life Insurance Policy,* is provided by National Viator Representatives, a viatical settlement information source, advisor, and broker. Users can access the publication online, download the document, or order a hard copy at 1-800-932-0050.

Living Will and Values History Project

http://www.euthanasia.org/lwvh.html

This site offers a Living Will package and Values History document, both available for download free-of-charge. Users can also receive hard copies for a nominal charge. The site also contains an extensive list of links to related sites.

Living Wills ⊗ ⊗

http://www.kepro.org/Bene_LivingWill.htm

Prepared by the Pennsylvania Medical Society, this site answers questions for the average patient regarding the development and use of a living will. It also provides a link to a free sample copy of a living will that can be completed and signed by individuals to be placed in their medical record.

National Chronic Care Consortium ⊗ ⊗ (some features fee-based)

http://www.ncccresourcecenter.org/index.html

The National Chronic Care Consortium is dedicated to transforming the delivery of chronic care services. Members of this group strive to make the delivery of chronic care more efficient and cost effective. The site provides information on conferences, contact details, and links to related sites. Members can take part in the Alzheimer's Project Developmental Group Discussion at the site and access other services.

Organ Donation ⊗ ⊗ ⊗

http://www.organdonor.gov

This government site answers frequently asked questions, dispels myths, and presents facts about organ donation. Visitors can download and print a donor card, and find links to related organizations on the Internet.

U.S. Living Will Registry ⊗ ⊗ ⊗

http://www.uslivingwillregistry.com

This free service electronically stores advance directives and makes them available directly to hospitals by telephone. Registration materials are available to download online or by calling 1-800-LIV-WILL.

USAhomecare.com ⊗ ⊗ ⊗

http://www.USAhomecare.com

USAhomecare.com is a consumer-oriented home care (home health and hospice) site. The site provides answers to common questions, a bookstore, links to related sites, news, contact information, and a directory of agencies offering home care or hospice services.

Directing Healthcare Concerns and Complaints

Congress.org ⊗ ⊗ ⊗

http://congress.org/main.html

This site offers a Capital directory, including members of Congress, the Supreme Court, state governors, and the White House. Users can also find comments on members of Congress by associations and advocacy groups, determine a bill's status through the site's search engine, send messages to Congress members, and find local congressional representatives.

Families USA ◎ ◎ ◎
http://www.familiesusa.org

Families USA is a national nonprofit, nonpartisan organization dedicated to the achievement of high-quality, affordable health, and long-term care for all Americans. The site offers a clearinghouse of information on Medicaid, Medicare, and General Managed Healthcare. Assistance and advice is provided on choosing an HMO, how to tell if a health policy or plan is good, and who to address if you have a healthcare complaint. Within the site, at www.familiesusa.org/medicaid/state.htm, a state-specific healthcare information guide is provided. This directory includes phone numbers to every state's Department of Insurance, which allows users to obtain reports on plans and information on complaint ratios.

Joint Commission of
Accreditation of Healthcare Organizations (JCAHO) ◎ ◎
http://www.jcaho.org/news/nb189.html

The JCAHO site lists a toll-free complaint hotline for patients, their families, and caregivers to express concerns about the quality of care at accredited healthcare organizations at this site. (The toll-free U.S. telephone number is 1-800-994-6610. The hotline is staffed between 8:30 a.m. and 5 p.m., central time, during weekdays.) The site also describes a mechanism for transmitting complaints via e-mail.

Medicare Rights Center (MRC) ◎ ◎ ◎
http://www.medicarerights.org

Medicare Rights Center is a national, nonprofit organization focused to ensure that seniors and people with disabilities on Medicare have access to quality, affordable healthcare. The site offers information on specific MRC programs, news, consumer publications, information on professional membership, and details on the Initiative for the Terminally Ill on Medicare. Visitors can also subscribe for a fee to a biweekly newsletter delivered by fax.

Quality Improvement Organizations ◎ ◎
http://www.qio.org

This site contains a directory of Peer Review Organizations (PRO) listed by state. These organizations monitor the care given to Medicare patients. Each state has a PRO that can decide whether care given to Medicare patients is reasonable, necessary, provided in the most appropriate setting, and meets standards of quality generally accepted by the medical profession. Peer Review Organizations can also be contacted to investigate beneficiary complaints.

State Insurance Commissioners ⚙ ⚙ ⚙

http://www.dtonline.com/insur/inlistng.htm

Deloitte and Touche Financial Counseling Services offers the addresses and phone numbers of each state's insurance commissioner at this site.

Elder and Extended Care

Administration on Aging ⚙ ⚙ ⚙

http://www.aoa.dhhs.gov

This site provides resources for seniors, practitioners, and caregivers, including news on aging, links to Web sites on aging, statistics about older people, consumer fact sheets, retirement and financial planning information, and help finding community assistance for seniors.

American Association for Retired Persons (AARP) ⚙ ⚙ ⚙

http://www.aarp.org

This nonprofit group is dedicated to the needs and rights of elderly Americans. Topics discussed at the site include caregiver support, community and volunteer organizations, Medicare, Medicaid, help with home care, finances, health and wellness, independent living, computers and the Internet, and housing options. Benefits and discounts provided to members are described, reference and research materials are available, and users can search the site by keyword.

American Association of Homes and Services for the Aging (AAHSA) ⚙ ⚙ ⚙

http://www.aahsa.org

This Association represents nonprofit organizations providing health care, housing, and services to the elderly. The site offers tips for consumers and family caregivers on choosing facilities and services, notices of upcoming events, press releases, fact sheets, an online bookstore, and links to sponsors, business partners, an international program, and other relevant sites.

Eldercare Locator ⚙ ⚙ ⚙

http://www.aoa.dhhs.gov/aoa/pages/loctrnew.html

The Eldercare Locator is a nationwide, directory assistance service designed to help older persons and caregivers locate local support resources for aging Americans. This site helps senior citizens find community assistance and Medicaid information. Interested parties can also contact the Eldercare Locator toll free at 1-800-677-1116.

Extendedcare.com ⊚ ⊚ ⊚ (some features fee-based)
http://www.elderconnect.com/asp/default.asp

This address offers information on choosing an extended care provider, a "Geriatric Library" of information resources, a glossary of terms related to extended care, a forum for asking questions of a participating physician, and information on over 60,000 care providers. Visitors can search for care providers by type of care and zip code, subscribe to an e-mail newsletter, and read archived newsletters and press releases. A tool for assessing an individual's care needs is also available. A professional section is available to users associated with registered hospitals.

Insure.com: Answers to Seniors'
Health Insurance Questions (on Medicare and Medicaid) ⊚ ⊚ ⊚
http://www.insure.com/health/ship.html

This site provides the phone number to each state's Health Insurance Advisory Program (SHIP). SHIP is a federally funded program found in all states under different names, helping elderly and disabled Medicare and Medicaid recipients understand their rights and options for healthcare. Services include assistance with bills, advice on buying supplement policies, explanation of rights, help with payment denials or appeals, and assistance in choosing a Medicare health plan.

End of Life Decisions

American Medical Association (AMA): Education
for Physicians on End-of Life Care (EPEC) ⊚ ⊚ ⊚ (free registration)
http://www.ama-assn.org/ethic/epec/index.htm

Supported by a grant from the Robert Wood Johnson Foundation, EPEC is a two-year program designed to educate physicians nationwide on "the essential clinical competencies in end-of-life care." Visitors will find an overview of the project's purpose, design, and scope, a call for EPEC training conference applications, previous conference details, a mailing list, and an annotated list of educational resource materials. Users must complete a free registration process to view educational materials.

Before I Die ⊚ ⊚ ⊚
http://www.pbs.org/wnet/bid

This address presents the Web companion to a public television program exploring the medical, ethical, and social issues associated with end-of-life care in the United States. Personal stories, a bulletin board, a glossary of terms, contact details for important support sources and organizations, and suggestions on forming a discussion group are available at the site. A program description, viewer's guide, outreach efforts and materials, and credits for the program are also provided.

CareOfDying.org: Supportive Care of the Dying ⊙ ⊙ ⊙

http://www.careofdying.org

This site is presented by a coalition of 13 Catholic healthcare associations and the Catholic Health Association, advocating for an improvement in supportive care for persons with life-threatening illnesses and their caregivers. Assessment tools available at the site include patient, family caregiver, bereaved family, and professional questionnaires, and a tool assessing competency. A quarterly newsletter, research report, and hints for conducting focus groups are also available. Links are listed to related resources, including information on an upcoming PBS end-of-life series, hosted by Bill Moyers.

Choice in Dying ⊙ ⊙

http://www.echonyc.com/~choice

Services offered by Choice in Dying include advance directives, counseling for patients and families, professional training, advocacy, and publications. Membership details, press releases, news, information on end-of-life issues, an online newsletter, state-specific advance directive documents, and a petition for end-of-life care are all found at this site. Visitors can also order publications and videos, and access links to related sites.

Decisions Near the End of Life ⊙ ⊙

http://www.edc.org/CAE/Decisions/dnel.html

Decisions Near the End of Life is a Continuing Medical Education program helps professional staff and patients of hospitals and nursing homes improve the way ethical decisions are made. The site describes typical program attendees, goals, format, leadership training, institutional profiles developed by the program, on-site programs, program components, and Continuing Medical Education credit details.

End of Life: Exploring Death in America ⊙ ⊙ ⊙

http://www.npr.org/programs/death

National Public Radio's "All Things Considered" presents transcripts of a recent series on death and dying and other resources at this excellent site. Contact information and links to valuable organizations and other support sources, a bibliography of important publications, texts related to death, dying, and healing, and a forum for presenting personal stories are found at this address.

George Washington University: Center to Improve Care of the Dying: Toolkit of Instruments to Measure End of Life ⊙ ⊙ ⊙

http://www.gwu.edu/~cicd/toolkit/toolkit.htm

Toolkits assessing the quality of end-of-life care are available at this address, providing healthcare institutions with information to "assess, improve, and enhance care for dying patients and their loved ones." Visitors can download a chart review instrument, surrogate questionnaires, and a patient questionnaire. Resources at the site assess quality of life, pain and other symptoms, depression and emotional symptoms, functional status, survival time and aggressiveness of care, continuity of care, spirituality, grief, caregiver and family experience, and patient and family member satisfaction with the quality of care.

Last Acts ⊙ ⊙ ⊙
http://www.lastacts.org

Designed to improve end-of-life care, Last Acts is devoted to "bring end-of-life issues out in the open and to help individuals and organizations pursue the search for better ways to care for the dying." The site presents information on Last Acts activities, a newsletter, press releases, and discussion forums. Links are available to details of recent news headlines, sites offering additional information resources, grant-making organizations, and a directory of Robert Wood Johnson Foundation end-of-life grantees.

Project on Death in America: Transforming the Culture of Dying ⊙ ⊙ ⊙
http://www.soros.org/death

The Project on Death and Dying in America supports initiatives in research, scholarship, the humanities, and the arts in transforming the American culture and experience of dying and bereavement. The Project also promotes innovations in care, public education, professional education, and public policy. Information is presented on the Project's Faculty Scholars Program, Professional Initiatives in Nursing, Social Work, and Pastoral Care, Arts and Humanities Initiative, Public Policy Initiative, Legal Initiative, and Community Initiative. Other resources described at the site include Grantmakers Concerned with Care at the End of Life, media resources, and other publications offered by the Project.

Hospice and Home Care

American Academy of Hospice and Palliative Medicine (AAHPM) ⊙ ⊙ ⊙
http://www.aahpm.org

This national nonprofit organization is comprised of physicians "dedicated to the advancement of hospice/palliative medicines, its practice, research, and education". Academy details, contact information, news, press releases, position statements, events and meetings notices, employment listings, and links to related sites are found at this address. Publications, Continuing Medical Education opportunities, and conference tapes are also available.

Growth House, Inc. ○ ○ ○

http://www.growthhouse.org

Growth House, Inc. offers a comprehensive resource for hospice and home care information at this site. General information, a listing of local hospice providers, online book reviews, and an index of reviewed resources for end-of-life care are available at the site.

Hospice Association of America (HAA) ○ ○ ○

http://www.hospice-america.org

Serving the needs of the most seriously ill patients with cancer and other diseases, the HAA offers a full menu of information about the field of hospice care, as well as a directory of home care and hospice state associations. Each localized association listing offers the name of the executive director, the address, telephone, fax, and e-mail contact.

Hospice Foundation of America ○ ○ ○

http://www.hospicefoundation.org

The Hospice Foundation of America offers a range of books and training services for hospice professionals and the general public. The Web site provides general information on hospice and specific types of grief management. There is also a listing of other Web resources and useful literature for both the healthcare provider and the patient.

Hospice Net ○ ○ ○

http://www.hospicenet.org

Hospice Net is dedicated to helping patients and families facing life-threatening illnesses. The site contains a listing of useful articles, FAQ sheets, caregiver information, and a listing of well-chosen links to other major Web resources.

HospiceWeb ○ ○ ○

http://www.hospiceweb.com/index.htm

This site contains general information, a listing of frequently asked questions, discussion board, hospice locator, and an extensive list of links to valuable sites. Links to other hospice organizations are categorized by state.

National Association for Home Care (NAHC) ○ ○ ○ (some features fee-based)

http://www.nahc.org

NAHC is a trade association representing more than 6,000 home care agencies, hospices, and home care aide organizations. The site offers news and Association announcements, a newsletter on pediatric home care, links to affiliates, international employment listings, legislative and regulatory information, statistics and technical papers, and directories of related state associations. Visitors can access a home care and hospice search tool for finding local service providers, and a consumer section offers information on choosing a home care provider, including descriptions of agencies providing home care, tips for finding information about agencies, and discussions of services, payment, patients' rights, accrediting agencies, and state resources. One section is restricted to members.

National Hospice Organization (NHO) ⊙ ⊙ ⊙
http://www.nho.org

The oldest and largest nonprofit public benefit organization devoted exclusively to hospice care, the NHO offers a comprehensive site providing information on all aspects of hospice care for the seriously and terminally ill, along with a state-by-state and city-by-city guide to hospice organizations in the United States. For each listing of a hospice facility, there is a telephone number and contact person.

Medical Insurance and Managed Care

Agency for Healthcare Research and
Quality (AHRQ): Checkup On Health Insurance Choices ⊙ ⊙ ⊙
http://www.ahcpr.gov/consumer/insuranc.htm

This discussion of health insurance choices informs consumers on topics including why individuals need insurance, sources of health insurance, group and individual insurance, making a decision of coverage, and managed care. Types of insurance described at the site include fee-for-service and "customary" fees, health maintenance organizations, preferred provider organizations, Medicaid, Medicare, disability insurance, hospital indemnity insurance, and long-term care insurance. The site also includes a checklist and worksheet to determine features important to an individual when choosing insurance. A glossary of terms is available for reference.

American Association of Health Plans Online ⊙ ⊙ ⊙
http://www.aahp.org/menus/index.cfm?CFID=221345&CFTOKEN=11327695

Located in Washington, D.C., the American Association of Health Plans represents more than 1,000 HMOs, PPOs, and other network-based plans. The site offers information on government and advocacy activities, public relations materials, reports and statistics, selected bibliographies listed by subject, information on services and products, conference details, and training program information. Consumer resources include information on choosing a health plan, descriptions of different types of health plans, women's health resources, and fact sheets about health plans. Users can search each specific area of the site for information by keyword.

drkoop.com Insurance Center ⊚ ⊚ ⊚

http://www.drkoop.com/hcr/insurance

This area of drkoop.com features an interactive Plan Profiler and Policy Chooser to help determine what type of plan is right for an individual consumer. An insurance library, glossary of insurance terms, and health insurance news updates are featured at the site.

Employer Quality Partnership (EQP) ⊚ ⊚

http://www.eqp.org

This site provides a guide to employees in selecting and understanding healthcare plans, provides assistance to employers in evaluating healthcare plans, and also guides employers on ways to improve the quality of their health plans. The site was developed by EQP, a volunteer coalition of employer organizations interested in promoting positive change in the healthcare marketplace and in educating employees regarding their employer-based healthcare plans.

Glossary of Managed Care and
Organized Healthcare Systems Terms ⊚ ⊚ ⊚

http://www.uhc.com/resource/glossary.html

Users will find and extensive list of managed care and organized healthcare terms and acronyms defined at this site.

Healthcare Financing Administration ⊚ ⊚ ⊚

http://www.hcfa.gov

This federal site provides a wealth of information on Medicare and Medicaid for both patients and healthcare professionals. It covers the basic features of each program and discusses laws, regulations, and statistics about federal healthcare programs. Information is also provided at the state level (state Medicaid), providing a list of sites with important state information.

Joint Commission of
Accreditation of Healthcare Organizations (JCAHO) ⊚ ⊚ ⊚

http://www.jcaho.org

The Joint Commission of Accreditation of Healthcare Organizations evaluates and accredits nearly 18,000 healthcare organizations and programs. Quality Check, a service offered by the Commission, allows consumers to check ratings and evaluations of accredited organizations at the site. Information is available for the general public, employers, healthcare purchasers, and unions; the international community; and healthcare professionals and organizations. The site also contains information on filing complaints, career opportunities, news, and links to related sites.

Managed Care Glossary ☻ ☻ ☻

http://mentalhelp.net/articles/glossary.htm

To be used for professional training purposes or as a general information source, this managed care glossary contains a continuously updated compilation of new terminology related to managed care with additional items in the field of information technology continuously being added. Physician and other healthcare professionals may want to bookmark this site to ensure a more complete understanding of modern health maintenance and preferred provider organization structure and service delivery.

Medical Insurance Resources ☻

http://www.nerdworld.com/trees/nw1654.html

This site offers a large index of medical insurance resources on the Internet. Links are provided to major insurance companies, and other related sites. Each link is accompanied by a brief explanation of what can be found at that particular site.

Medicare ☻ ☻ ☻

http://www.medicare.gov

The Health Care Financing Administration (HCFA) administers Medicare, the nation's largest health insurance program, which covers 39 million Americans. This site answers Medicare questions regarding eligibility, additional insurance, Medicare amounts, and enrollment. Consumer information includes answers to frequently asked questions on Medicare and helps regarding health plan options. Those interested in additional information can call 1-800-MEDICARE to receive additional help in organizing Medicare health options.

National Committee for Quality Assurance (NCQA) ☻ ☻ ☻

http://www.ncqa.org/Pages/Main/index.htm

The National Committee for Quality Assurance (NCQA) is a private, nonprofit organization dedicated to assessing and reporting on the quality of managed healthcare plans. These activities are accomplished through accreditation and performance measurement of participating plans. Almost half the HMOs in the nation, covering three-quarters of all HMO enrollees, are involved in the NCQA accreditation process. A set of more than 50 standardized performance measures called the Health Plan Employer Data and Information Set (HEDIS), is used to evaluate and compare health plans. The NCQA Web site allows the user to search the accreditation status list. The search results will include the accreditation status designation and a summary report of the strengths and weaknesses of the plan entered. NCQA accreditation results allow users to evaluate healthcare plans in such key areas as quality of care, member satisfaction, access, and service.

Quotesmith.com ⊙ ⊙ ⊙

http://www.quotesmith.com

Visitors to this site can access current quotes for individual, family, and small group medical plans. Instant quotes on dental and term life insurance are also available.

U.S. News and World Report: America's Top HMOs ⊙ ⊙ ⊙

http://www.usnews.com/usnews/nycu/health/hetophmo.htm

This site helps consumers to rate their managed care plan by ranking HMOs by state. Other useful tools include an HMO glossary, a medical dictionary, a best hospitals finder, and a list of the 40 highest rated HMOs in the United States. Fitness tips, articles related to HMOs, and a forum for answering health professionals are all found at this site.

Yahoo! Life and Health Insurance Center ⊙ ⊙ ⊙

http://insurance.yahoo.com/life.html

The Yahoo insurance center is an excellent starting point for locating insurance information. Yahoo provides answers to frequently asked questions, a glossary of common terms, and quick estimates on the cost of a health insurance policy. An extensive list of links to related sites and a list of current articles of interest are available.

13.4 Nutrition and Physical Wellness

American Dietetic Association ⊙ ⊙ ⊙ (fee-based)

http://www.eatright.org

The American Dietetic Association presents an ideal site for consumers, students, and dietetic professionals. This site has information on nutrition resources, government affairs, current issues and publications, job opportunities, and a public relations team to answer media questions. Users can contact other dietitians through the site. A search engine and a site map are provided to ease in the searching process. There are also links to consumer education and public policy sites; dietetic associations and networking groups; dietetic practice groups; food; food service and culinary organizations; and medical, health, and other professional organizations.

AOL's Health Webcenter ⊙ ⊙ ⊙

http://www.aol.com/webcenters/health/diet.adp

AOL's Health Webcenter contains well-organized links to a variety of health related sites organized by topic. The site focuses on consumer needs, providing information on topics including illness and treatment; fitness and sports medicine; health and beauty; and women's, men's, children's, and seniors health. A health assessment and drug information search tool, vitamin guide, pregnancy calendar, calorie counter, and body-mass calculator are additional features of the site.

Arbor Nutrition Guide ◎ ◎ ◎

http://www.netspace.net.au/%7Ehelmant/search.htm

The Arbor Nutrition Guide covers all areas of nutrition including applied and clinical nutrition. The site provides links to information on dietary guidelines, special diets, sports nutrition, individual vitamins and minerals, and cultural nutrition. There are also links relating to food science, such as food labeling in other countries, food regulation, food additives, science journals, phytochemistry, and other related topics.

Austin Nutritional Research ◎ ◎ ◎

http://www.realtime.net/anr/referenc.html

This megasite provides links to various organizations and institutions worldwide regarding health and nutrition. Sites include those of professional organizations, research centers, and alternative therapy sources.

Health Resource Links ◎ ◎ ◎

http://www.rxmed.com/healthresourcelinks.html

This site provides links to many professional health-related associations and government agencies. Prescribing information, patient handouts, travel health resources, employment opportunities, medical supply resources, and investment information are all included at this comprehensive site.

International Food Information Council ◎ ◎ ◎

http://ificinfo.health.org

The International Food Information Council presents resources at this site including current issues, up to date information for the media, food safety and nutrition facts, and extensive links to government affairs and agencies. The site also serves as a reference tool for educators, and provides users with a site search engine for locating specific information.

Nutrition & Health Linkstation ◎ ◎ ◎

http://www.amazingstocks.com/nutrition/

The Nutrition & Health Linkstation provides links to recipes, discussion groups, nutrient analysis programs, and energy calculators. The site also offers direct searches of government health organizations, associations, national health research pages, world health research pages, and pharmacy and medicine sites.

Public Health Nutritionists' Home Page ◉ ◉ ◉

http://Weber.u.washington.edu/~phnutr/Internet/nutrlist.html

The Public Health Nutritionists' Home Page is an extensively compiled site for public health and nutrition organized by the School of Public Health and Community Medicine at the University of Washington. This site provides access to many resources, including applied nutrition, cardiovascular disease, food security, vegetarianism, growth charts, breast feeding and infant feeding. Access to the UNICEF gopher server is available to learn more about the United Nations program. Information on educational programs and newsletters are also available.

ThinkQuest Library of Entries ◉ ◉ ◉

http://library.thinkquest.org/library/list.cgi?c=HEALTH_%26_SAFETY

Click on "Food and Nutrition" at this site to access in-depth information for adults, teens, and children on food and nutrition. The links provide access to information on RDA, BMI, personal caloric needs, eating out, specific sites for teens, and general information on more specific health and nutrition topics.

Tufts University Nutrition Navigator ◉ ◉ ◉

http://navigator.tufts.edu

This site, presented by the Center on Nutrition Communication, School of Nutrition Science and Policy at Tufts University, is an up-to-date, rated guide to other nutrition sites. It provides information on general nutrition for parents, kids, women, health professionals, and journalists. One section is devoted to sites providing information about special dietary needs. A search engine is provided at the site for more specific resources.

U.S. Department of Health and Human Services (HHS) ◉ ◉ ◉

http://www.dhhs.gov

The Department of Health and Human Services (HHS) is the United States government's principal agency for protecting the health of all Americans and providing essential human services, especially for those who are least able to help themselves. HHS Operating Divisions include National Institutes of Health, Food and Drug Administration, Centers for Disease Control and Prevention, Agency for Toxic Substances and Disease Registry, Indian Health Service, Health Resources and Services Administration, Substance Abuse and Mental Health Services Administration, and the Agency for Health Care Policy and Research. This site provides news and public affairs information related to HHS, a site search engine, and notices of new site features.

University of Pennsylvania Library ⊙ ⊙ ⊙

http://www.library.upenn.edu

The University of Pennsylvania Library presents an informative site containing information on health disciplines and topics. The site provides access to databases as well as lists of associations, government organizations, and other search tools. Links to alternative medicine sites are also available.

USDA Nutrient Values ⊙ ⊙

http://www.rahul.net/cgi-bin/fatfree/usda/usda.cgi

Visitors can utilize the search engine housed at this site to find the recommended daily allowance (RDA) nutrient values of over 5,000 food items for three different serving sizes in men averaging 174 pounds, and women averaging 138 pounds, between the ages of 25 and 50.

13.5 **Online Drug Stores**

Corner Drugstore Specialties ⊙ ⊙

http://www.cornerdrug.com

Corner Drugstore Specialties provides customers with a catalog of pharmacy products that includes nonprescription drugs, vitamins, personal care items, and other products typically found in a convenience store or pharmacy.

CVS Pharmacy ⊙ ⊙ ⊙

http://www.cvs.com

This site offers customers a way to order prescription and nonprescription drugs along with other pharmacy items. The prescription section offers an extensive description of the purpose of the drug, side effects, precautions, drug interactions, and other prescribing information. All prescription orders are verified by the pharmacy and will be sent by either the U.S. Postal Service or UPS. Non-prescription drugs, vitamins, first aid, home care, and personal care items are also available.

Drug Emporium ⊙ ⊙

http://www.drugemporium.com

This Web site offers customers a wide variety of products including over-the-counter medicine, personal care items, vitamins, and electronics. Prescription medicine is also available. New patients must register by filling out an online form and provide a way to contact their doctors for prescription information. Prescriptions are processed by a registered pharmacist. Orders are shipped via UPS and shipping costs are added to the bill.

Drugstore.com ⊗ ⊗ ⊗

http://www.drugstore.com

As one of the first online drugstores, Drugstore.com has developed an extensive and informative site that provides prescription and nonprescription medicine, personal care products, vitamins, and other products. There are also articles on solutions to some health and beauty problems, an opportunity to ask a Drugstore.com pharmacist questions, and opinions on products from customers.

Home Pharmacy ⊗ ⊗

http://www.homepharmacy.com

Home Pharmacy is an online drugstore that provides a variety of healthcare products at a relatively low cost. Products can be sent by standard shipping or by Federal Express.

Merck-Medco Managed Care Online ⊗ ⊗ ⊗

http://www.merck-medco.com

An online pharmacy, the Merck-Medco site provides information on member services; a newsletter, *Optimal Health* with current health news; medication information and articles for healthy aging; client and provider services, including a list of selected FDA-approved prescription medications; a newsroom containing news releases on Merck-Medco and prescription drug-care; and important drug-related consumer announcements.

Online Drugstore.com ⊗ ⊗

http://www.onlinedrugstore.com/Temp/default.htm

Prescription products at a low cost can be ordered from this service by phone, mail, or e-mail. Visitors can compare prices offered by competitors, access a list of products, and find a more detailed description of the service.

Planet Rx ⊗ ⊗ ⊗

http://www.planetrx.com

Planet Rx, one of the first online drugstores, offers customers a variety of products and information resources. Prescription and nonprescription drugs, personal care items, beauty and spa products, and medical supplies are available. The site also offers articles on health problems and possible treatments, and opinions on products from customers.

Safeweb Medical ⊗ ⊗

http://drugstore.virtualave.net

The Safeweb Medical Web site provides selected popular prescription drugs and online consultations. The customer receives orders 24–48 hours after doctors approve a prescription.

Self Care ○ ○ ○

http://www.selfcare.com

This Web site has sections for beauty and spa items, nonprescription drugs and medicinal supplies, alternative therapies, nutrition and fitness products, and home care merchandise. Descriptions of products are also available. Orders are sent by standard shipping, priority air delivery, or express air delivery.

Verified Internet Pharmacy Practice Sites (VIPPS) Program ○ ○ ○

http://www.nabp.net/vipps/intro.asp

The Verified Internet Pharmacy Practice Sites (VIPPS) Program of the National Association of Boards of Pharmacy (NABP) was developed in 1999 out of public concern for the safety of pharmacy practices on the Internet. This site contains a menu with links providing information on the criteria for VIPPS certification; a VIPPS list (which includes the pharmacy name and Web site address); VIPPS definitions; and links to Web sites of state boards of pharmacy, state medical boards, federal agencies, and professional organizations.

14. RARE DISORDERS

eMedguides.com provides the following glossary of Rare Disorders as a reference tool. The material found in this section is copyrighted by the National Organization for Rare Disorders, Inc. (NORD). All abstracts are provided for informational purposes only, and not with the intent of rendering medical advice, which should only be obtained from a physician. Every effort was made to ensure that the details for each entry are as current as possible; however, all abstract information is subject to change without notice.

14.1 National Organization for Rare Disorders Oncology and Hematology Glossary

The National Organization for Rare Disorders (NORD) is a unique federation of voluntary health agencies, individuals, and medical professionals dedicated to the identification, treatment, and cure of rare "orphan" diseases. There are more than 6,000 of these serious health conditions, most of which are genetically caused. Each orphan disease affects fewer than 200,000 Americans, but combined, they affect more than 25 million people in the United States.

NORD came together during the late 1970s as an informal coalition of voluntary health agencies that were determined to solve the "orphan drug" dilemma. Each of the rare disease charities spent considerable effort raising funds to support research on "their" disease. However, as the cost of pharmaceutical development escalated, it became apparent that when academic scientists actually discovered a new treatment for a rare disorder, pharmaceutical companies did not want to make it commercially available. Thus, treatments for rare diseases became known as "drugs of limited commercial value," or "orphan drugs."

The "Orphan Drug Act" created financial incentives to entice pharmaceutical companies into developing orphan drugs. These incentives include seven years of exclusive marketing rights and a tax credit for the cost of clinical research. The FDA Office for Orphan Products Development also provides clinical research grants to academic scientists and small pharmaceutical companies for pivotal clinical trials.

After the law was enacted in 1983, NORD formalized its associations and incorporated as a nonprofit voluntary health agency serving the common needs of people with all rare diseases through programs of education, advocacy, research, and service. To this end, NORD became an international clearinghouse for information about rare disorders with a goal of creating understandable information for patients and families.

Education Programs

National Organization for Rare Disorders, Inc. (NORD): Rare Disease Database

During the struggle to pass the Orphan Drug Act, media attention highlighted the many problems people with rare diseases face in their daily lives. These patients contacted NORD and asked for assistance. Most importantly, orphan disease patients needed understandable information about their disease including the location of support groups (when they exist), and of clinical trials in which they might want to participate.

NORD's Rare Disease Database (RDB) can be accessed through NORD's Internet site, www.rarediseases.org. The database contains information on over 1,100 diseases written in layman's terminology, including: General Description (abstract), Synonyms, Symptoms, Causes (etiology), Affected Population (epidemiology), Related Disorders (for differential diagnosis), Standard Treatments, Investigational Treatments, Resources (contacts for further information), and References (bibliography). The database can be searched using the disease name, synonyms, or symptoms.

Several other databases can be accessed through the NORD home page at the URL http://www.rarediseases.org, including:

Organization Database

This database lists approximately 1,200 disease-specific organizations and support groups, registries, clinics, Web sites, umbrella organizations, and service agencies. Information includes addresses, phone and fax numbers, Web addresses, publications, and services available through each agency. Most are American agencies, but Canadian and European rare disease organizations are also listed.

Orphan Drug Designation Database

The FDA has designated almost 1,000 pharmaceuticals as "orphan drugs." This database of approved and investigational orphan products lists officially designated orphan drugs, the indications for which they are approved, and ways in which to contact the manufacturers of these orphan drugs. The database is searchable by the name of the product, manufacturer, or the name of the disease.

Medical Equipment Exchange

Many patients do not have insurance with reimbursement benefits for durable medical equipment such as wheelchairs. This database contains ads placed by people who no longer need medical equipment and who are willing to sell, trade, or give the equipment away for free.

Other NORD Programs

Aside from its primary program of education and information, NORD acts as an advocate for programs and government services that benefit people with all rare diseases. NORD also supports biomedical research at academic institutions through clinical research grants. Donors can give for clinical research on all rare diseases, or restrict their gift to a specific rare disease.

NORD also provides services to rare disease patients and families including a Networking Program that links together the families of patients with the same diagnoses.

At NORD's Annual Conference, families from throughout the United States come together to learn about the latest medical advancements in rare disease research, how to obtain services and benefits aimed at people with disabilities, coping mechanisms for patients and caregivers, etc. NORD also assists in locating free or low cost transportation for patients who must travel to distant medical facilities. Additionally, NORD administers several Medication Assistance Programs for pharmaceutical manufacturers, providing several free orphan drugs to uninsured and underinsured patients who cannot afford to purchase them.

NORD Is Here To Help

NORD's various programs and services have been created to serve the orphan disease community, patient organizations, and medical professionals who care for rare disease patients. Numerous surveys have shown that people with rare diseases go undiagnosed or misdiagnosed for extensive periods of time. Once diagnosed, they often have great difficulty locating information that they can understand and apply to their daily lives. Isolation and despair are common until they can obtain appropriate information. For some people, contacting others who have shared similar experiences is critically important. Most importantly, all people with rare diseases need hope that comes from knowledge that research is being pursued on their disease. If they wish to participate in a clinical research program, it is essential that patients can identify the location of clinical trials.

We invite you to contact NORD through the Web site www.rarediseases.org, by phone 203-746-6518 (or recorded Help-Line: 1-800-999-6673), or via mail at: NORD, P.O. Box 8923, New Fairfield, CT 06812.

14.2 Rare Disorders Glossary

Acanthosis Nigricans
http://www.rarediseases.org/lof/lof.html#B
Acanthosis Nigricans is a rare skin disorder characterized by skin lesions that become thick (hyperkeratotic) and have a brownish-gray color (hyperpigmentation). Four types of Acanthosis Nigricans are recognized. Miescher Syndrome is an inherited benign form of Acanthosis Nigricans. Gougerot-Carteaud Syndrome is a benign, possibly inherited form of the disease that usually occurs in young adult females. Pseudoacanthosis Nigricans is a benign juvenile form that is associated with obesity and/or endocrine disorders. An adult form of Acanthosis Nigricans, known as Malignant Acanthosis, is frequently associated with cancer in another part of the body.

Synonyms:

Miescher's Type I Syndrome, Benign Acanthosis Nigricans, Insulin Resistant Acanthosis Nigricans, Benign Keratosis Nigricans, Pseudoacanthosis Nigricans, Gougerot-Carteaud Syndrome, Confluent Reticular Papillomatosis, Malignant Acanthosis, Keratosis Nigricans

Acoustic Neuroma

http://www.rarediseases.org/lof/lof.html#B

Acoustic Neuroma is a benign (noncancerous) tumor of the 8th cranial nerve. This nerve lies within the ear (auditory) canal, and is associated with hearing loss and sending balance information from the inner ear to the brain.

Synonyms:

Acoustic Neurilemoma, Bilateral Acoustic Neuroma, Cerebellopontine Angle Tumor, Fibroblastoma, Perineural, Neurinoma of the Acoustic Nerve, Neurofibroma of the Acoustic Nerve, Schwannoma of the Acoustic Nerve

AIDS (Acquired Immune Deficiency Syndrome)

http://www.rarediseases.org/lof/lof.html#B

AIDS is an infectious disorder that suppresses the normal function of the immune system. It is caused by the human immunodeficiency virus (HIV), which destroys the body's ability to fight infections. Specific cells of the immune system that are responsible for the proper response to infections (T cells) are destroyed by this virus. Characteristically, a person infected with HIV initially experiences no symptoms for a long period of time. This may be followed by the development of persistent generalized swelling of the lymph nodes (AIDS-related lymphadenopathy). Eventually most patients infected with HIV experience a syndrome of symptoms that includes excessive fatigue, weight loss, and/or skin rashes.

The later stages of HIV infection are characterized by the progressive depression of T-cells and infections that can even occur during a course of antibiotic therapy for another infection (superinfections). People with AIDS are particularly vulnerable to "opportunistic infections" from bacteria that other people normally fight off. Pneumocystis carinii, which causes severe inflammation of the lungs (pneumonia), is a common infection that affects people with AIDS. Cancers (malignant neoplasms), and a wide variety of neurological abnormalities, most notably the AIDS dementia complex, may also be present. These neurological symptoms appear to be a direct result of HIV infection of the nervous system.

Synonyms:

AIDS related complex, ARC, AIDS Prodrome, Wasting/Lymph Node Syndrome, Mini-AIDS, Acquired Immune Deficiency Syndrome, AIDS-Related Complex (ARC)

Ameloblastoma

http://www.rarediseases.org/lof/lof.html#B

Ameloblastoma is a very rare disorder of the jaw and sinuses. Major symptoms may include cysts or tumors in the dental area. They may also occur in the sinuses, nose and/or eye sockets. In some cases, the ameloblastoma may become malignant and spread to other areas of the body.

Synonyms:

Adamantinoma, Mandibular Ameloblastoma, Maxillary Ameloblastoma, Odontogenic Tumor

Amyloidosis

http://www.rarediseases.org/lof/lof.html#B

Amyloidosis is the term applied to a group of metabolic disorders in which amyloid (a fibrous protein) accumulates in tissues of the body. The excessive accumulation of amyloid causes the affected organ to malfunction. The accumulation may be localized, general, or systemic. There are various systems used to classify the different forms of the disorder. The most widely used classification system is based on the chemical properties of the fiber-like structures within amyloid (fibrils).

The most common form of Amyloidosis is AL or light-chain-related (Primary Amyloidosis). This form of the disease may occur independently of other disease, or in the presence of multiple tumors arising from the bone marrow (myeloma). This form of the disorder generally effects the tongue, thyroid gland, intestinal tract, liver, and spleen. Cardiac involvement may result in congestive heart failure.

AA Amyloidosis, or Secondary Amyloidosis, is most often discovered during the course of a chronic inflammatory disease, such as rheumatoid arthritis, chronic infections, or familial Mediterranean fever. AA Amyloidosis commonly impairs the proper functioning of the kidneys, liver, and spleen. The adrenal glands, lymph nodes, and vascular system may be affected as well. The skin inflammation that occurs with recurrent injections that are given to treat some inflammatory diseases seems to induce AA Amyloidosis. Malfunctioning of the kidneys, as in nephrotic syndrome and kidney (renal) failure, causes the most fatalities in AA Amyloidosis. This type of Amyloidosis is reported in approximately one percent of cases of chronic inflammatory diseases in the United States.

Amyloidosis of Aging commonly affects the heart. Sometimes this form of Amyloidosis also affects the pancreas and brain.

Hemodialysis-Associated Amyloidosis is seen in patients who have experienced long-term hemodialysis (a procedure in which impurities or wastes are removed from the blood due to the malfunctioning of the kidneys).

Familial Amyloidosis is found in a series of genetically transmitted diseases that typically affect the kidney, heart, skin, and other areas of the body.

Synonyms:

Systemic Amyloidosis, Secondary Amyloidosis, Hereditary Amyloidosis, Transthyretin Methionine-30 Amyloidosis (Type I), Indiana Type Amyloidosis (Type II), Danish Cardiac Type Amyloidosis (Type III), Iowa Type Amyloidosis (Type IV), Finnish Type Amyloidosis (Type V), Icelandic Type Amyloidosis (Type VI), Ohio Type Amyloidosis (Type VII), Familial Visceral Amyloidosis (Type VIII), Familial Lichen Amyloidosis (Type IX), Appalachian Type Amyloidosis, Analine 60 Amyloidosis, Ashkenazi Type Amyloidosis, Isoleucine 33 Amyloidosis, Corneal Amyloidosis, Amyloid Corneal Dystrophy, Familial Cutaneous Amyloidosis, Hemodialysis-Related Amyloidosis, A Beta-2-Microglobulin Amyloidosis, Amyloid Arthropathy of Chronic Hemodialysis Amyloidosis, Illinois Type Amyloidosis, Prealbumin Tyr-77 Amyloidosis, Abercrombie Syndrome, Amyloidosis of Familial Mediterranean Fever, Atypical Amyloidosis, Cardiopathic Amyloidosis, Hereditary Nephropathic Amyloidosis, Idiopathic Amyloidosis, Lichen Amyloidosis, Macular Amyloidosis, Neuropathic Amyloidosis, Paramyeloidosis, Pericollagen Amyloidosis, Portuguese Type Amyloidosis, Primary Amyloidosis, Primary Cutaneous Amyloidosis, Primary Nonhereditary Amyloidosis, Secondary Generalized Amyloidosis, Waxy Disease

Anemia, Fanconi's

http://www.rarediseases.org/lof/lof.html#B

Fanconi's Anemia is an inherited condition that leads to a deficiency of certain blood cells that are produced by the bone marrow. This disorder occurs mainly in children and is characterized by abnormalities of the heart, kidneys, and skeleton. Skin color (pigmentation) changes may also occur. In both types of Fanconi's Anemia (Type I and Type II) the symptoms are the same. Although the location of the defective gene that causes Fanconi's Anemia is unknown, it is thought that the gene that causes each type of Fanconi's Anemia is at a different location on the chromosome.

Synonyms:

Fanconi's Anemia, Type I (FA1), Fanconi's Anemia, Complementation Group A (FANCA); FAA, Fanconi Pancytopenia, Fanconiís Anemia, Estren-Dameshek Variant, Fanconi's Anemia, Complementation Group B (FANCB); FACB, Aplastic Anemia with Congenital Anomalies, Congenital Pancytopenia, Constitutional Aplastic Anemia, Fanconi Panmyelopathy, Fanconiís Anemia, Complementation Group C (FANCC); FAC, Fanconiís Anemia, Complementation Group D (FANCD); FACD, Fanconiís Anemia, Complementation Group E (FANCE); FACE, Fanconi's Anemia, Complementation Group F (FANF); FACF, Fanconi's Anemia, Complementation Group G (FANG); FACGFanconi's Anemia, Complementation Group H (FANH); FACH

Anemia, Pernicious

http://www.rarediseases.org/lof/lof.html#B

Pernicious Anemia is a rare blood disorder characterized by the inability of the body to properly utilize vitamin B12 (a cobalamin), which is essential for the development of red blood cells. The symptoms of Pernicious Anemia may include weakness, fatigue, an upset stomach, an abnormally rapid heartbeat (tachycardia), and/or chest pains. Recurring episodes of anemia (megaloblastic) and an abnormal yellow coloration of the skin (jaundice) are also common. Pernicious Anemia is thought to be an autoimmune disorder, and certain people may have a genetic predisposition to this disorder.

The three recognized forms of Pernicious Anemia include: Congenital Pernicious Anemia, Juvenile Pernicious Anemia, and Adult Onset Pernicious Anemia. The subdivisions are based on the age at onset and the precise nature of the defect causing impaired B12 utilization (e.g., absence of intrinsic factor).

Synonyms:
Congenital Pernicious Anemia due to Defect of Intrinsic Factor, Gastric Intrinsic Factor, Failure of Secretion, Enterocyte Cobalamin Malabsorption, Enterocyte Intrinsic Factor Receptor, Defect of, Adult Onset Pernicious Anemia, Juvenile Intestinal Malabsorption of Vit B12, Addison's Anemia, Addison-Biermer Anemia, Addisonian Pernicious AnemiaPrimary Anemia

Astrocytoma, Benign
http://www.rarediseases.org/lof/lof.html#B
Benign astrocytomas are abnormal growths or tumors that occur in the brain and spinal cord. They are composed of star-shaped neurological cells called astrocytes. Astrocytomas may be benign (noncancerous) or malignant (cancerous), and either type can be disabling. The bones of the skull prevent the brain from expanding outward as the tumor grows and takes up space. Consequently, healthy brain tissue is compressed, causing symptoms controlled by the area of the brain that is compressed. Because of the pressure either type of astrocytoma (benign or malignant) exerts upon the brain and the resulting symptoms, the distinction between benign (noncancerous) and malignant (cancerous) tumors of the brain is less critical than for tumors occurring elsewhere in the body.

Benign astrocytomas are usually more slow growing than the malignant forms. Astrocytomas can occur anywhere in the brain or spinal cord, with the subcortical (beneath the brain covering) white matter (fibrous tissue) of the brain hemispheres being the most common location in adults. The brain stem, cerebellum, and optic nerve are the most common locations of benign astrocytomas in children.

Synonyms:
Astrocytoma Grade I (Benign), Astrocytoma Grade II (Benign), Intracranial Neoplasm

Astrocytoma, Malignant
http://www.rarediseases.org/lof/lof.html#B
Malignant Astrocytoma is an infiltrating, primary brain tumor, with tentacles that may invade surrounding tissue. This provides a butterfly-like distribution pattern through the white matter of the cerebral hemispheres. The tumor may invade a membrane

covering the brain (the dura), or spread via the spinal fluid through the ventricles of the brain. Spread of the tumor (metastasis) outside the brain and spinal cord is rare.

Synonyms:

Anaplastic Astrocytoma, Astrocytoma, grades 3-4, Giant Cell Glioblastoma, Astrocytoma, Spongioblastoma Multiforme

Ataxia Telangiectasia

http://www.rarediseases.org/lof/lof.html#B

Ataxia Telangiectasia, also known as Louis Bar Syndrome, is an inherited progressive form of cerebellar ataxia that usually begins during infancy. It involves progressive loss of coordination of the limbs, head, and eyes, and decreased immune responses against infections. During the course of the disorder, dilated blood vessels (telangiectasias) appear in the eyes and skin. Individuals with this form of ataxia are more susceptible to sinus and lung infections and may also develop tumors (neoplasia). Ataxia Telangiectasia may be misdiagnosed as Friedreich's Ataxia until telangiectasias appear. (Friedreich's Ataxia is a hereditary neuromuscular syndrome characterized by slow degenerative changes of the spinal cord and the brain.)

Synonyms:

AT, Cerebello-Oculocutaneous Telangiectasia, Immunodeficiency with Ataxia Telangiectasia, Louis-Bar Syndrome

Bloom Syndrome

http://www.rarediseases.org/lof/lof.html#B

Bloom Syndrome is a rare inherited disorder characterized by short stature, multiple small dilated blood vessels on the face (facial telangiectasia), increased sensitivity to light (photosensitivity), and susceptibility to infections. Later in life, some individuals with Bloom Syndrome may be at an increased risk for certain malignancies. Bloom Syndrome is inherited as an autosomal recessive genetic trait.

Synonyms:

Bloom-Torre-Mackacek Syndrome, BS, Dwarfism, Levi's Type, Short Stature and Facial TelangiectasisShort Stature, Telangiectatic Erythema of the Face

Bowen's Disease

http://www.rarediseases.org/lof/lof.html#B

Bowen's Disease is characterized by a precancerous, slow growing skin malignancy. The major symptom is a red-brown, scaly or crusted patch on the skin which resembles psoriasis or dermatitis. It may occur on any part of the skin or in the mucous membranes.

Synonyms:

Intraepidermal Squamous cell Carcinoma, Precancerous Dermatosis

Brain Tumors, General

http://www.rarediseases.org/lof/lof.html#B

Brain Tumors are abnormal growths in the brain that can be either cancerous (malignant) of noncancerous (benign). The effects on the brain of malignant and benign brain tumors are very similar and can cause the same types of problems depending upon the type of tumor and where it is located in the brain.

Synonyms:

Brain Tumors, Benign, Brain Tumors, Malignant, Benign Tumors of the Central Nervous System, Intracranial Tumors, Primary Tumors of Central Nervous System, Malignant Tumors of the Central Nervous System

Cancers, Skin, General

http://www.rarediseases.org/lof/lof.html#B

There are many different types of skin cancer. Combined together, all types of skin cancer represent the most prevalent type of cancer. Most skin cancers are characterized by changes in the color or texture of the skin, but some types begin under the skin where they can spread to other parts of the body. Malignant melanoma is the most dangerous of this type of skin cancer.

Synonyms:

Melanoma, Malignant, Squamous Cell Carcinomas, Acral Lentiginious Melanoma, Juvenile Melanoma, Kaposi's Sarcoma, Malignant Lentico Melanoma, Skin Cancer, Non-Melanoma, Basal Cell Carcinoma

Carcinoid Syndrome

http://www.rarediseases.org/lof/lof.html#B

Carcinoid Syndrome is a rare, malignant disease affecting the small bowel, stomach, and/or pancreas. Slow growing tumors can spread (metastasize) to the liver, lungs, and ovaries. Major symptoms include flushing, diarrhea, and wheezing. The exact cause of Carcinoid Syndrome is not known.

Synonyms:

Carcinoid Tumors, Endocrine Tumors, Carcinoid Type Malignant Carcinoid Syndrome, Metastatic Carcinoid Tumor

Carcinoma, Renal Cell

http://www.rarediseases.org/lof/lof.html#B

Renal Cell Carcinoma is a rare malignant kidney disorder. Major symptoms may include loss of kidney function, fever, weight loss, blood problems, high levels of calcium in the system, high blood pressure, blood clots, and congestive heart failure. However, the most common feature of the syndrome is the passing of blood in the urine (hematuria).

Grawitz Tumor, Hypernephroma, Nephrocarcinoma, RCC, Renal Adenocarcinoma

Carcinoma, Squamous Cell

http://www.rarediseases.org/lof/lof.html#B

Squamous Cell Carcinoma is among the most common types of skin cancer. It usually develops on the tissue of the skin and mucous lining of the body cavities (epithelium), but may occur anywhere on the body. With appropriate treatment, it is usually curable. Squamous Cell Carcinoma most commonly affects individuals who are exposed to large amounts of sunlight. Susceptibility is related to the amount of melanin pigment in the skin, and light-skinned persons are most vulnerable.

Synonyms:
Bowen's Disease, Carcinoma, Epirmoid Intradermal, Skin Cancer, Squamous Cell Type

Castleman's Disease

http://www.rarediseases.org/lof/lof.html#B

Castleman's Disease is a rare disorder characterized by non-cancerous (benign) growths (tumors) that may develop in the lymph node tissue throughout the body (i.e., systemic disease [plasma cell type]). Most often, they occur in the chest, stomach, and/or neck (i.e., localized disease [hyaline-vascular type]). Less common sites include the armpit (axilla), pelvis, and pancreas. Usually the growths represent abnormal enlargement of the lymph nodes normally found in these areas (lymphoid hamartoma). There are two main types of Castleman's Disease: hyaline-vascular type and plasma cell type. The hyaline vascular type accounts for approximately 90 percent of the cases. Most individuals exhibit no symptoms of this form of the disorder (asymptomatic) or they may develop non-cancerous growths in the lymph nodes. The plasma cell type of Castleman's Disease may be associated with fever, weight loss, skin rash, early destruction of red blood cells, leading to unusually low levels of circulating red blood cells (hemolytic anemia), and/or abnormally increased amounts of certain immune factors in the blood (hypergammaglobulinemia).

A third type of Castleman's Disease has been reported in the medical literature. This type may affect more than one area of the body (multicentric or generalized Castleman's Disease). Many individuals with Multicentric Castleman's Disease may exhibit an abnormally large liver and spleen (hepatosplenomegaly). Researchers' opinions in the medical literature differ as to whether Multicentric Castleman's Disease is a distinct entity or a multicentric form of the plasma cell type of Castleman's Disease.

Synonyms:
Angiofollicular Lymph Node Hyperplasia, Angiomatous Lymphoid, Castleman Tumor, Giant Benign Lymphoma, Hamartoma of the Lymphatics, Giant Lymph Node Hyperplasia

Chediak Higashi Syndrome

http://www.rarediseases.org/lof/lof.html#B

Chediak-Higashi Syndrome is a rare inherited form of albinism characterized by a decrease in the amount of skin coloration (decreased pigmentation) and visual difficulties. Albinism is a group of rare inherited disorders associated with the absence at birth of color in the skin, hair, and/or eyes. White blood cell (leukocyte) abnormalities associated with Chediak-Higashi Syndrome result in immune deficiencies. Affected individuals may have an increased susceptibility to infections and certain cancers.

Synonyms:

Begnez-Cesar's Syndrome, Chediak-Steinbrinck-Higashi Syndrome, CHS, Leukocytic Anomaly Albinism, Natural Killer Lymphocytes, Defect in, Oculocutaneous Albinism, Chediak-Higashi Type

Common Variable Immunodeficiency

http://www.rarediseases.org/lof/lof.html#B

Common Variable Immunodeficiency (CVI) is a group of rare genetic (primary) immunodeficiency disorders in which abnormalities in immune cell development (maturation) result in a decreased ability to appropriately produce antibodies in response to invading microorganisms, toxins, or other foreign substances. The symptoms of CVI usually become apparent during the second to the fourth decade of life.

The term "Common Variable Immunodeficiency" is used to designate an immune defect in which there is a substantial reduction of the level of immunizing agents (immunoglobulins) in the fluid portion of the blood (serum). According to the medical literature, most individuals with CVI share common, distinctive symptoms, and physical findings (phenotype) due to decreased levels of all major classes of immunoglobulins in blood serum (panhypogammaglobulinemia). Defective production of certain antibodies in response to invading microorganisms (antibody deficiency) and recurrent bacterial infections are also characteristic of CVI. Such infections often affect the upper and lower respiratory tracts and the gastrointestinal (digestive) system.

In some cases, individuals with CVI have an increased tendency to develop certain diseases characterized by abnormal tissue growths (neoplasms) that may be benign or malignant. In addition, some individuals with CVI may have an unusual susceptibility to certain autoimmune diseases. These disorders occur when the body's natural defenses against invading microorganisms mistakenly attack healthy tissue. The range and severity of symptoms and findings associated with CVI may vary from case to case.

It is thought that CVI may result from a combination of genetic defects or from different disease genes (heterogenous). In many cases, there is no clear pattern of inheritance. However, in successive generations of some affected families (kindreds), there is evidence that CVI may be inherited as an autosomal recessive genetic trait. In addition, a rare acquired form of the disorder has been described in the medical literature.

Synonyms:

Acquired Hypogammaglobulinemia, Common Variable Hypogammaglobulinemia, CVI, CVID, Late-Onset Immunoglobulin Deficiency

Cystic Hygroma
http://www.rarediseases.org/lof/lof.html#B

Cystic Hygroma is an inborn tumor of the lymphatic system that, in some rare cases, may be inherited as an autosomal recessive genetic trait. This progressive disorder is characterized by a large sac filled with lymph fluid protruding from the skull at the nape of the neck. The hygroma is thought to be caused by a failure of the lymph system to properly connect with the blood vessels in the neck and thus with the appropriate blood circulation system.

Synonyms:

Cystic Lymphangioma, Familial Nuchal Bleb, FCH, Fetal Cystic Hygroma, Hygroma Colli

Drash Syndrome
http://www.rarediseases.org/lof/lof.html#B

Drash Syndrome is a very rare disorder that typically appears for no apparent reason (sporadically). In rare cases, it may be inherited as an autosomal dominant genetic trait. This disorder usually appears early in life. In its complete form, it is characterized by the combination of abnormal kidney function, genital abnormalities (pseudohermaphroditism), and a cancerous tumor of the kidney called a Wilms' tumor. Some affected individuals may have the incomplete form of Drash Syndrome, which consists of abnormal kidney function with either genital abnormalities (pseudohermaphroditism) or Wilms' tumor. This disorder predominantly affects males but a few female cases have been reported.

Synonyms:

Denys-Drash Syndrome, Nephropathy-Pseudohermaphroditism-Wilms Tumor, Pseudohermaphroditism-Nephron Disorder-Wilm's Tumor, Wilms Tumor and Pseudohermaphroditism, Wilms Tumor-Pseudohermaphroditism-Nephropathy, Wilms Tumor-Pseuodohermaphroditism-Glomerulopathy

Dysplastic Nevus Syndrome
http://www.rarediseases.org/lof/lof.html#B

Dysplastic Nevus Syndrome is a malignant genetic skin disorder characterized by mole-like tumors. These tumors may appear in different sizes, shapes, and shades of color (usually reddish-brown to pink). The tumors have a variable ability for spreading to adjacent parts of the skin, or through the blood and lymph circulation to other organs. Dysplastic Nevus Syndrome may later evolve into Malignant Melanoma, a common form of skin cancer.

Synonyms:
B-K Mole Syndrome, CMM, Cutaneous Malignant Melanoma, Hereditary, DNS, Hereditary, Familial Atypical Mole-Malignant Melanoma Syndrome, FAMMM, HCMM, Malignant Melanoma, Dysplastic Nevus Type

Exostoses, Multiple
http://www.rarediseases.org/lof/lof.html#B

Multiple Exostoses is a rare disorder that is inherited as an autosomal dominant genetic trait. This disorder is characterized by multiple bony growths or tumors (exostoses) that are covered by cartilage. The bone tumors continue to grow until shortly after puberty and may cause deformities especially of the ankle, knee, and wrist.

Synonyms:
Diaphyseal Aclasis, EXT, External Chondromatosis Syndrome, Multiple Cartilaginous Exostoses, Multiple Exostoses, Multiple Exostoses Syndrome, Multiple Osteochondromatosis

Fibromatosis, Congenital Generalized
http://www.rarediseases.org/lof/lof.html#B

Congenital Generalized Fibromatosis is a rare disorder characterized by multiple noncancerous tumors. It is an invasive and recurring disorder that can involve the bones, internal organs, skin, and muscles. These tumors are usually present at, or may occur, within a few months of birth.

Synonyms:
CGF, Myofibromatosis

Gardner Syndrome
http://www.rarediseases.org/lof/lof.html#B

Gardner Syndrome is a rare inherited disorder characterized by multiple growths (polyps) in the colon, extra teeth (supernumerary), bony tumors of the skull (osteomas), and fatty cysts (epithelial) and/or fibrous tumors in the skin (fibromas or epithelial cysts). Gardner Syndrome is a variant of Familial Polyposis, which is a group of disorders characterized by the growth of multiple polyps in the colon.

Synonyms:
Bone Tumor-Epidermoid Cyst-Polyposis, Familial Adenomatous Polyposis with Extraintestinal Manifestations, FAPG, GRS, Intestinal Polyposis III, Oldfield Syndrome, Polyposis, Gardner TypePolyposis-Osteomatosis-Epidermoid Cyst Syndrome

Glioblastoma Multiforme

http://www.rarediseases.org/lof/lof.html#B

Glioblastoma multiforme is a highly malignant, rapidly infiltrating, primary brain tumor, with tentacles that may invade surrounding tissue. This provides a butterfly-like distribution pattern through the white matter of the cerebral hemispheres. The tumor may invade a membrane covering the brain (the dura), or spread via the spinal fluid through the ventricles of the brain. Spread of the tumor (metastasis) outside the brain and spinal cord is rare.

Synonyms:

Giant Cell Glioblastoma, Multiforme, Spongioblastoma Multiforme,Glioblastoma

Granulomatosis, Lymphomatoid

http://www.rarediseases.org/lof/lof.html#B

Lymphomatoid Granulomatosis is a rare, progressive, vascular disease characterized by infiltration and destruction of the veins and arteries by lesions. These lesions can affect various parts of the body, especially the lungs. It can be a benign or malignant condition.

Synonyms:

Benign Lymph Angiitis and Granulomatosis, Malignant Lymph Angiitis and Granulomatosis, Pulmonary Angiitis, Pulmonary Wegener's Granulomatosis

Granulomatous Disease, Chronic

http://www.rarediseases.org/lof/lof.html#B

Chronic Granulomatous Disease is a very rare inherited primary immune deficiency disorder that affects certain white blood corpuscles (lymphocytes). It is characterized by widespread granulomatous tunor-like lesions, and an inability to resist repeated infectious diseases. Life-threatening infections of the skin, lungs, and bones may occur along with swollen areas of inflamed tissues known as granulomas.

Synonyms:

CGD, Chronic Dysphagocytosis, Granulomatosis, Chronic, Familial, Granulomatosis, Septic, Progressive, Fatal Granulomatous Disease of Childhood, Impotent Neutrophil Syndrome, Congenital Dysphagocytosis

Hemangioma Thrombocytopenia Syndrome

http://www.rarediseases.org/lof/lof.html#B

Hemangioma-Thrombocytopenia Syndrome (also known as Kasabach-Merritt Syndrome) is a rare disorder characterized by an abnormal blood condition in which the low number of blood platelets causes bleeding (thrombocytopenia). The thrombocytopenia is found in association with a benign tumor consisting of large, blood-filled spaces (cavernous hemangioma). The exact cause of this disorder is not known.

Synonyms:

Kasabach-Merritt Syndrome, Thrombocytopenia-Hemangioma Syndrome

Hodgkin's Disease

http://www.rarediseases.org/lof/lof.html#B

Hodgkin's Disease is a form of cancer of the lymphatic system, especially the lymph nodes. Tumors occur in the lymph nodes (places where lymphatic vessels unite) and/or the area around the nodes. Fever, night sweats, and weight loss may occur along with swollen lymph nodes.

Synonyms:

Hodgkin Disease, Hodgkin's Lymphoma

Kikuchi's Disease

http://www.rarediseases.org/lof/lof.html#B

Kikuchi's Disease is a rare noncancerous disorder in which there are lesions that typically affect the lymph nodes in the neck of young adults. This disorder is often mistaken for malignant Lymphoma because the symptoms are very similar. The lesions, or tissue abnormalities in this disorder cause the lymph nodes to become enlarged, inflamed, and painful. The exact cause of Kikuchi's Disease is not known.

Synonyms:

Histiocytic Necrotizing Lymphadenitis, HNL, Kikuchi's Histiocytic Necrotizing Lymphadenitis, Kikuchi-Fujimoto Disease, Necrotizing Lymphadenitis

Leukemia, Chronic Lymphocytic

http://www.rarediseases.org/lof/lof.html#B

Chronic Lymphocytic Leukemia is a malignant blood disorder in which there is an increased number of white blood cells formed in the lymphoid tissue. This uncontrolled buildup and enlargement of lymphoid tissue can occur in various sites of the body such as the lymph nodes, spleen, bone marrow, and lungs. There are many different forms of Leukemia which are all characterized by an overabundance of white blood cells. In Chronic Lymphocytic Leukemia the disease occurs in the lymphoid tissue.

The lymph vessels, which return fluids to the circulatory system, and the lymph nodes, which are a mass of tissue separated into compartments by connective tissue, make up the immune system. The lymph nodes serve as filters, removing foreign particles, tissue debris, and bacterial cells from the circulation. When this system is not working properly, the body's defenses cannot fight off foreign particles.

In the majority of cases, Chronic Lymphocytic Leukemia is the result of a rapid production of B lymphocyte cells (a short-lived type of white blood cell that is responsible for the production of vertebrate serum proteins that include antibodies). A small percentage of Chronic Lymphocytic Leukemia cases stem from the overproduction of T lymphocyte cells (a type of white blood cell that have a long life and are important in the resistance of disease).

Synonyms:
CLL

Leukemia, Chronic Myelogenous

http://www.rarediseases.org/lof/lof.html#B

Chronic myelogenous leukemia is characterized by an excessive amount of white blood cells in the bone marrow, spleen, liver, and blood. As the disease progresses, the leukemic cells invade other areas of the body including the intestinal tract, kidneys, lungs, gonads, and lymph nodes.

There are two phases to chronic myelogenous leukemia. The first phase, or chronic phase, is characterized by an overproduction of white blood cells. An advanced phase is called the acute phase or blast crisis. At this point, over 50 percent of the cells in the bone marrow are immature malignant cells (blast cells or promelocytes). In the acute phase, the leukemia is very aggressive and does not respond well to therapy. Approximately 85 percent of all individuals with chronic myelogenous leukemia enter the acute phase.

Synonyms:
CGL, Chronic Granulocytic Leukemia, Chronic Myelocytic Leukemia, Chronic Myeloid Leukemia, GML

Leukemia, Hairy Cell

http://www.rarediseases.org/lof/lof.html#B

Hairy cell leukemia is a rare type of blood cancer characterized by the presence of abnormal mononuclear blood cells called "hairy cells," and by a deficiency of other blood cell elements (pancytopenia), including an abnormal decrease of certain white blood cells (neutrophils [neutropenia]) and certain red blood cells (platelets [thrombocytopenia]). Affected individuals usually exhibit fatigue, weakness, fever, weight loss, and/or abdominal discomfort due to an abnormally enlarged spleen (splenomegaly). In addition, affected individuals may have a slightly enlarged liver (hepatomegaly) and may be unusually susceptible to bruising and/or severe infection. The exact cause of hairy cell leukemia is not known.

Synonyms:
Leukemic Reticuloendotheliosis, HCL

Lymphadenopathy, Angioimmunoblastic with Dysproteinemia

http://www.rarediseases.org/lof/lof.html#B

Angioimmunoblastic Lymphadenopathy with Dysproteinemia (AILD) is a progressive immune system disorder possibly caused by viral infections, chronic stimulation of immune responses, or drug treatments prescribed for other conditions. This disorder occurs mostly among persons over 50 years of age. Fever, chills, sweating, a general feeling of discomfort, weight loss, and/or skin rashes are the major symptoms. In some cases, AILD may evolve into a severe form of lymphoma (a type of cancer).

Synonyms:

AILD, Immunoblastic Lymphadenopathy

Lymphangioma, Cavernous

http://www.rarediseases.org/lof/lof.html#B

Cavernous Lymphangioma is a congenital disorder of the lymph vessels. It is characterized by a mass of lymphoid tissue under the skin. Lymphangioma is usually present at birth but may develop later in life as well.

Synonyms:

Chylangioma

Lymphoma, Gastric, Non-Hodgkins Type

http://www.rarediseases.org/lof/lof.html#B

Non-Hodgkins Type Gastric Lymphoma is a rare form of stomach cancer characterized by unrestrained growth of certain lymphoid cells of the stomach. This form of cancer is thought to arise from certain white blood cells (lymphocytes) within lymphoid tissue of the stomachís mucous membrane (mucosa). Non-Hodgkins Type Gastric Lymphoma may be a primary disease process (primary lymphoma) or may develop due to another underlying lymphoma. Symptoms and findings associated with Non-Hodgkins Type Gastric Lymphoma may include pain, bleeding, obstruction of, and/or the development of a hole in the wall of the stomach (perforation). In many affected individuals, an abnormal mass may be felt (palpable) in the upper middle (epigastric) region of the abdomen. Non-Hodgkins Type Gastric Lymphoma affects males more often than females and usually appears to occur during middle age. According to the medical literature, Non-Hodgkins Type Gastric Lymphoma tends to occur an average of approximately 10 years earlier than gastric adenocarcinoma, a more common form of stomach cancer.

Synonyms:

Non-Hodgkins Gastric Lymphoma, Stomach Lymphoma, Non-Hodgkins Type

Lynch Syndromes

http://www.rarediseases.org/lof/lof.html#B

The Lynch Syndromes are rare hereditary disorders that usually cause cancer to develop either in the colorectal area or in other sites. Primary cancers may develop in the female genital tract, stomach, brain, breasts, or urological system. The cancers of the colorectal area associated with the Lynch Syndromes usually develop at a younger age than is normally found in other persons with colorectal cancer.

Synonyms:

Lynch Syndrome I, Hereditary Site Specific Cancer, Lynch Syndrome II, Cancer Family Syndrome, Lynch Type, Hereditary Nonpolyposis Colorectal Cancer (Lynch Syndrome I and II), Hereditary Nonpolyposis Colorectal Carcinoma

Medulloblastoma

http://www.rarediseases.org/lof/lof.html#B

A Medulloblastoma is a tumor in the cerebellum (a part of the brain), located in the lower rear portion of the skull (posterior fossa). About half of medulloblastomas are confined to the connecting bridge between the two halves of the cerebellum (vermis), and the other half actually invade the cerebellum or the brainstem (pons and medulla).

Melanoma, Malignant

http://www.rarediseases.org/lof/lof.html#B

Malignant Melanoma is a common skin cancer that arises from the melanin cells of the upper layer of the skin (epidermis) or from similar cells that can be found in moles (nevi). This type of skin cancer may send down roots into deeper layers of the skin. Some of these microscopic roots can spread (metastasize) causing new tumor growths in vital organs of the body.

Synonyms:

Acral Lentiginous Melanoma, Juvenile Melanoma, Malignant, Malignant Lentigo (Melanoma), Melanoblastoma, Melanocarcinoma, Melanoepithelioma, Melanoma, Melanosarcoma, Melanoscirrhus, Melanotic Carcinoma, Nevus Pigmentosa

Meningioma

http://www.rarediseases.org/lof/lof.html#B

Meningiomas are benign, slow-growing tumors, classified as brain tumors, but actually growing in the three protective membranes that surround the brain (meninges). Sometimes they cause thickening or thinning of adjoining skull bones. Meningiomas do not spread to other areas of the body.

Synonyms:

Arachnoidal Fibroblastoma, Dural Endothelioma Leptomeningioma, Meningeal Fibroblastoma, Frontal Tumor, Meningioma, Temporal Tumor, Meningioma Parietal Tumor, Meningioma

Mycosis Fungoides

http://www.rarediseases.org/lof/lof.html#B

Mycosis Fungoides is a rare form of T-cell lymphoma of the skin (cutaneous); the disease is typically slowly progressive and chronic. In individuals with Mycosis Fungoides, the skin becomes infiltrated with plaques and nodules that are composed of lymphocytes. In advanced cases, ulcerated tumors and infiltration of lymph nodes by diseased cells may occur. The disorder may spread to other parts of the body including the gastrointestinal system, liver, spleen, or brain.

Synonyms:

Vidal-Brocq Mycosis Fungoides, Granuloma Fungoides

Neurofibromatosis Type 1 (NF-1)

http://www.rarediseases.org/lof/lof.html#B

Neurofibromatosis Type 1 (NF-1) is a rare inherited disorder of the nervous system and is characterized by the development of tumors on the covering of nerves. The symptoms of Neurofibromatosis Type 1 include brown spots (cafe-au-lait) and freckles on the skin, as well as multiple benign tumors on the covering of nerves. These tumors can grow on any nerve and may appear at any time, including childhood, adolescence, or adulthood. Neurofibromatosis Type 1 is inherited as an autosomal dominant genetic trait. Approximately 50 percent of individuals with NF-1 do not have a family history of Neurofibromatosis; these cases represent spontaneous genetic changes (mutations).

The term "Neurofibromatosis" is also used in a general way to describe two genetically distinct disorders: Neurofibromatosis Type 1 (NF-1) and Neurofibromatosis Type 2 (NF-2). Neurofibromatosis Type 2 is characterized by benign tumors on both auditory nerves (acoustic neuromas of 8th cranial nerves) and tumors primarily on the central nervous system (brain and spine). Acoustic Neuromas generally cause a loss of hearing.

Synonyms:

Segmental Neurofibromatosis, Neurofibroma, Multiple Neurofibromatosi-Pheo-chromocytoma-Duodenal Carcinoid Syndrome, NF-1, Peripheral Neurofibromatosis Recklinghausen's Phakomatosis Von Recklinghausen's Disease, Von Recklinghausen's Neurofibromatosis

Neurofibromatosis Type 2 (NF-2)

http://www.rarediseases.org/lof/lof.html#B

Neurofibromatosis Type 2 (NF-2) is a rare inherited disorder characterized by the development of benign tumors on both auditory nerves (acoustic neuromas). Other tumors of the central nervous system may also develop (e.g., neurofibromas, meningiomas, gliomas, and/or schwannomas). Symptoms may include balance problems, ringing in the ears (tinnitis), and/or hearing loss. Neurofibromatosis Type 2 is inherited as an autosomal dominant genetic trait.

The term "Neurofibromatosis" is also used in a general way to describe two genetically distinct disorders: Neurofibromatosis Type 1 (NF-1) and Neurofibromatosis Type 2 (NF-2). Neurofibromatosis Type 1 is characterized by the development of multiple benign tumors on the covering of nerve fibers.

Synonyms:

Bilateral Acoustic Neurofibromatosis, Central Form, Neurofibromatosis, NF-2, Vestibular Schwannoma Neurofibromatosis

Ollier Disease

http://www.rarediseases.org/lof/lof.html#B

Ollier disease is a rare skeletal disorder characterized by abnormal bone development (skeletal dysplasia). This disorder is present at birth (congenital); however, it may not be apparent until early childhood when certain symptoms, such as deformities or improper limb growth, are observed. Ollier disease primarily affects the long bones and cartilage in the joints of the arms and legs, specifically the area where the shaft and head of a long bone meet (metaphyses). The pelvis is often involved; in rare cases, the ribs, breast bone (sternum), and/or skull may also be affected. Deformities may also develop in the wrists and ankles.

In Ollier disease an overgrowth of cartilage in the long bones of the arms and legs results in abnormal bone growth and thinning of the outer layer (cortex) of the bone. These masses of cartilage are benign (non-cancerous) tumors known as enchondromas. The growth of enchondromas can occur anytime. After puberty these growths stabilize as cartilage is replaced by bone. In rare cases, the enchondromas may undergo malignant changes (e.g., chondrosarcomas). The exact cause of Ollier disease is not known although some cases may be inherited as an autosomal dominant genetic trait.

Synonyms:

Multiple Enchondromatosis, Multiple Cartilaginous Enchondroses, Ollier Osteochondromatosis, Unilateral Chondromatosis

Paget's Disease of the Breast

http://www.rarediseases.org/lof/lof.html#B

Paget's Disease of the Breast is a very rare form of cancer. It is characterized by skin changes resembling eczema around the nipple and breast. It may also occur in the skin areas of the genitals and rectum. When it spreads to these areas of the body Paget's Disease of the Breast is called Extramammary Paget's Disease. Paget's Disease of the Breast often signals the existence of other internal cancer. It can occur in men as well as women. Paget's Disease of the Breast is not Paget's Disease of the bones.

Synonyms:

Adenocarcinoma of the Nipple, Extramammary Paget's Disease, Mammary or Extramammary Paget's Disease, Nipple Cancer, Paget's Disease of the Nipple

Pancreatic Islet Cell Tumor

http://www.rarediseases.org/lof/lof.html#B

Pancreatic Islet Cell Tumors appear in one of two forms. They may be nonfunctioning or functioning tumors. Nonfunctioning tumors may cause obstruction in the shortest part of the small intestine (duodenum) or in the biliary tract, which connects the liver to the duodenum and includes the gall bladder. These nonfunctioning tumors may erode and bleed into the stomach and/or the intestines, or they may cause an abdominal mass.

Functioning tumors secrete excessive amounts of hormones, which may lead to various syndromes including low blood sugar (hypoglycemia), multiple bleeding ulcers (Zollinger-Ellison Syndrome), pancreatic cholera (Verner-Morrison Syndrome), carcinoid syndrome, or diabetes.

Islet cells are small, isolated masses of cells that make up the Islet of Langerhans in the pancreas. When functioning normally, they secrete the protein hormones insulin and glucagon. Tumors composed of irregular islet cells may occur alone or in a group of many tumors. Approximately 90% of islet-cell tumors are noncancerous (benign). They usually range in size from 0.5 to 2 cm in diameter.

Synonyms:

Encephalopathy, Hypoglycemic, Multiple Endocrine Adenomatosis

Peutz-Jeghers Syndrome

http://www.rarediseases.org/lof/lof.html#B

Peutz-Jeghers Syndrome is a rare inherited disorder characterized by multiple benign nodular growths (hamartomas) on the mucous lining of the intestinal wall. Affected individuals also have dark skin discolorations, especially around the lips and mucous membranes of the mouth.

Synonyms:

Hutchinson-Weber-Peutz Syndrome, Intestinal Polyposis II, Intestinal Polyposis-Cutaneous Pigmentation Syndrome, Jegher's Syndrome, Lentigio-Polypose-Digestive Syndrome, Melanoplakia-Intestinal Polyposis, Peutz-Touraine Syndrome, PJS, Polyposis, Hamartomatous Intestinal, Polyps and Spots Syndrome

POEMS Syndrome

http://www.rarediseases.org/lof/lof.html#B

POEMS Syndrome is an acronym for Polyneuropathy (a disease of many nerves), Organomegaly (the enlargement of an organ), Endocrinopathy (a functional disorder of an endocrine gland), M protein (monoclonal immunoglobin, a type of antibody), and Skin changes. The exact cause of POEMS Syndrome is not known.

Synonyms:

Crow-Fukase Syndrome, PEP Syndrome, Shimpo's Syndrome, Takatsuki's Syndrome

Polyposis, Familial

http://www.rarediseases.org/lof/lof.html#B

Familial Polyposis is a group of rare inherited disorders of the gastrointestinal system. Initially the disorder is characterized by benign growths (adenomatous polyps) in the mucous lining of the gastrointestinal tract. If left untreated, affected individuals usually develop cancer of the colon and/or rectum.

Synonyms:

ACR (Adenomatosis of the Colon and Rectum, Adenomatous Polyposis, Familial, Familial Adenomatous Colon Polyposis, Familial Polyposis Coli FAP, Intestinal Polyposis I, Multiple Familial Polyposis

Pseudotumor Cerebri

http://www.rarediseases.org/lof/lof.html#B

Pseudotumor Cerebri is a condition characterized by increased pressure inside the skull (intracranial pressure), headache, nausea, vomiting, and swelling of the optic disk (papilledema), which is the portion of the optic nerve that enters the eye and joins the nerve-rich membrane lining the eye (retina). (The optic nerves are the pair of nerves [second cranial nerves] that transmit impulses from the retinas to the brain.) In some cases, papilledema may cause progressive visual loss and/or impairment of one of the cranial nerve pairs (sixth cranial nerves [nervus abducens]) arising from the brain (cranial nerve palsy). The sixth cranial nerves control the muscles (lateral rectus muscles) that turn the eyes outward. Although the symptoms and findings associated with Pseudotumor Cerebri are similar to those that may occur due to certain brain tumors, no tumor is involved in individuals with Pseudotumor Cerebri.

Pseudotumor Cerebri most commonly occurs in young, obese females. In most cases, the exact cause of Pseudotumor Cerebri is unknown. However, in some cases, the condition appears to occur in association with pregnancy, use of sex hormones, certain parathyroid or adrenal gland disorders, or other underlying disorders, conditions, or other factors.

Synonyms:

Benign Intracranial Hypertension, Idiopathic Intracranial Hypertension

Radiation Syndromes

http://www.rarediseases.org/lof/lof.html#B

Radiation syndromes describe the harmful effects—acute, delayed, or chronic—produced by exposure to ionizing radiations. Tissues vary in response to immediate radiation injury according to the following descending order of sensitivity: (1) lymph cells, (2) reproductive organs, (3) proliferating cells of the bone marrow, (4) epithelial cells of the bowel, (5) top layer (epidermis) of the skin, (6) liver cells, (7) epithelium of the little lung sacs (alveoli) and bile passages, (8) kidney epithelial cells, (9) endothelial cells of the membranes around the lungs, lining the chest cavity (pleura) and the abdominal cavity (peritoneum), (10) nerve cells, (11) bone cells, (12) muscle and connective tissue. Generally, the more rapid the turnover of the cell, the greater the radiation sensitivity.

Synonyms:

Radiation Disease, Radiation Effects, Radiation Illness, Radiation Injuries, Radiation Reaction, Radiation Sickness

Retinoblastoma

http://www.rarediseases.org/lof/lof.html#B

Retinoblastoma is an extremely rare malignant tumor that develops in the nerve-rich layers of one eye or both eyes, most commonly in children under the age of three years. The most typical finding associated with retinoblastoma is the appearance of a distinctive white mass in the pupil area behind the lens of the eye or so called "cat's eye reflex" (leukokoria). In addition, the eyes may appear crossed (strabismus). In some affected children, the eye(s) may become red and/or painful. The presence of the tumor may cause a rise in the pressure in the eyeball (glaucoma). In most cases, retinoblastomas occur spontaneously for no apparent reason (sporadic); however, approximately 20 percent of cases are transmitted as an autosomal dominant genetic trait.

Synonyms:

Retina, Glioma

Sarcoma, Ewing's

http://www.rarediseases.org/lof/lof.html#B

Ewing's Sarcoma is a malignant tumor of bone (i.e., primitive small round cell tumor) that may invade surrounding soft tissues. In many cases, Ewing's Sarcoma affects the shafts of the long bones (diaphyses) of the legs or arms. Ewing's Sarcoma may also develop in bones of the foot, the hand, the spinal column (vertebrae), the pelvis, the lower jaw (mandible), the skull, and/or other locations. Individuals with Ewing's Sarcoma often experience associated pain and swelling, fever, and abnormally increased levels of circulating white blood cells (leukocytosis). Ewing's Sarcoma affects males more often than females and usually develops between the ages of 10 and 20 years. The exact cause of Ewing's Sarcoma is not known.

Tongue Carcinoma

http://www.rarediseases.org/lof/lof.html#B

Tongue Carcinoma is an oral cancer that is characterized by an ulcerating malignant tumor, usually on the side of the tongue, consisting of scaly (squamous) cells. The tumor may spread to the lymph nodes on the same side of the neck.

Synonyms:
Cancer of the Tongue, Carcinoma of the Tongue

Tuberous Sclerosis

http://www.rarediseases.org/lof/lof.html#B

Tuberous Sclerosis is a rare genetic multisystem disorder characterized by the appearance of characteristic benign tumors in various areas of the body, seizures, and mental retardation. Other findings and symptoms may include developmental delays; characteristic skin lesions (e.g., adenoma sebaceum); lesions in the eyes (ocular); uncontrollable involuntary muscle spasms (myoclonic jerking); and/or learning disabilities. The range and severity of associated symptoms and findings may vary greatly from case to case. Tuberous Sclerosis is inherited as an autosomal dominant genetic trait. Two genes have been identified that may cause this disorder. One disease gene, the TSC1 gene, is located on the long arm of chromosome 9 (9q34). The other gene, the TSC2 gene, has been located on the short arm of chromosome 16 (16p13.3). Approximately 65 percent of the cases of Tuberous Sclerosis occur as a result of a spontaneous genetic change (new mutation).

Synonyms:
Bourneville Pringle Syndrome, Epiloia, Phakomatosis TS, TSC1, TSC2, Tuberose Sclerosis, Tuberous Sclerosis Complex, Tuberous Sclerosis-

Tyrosinemia, Hereditary

http://www.rarediseases.org/lof/lof.html#B

Tyrosinemia is a rare inborn error of metabolism involving the amino acid tyrosine associated with a lack of the enzyme fumarylacetoacetase parahydroxyphenylpyruvic acid (p-HPPA) oxidase. The disorder is characterized by elevated levels of tyrosine and its metabolites (including succinylacetone) in the urine. It causes developmental delay and profound liver dysfunction, kidney problems, and liver cell cancer. There are often neurologic problems causing peripheral nerve palsy and paralysis.

Synonyms:
Acute Form Hereditary Tyrosinemia, Chronic Form Hereditary Tyrosinemia, Tyrosinemia, Hereditary, Hepatorenal Type Tyrosyluria

Von Hippel-Lindau Disease

http://www.rarediseases.org/lof/lof.html#B

Von Hippel-Lindau Disease is a rare inherited multi-system disorder characterized by the abnormal growth of blood vessels in certain parts of the body (angiomatosis). Very small blood vessels (capillaries) "knot" together to form benign growths known as angiomas. These may develop in the retinas of the eyes (retinoangioma) or in the brain (cerebellar hemangioblastoma). Benign growths may also occur in other parts of the brain, spinal cord, the adrenal glands (pheochromocytoma), and other parts of the body. The symptoms of von Hippel-Lindau Disease vary greatly and depend on the size and location of the growths. People with von Hippel-Lindau Disease are also genetically predisposed to certain types of malignant tumors (i.e., renal cell carcinoma).

Synonyms:

Angiomatosis Retinae, Angiophakomatosis Retinae et Cerebelli, Cerebelloretinal Hemangioblastomatosis, Hippel Disease, Hippel-Lindau Syndrome, HLS, Lindau Disease, Retinocerebellar Angiomatosis, VHL

WAGR Syndrome

http://www.rarediseases.org/lof/lof.html#B

WAGR Syndrome is a rare genetic syndrome in which there is a predisposition to several distinct disorders. The acronym WAGR stands for Wilms' Tumor, Aniridia, Gonadoblastoma, and Mental Retardation. A combination of two or more of these symptoms must be present for an individual to be diagnosed with WAGR Syndrome. The clinical picture varies, depending upon the combination of symptoms present. The only feature that has been present in all documented cases of WAGR Syndrome, with only one known exception, is the partial or complete absence of the colored portion of the eye or iris (Aniridia). Mental retardation, Wilms' Tumor (the most common form of kidney cancer in children), and/or cancer of the cells that form the testes in males or the ovaries in females (Gonadoblastoma) may or may not be present in affected individuals.

WAGR Syndrome is most often caused by a spontaneous genetic change during early embryonic development (de novo) that occurs for unknown reasons (sporadic). In a small number of cases, chromosomal abnormalities may be present in the parents of children with WAGR Syndrome. In these very rare cases, the syndrome may have been inherited as an autosomal dominant genetic trait.

Synonyms:

Aniridia-Wilms' Tumor Association, AWTA, Aniridia-Ambiguous Genitalia-Mental Retardation, AGR Triad, Aniridia-Wilms' Tumor-Gonadoblastoma, WAGR Complex, Wilms' Tumor-Aniridia-Genitourinary Anomalies-Mental Retardation Syndrome, Wilms' Tumor-Aniridia-Gonadoblastoma-Mental Retardation Syndrome

Wilms' Tumor

http://www.rarediseases.org/lof/lof.html#B

Wilms' Tumor is the most common form of kidney cancer in children, accounting for six to eight percent of all childhood cancers. The exact cause is not known, although it is thought to be inherited in some cases. An abdominal swelling is the most common symptom usually leading to early detection of the disease. Wilms' Tumor can often be treated successfully depending on the stage of the tumor at detection and the age and general health of the child.

Synonyms:

Embryoma Kidney, Embryonal Adenomyosarcoma Kidney, Embryonal Carcinosarcoma Kidney, Embryonal Mixed Tumor Kidney, Nephroblastoma

X-linked Lymphoproliferative Syndrome

http://www.rarediseases.org/lof/lof.html#B

X-linked Lymphoproliferative Syndrome (XLP) is an extremely rare inherited (primary) immunodeficiency disorder characterized by a defective immune system response to infection with the Epstein-Barr virus (EBV). This herpes virus is common among the general population and causes infectious mononucleosis (IM), usually with no long-lasting effects. However, in individuals with X-Linked Lymphoproliferative Syndrome, exposure to EBV may result in severe, life-threatening infectious mononucleosis; abnormally low levels of antibodies in the blood and body secretions (hypogammaglobulinemia), resulting in increased susceptibility to various infections; malignancies of certain types of lymphoid tissue (B-cell lymphomas); and/or other abnormalities. The range of symptoms and findings associated with XLP may vary from case to case. In addition, the range of effects may change in an affected individual over time. In most cases, individuals with XLP experience an onset of symptoms anytime from approximately six months to 10 years of age.

Approximately half of individuals with X-linked Lymphoproliferative Syndrome experience severe, life-threatening mononucleosis characterized by fever, inflammation and soreness of the throat (pharyngitis), swollen lymph glands, enlargement of the spleen (splenomegaly), enlargement of the liver (hepatomegaly), and/or abnormal functioning of the liver, resulting in yellowing of the skin, mucous membranes, and whites of the eyes (jaundice or icterus). In some cases, individuals who experience life-threatening mononucleosis infection may subsequently have an abnormal increase (i.e., proliferation) of certain white blood cells (lymphocytes and histiocytes) in particular organs, severe liver damage and/or failure, damage to the blood-cell generating bone marrow (hematopoietic marrow cells) that may result in aplastic anemia, and/or other symptoms that may result in life-threatening complications in affected children or adults. Aplastic anemia is characterized by a marked deficiency of all types of blood cells (pancytopenia) including low levels of red blood cells, certain white blood cells, and platelets, specialized red blood cells that function to assist appropriate blood clotting. In individuals with XLP, a decrease in platelets (thrombocytopenia) results in increased susceptibility to bruising and excessive bleeding (hemorrhaging). Because X-linked Lymphoproliferative Syndrome is inherited as an X-linked recessive genetic trait, the disorder is usually fully expressed in males only.

Synonyms:

Duncan Disease, EBV Susceptibility (EBVS), Epstein-Barr Virus-Induced Lymphoproliferative Disease in Males, Immunodeficiency-5 (IMD5), X-Linked Progressive Combined Variable Immunodeficiency, Purtilo Syndrome, XLP

Xeroderma Pigmentosum

http://www.rarediseases.org/lof/lof.html#B

Xeroderma Pigmentosum (XP) is a group of rare inherited skin disorders that is characterized by a heightened reaction to sunlight (photosensitivity) with skin blistering occurring after exposure to the sun. In some cases, pain and blistering may occur immediately after contact with sunlight. Acute sunburn and persistent redness or inflammation of the skin (erythema) are also early symptoms of Xeroderma Pigmentosum. In most cases, these symptoms may be apparent immediately after birth or occur within the next three years. In some rare cases, symptoms may not be apparent until later in childhood. Other symptoms of Xeroderma Pigmentosum may include discolorations of the skin, weak and fragile skin, and/or scarring of the skin.

Xeroderma Pigmentosum affects the eyes as well as the skin, has been associated with several forms of cancer, and may occur along with dwarfism, mental retardation, and/or delayed development.

There are several types of Xeroderma Pigmentosum. Each type is categorized according to the capacity of the body to repair the DNA damaged by ultraviolet light. Any of the symptoms of the classic form of Xeroderma Pigmentosum may occur in any of these subdivisions. These types are: XP, Type A (XPA-Classical); XP, Type B (XPB); XP, Type C (XPC); XP, Type D (XPD); XP, Type E (XPE); XP, Type F (XPF); XP, Type G (XPG); and XP, Dominant Type. In most cases, Xeroderma Pigmentosum is inherited as an autosomal recessive genetic trait.

Synonyms:

Kaposi Disease (not Kaposi Sarcoma), XP, Xeroderma Pigmentosum, Type A, I, XPA, Classical Form, Xeroderma Pigmentosum, Type B, II, XPB, Xeroderma Pigmentosum, Type C, III, XPC, Xeroderma Pigmentosum, Type D, IV, XPD, Xeroderma Pigmentosum, Type E, V, XPE, Xeroderma Pigmentosum, Type F, VI, XPF, Xeroderma Pigmentosum, Type G, VII, XPG, Xeroderma Pigmentosum, Dominant Type, Xeroderma Pigmentosum, Variant Type, XP-V

Zollinger-Ellison Syndrome

http://www.rarediseases.org/lof/lof.html#B

Zollinger-Ellison Syndrome is an unusual ulcerative condition characterized by small tumors (usually of the pancreas) that secrete a hormone that produces excess amounts of stomach (gastric) juices. These tumors can also appear in the lower stomach wall, spleen, or lymph nodes close to the stomach. Large amounts of gastric acid can be found in lower stomach areas where ulcers can form. Ulcers can appear suddenly even in areas where they are rarely found, may persist following treatment, and can be accompanied by diarrhea. Prompt medical treatment of these ulcers is necessary to prevent complications such as bleeding and perforation.

Synonyms:

Gastrinoma, Pancreatic Ulcerogenic Tumor Syndrome, Partial Multiple Endocrine Adenomatosis, Z-E Syndrome

15. WEB SITE AND TOPICAL INDEX

O

William S. Graham Foundation for
  Melanoma Research, Inc., 266
Wilms' Tumor, 331, 482
Wistar Institute's Albert R. Taxin Brain
  Tumor Research Center, 318
Women's Cancer Center, 159
Women's Cancer Information Project,
  160
Women's Cancer Network (WCN), 160
World Health Organization (WHO)
  Statistical Information System, 371
World Marrow Donor Association
  (WMDA), 194, 248
World Oncology Network (WON), 157
World Standard Drug Database, 388
World Wide Web Virtual Library
  Biotechnology, 400

X

Xeroderma Pigmentosum, 483
X-linked Lymphoproliferative Syndrome,
  482
X-ray Imaging, 126

Y

Yahoo!, 385, 435
Yahoo! Life and Health Insurance
  Center, 448
Yahoo! News
  Health Headlines, 340
Yale Center for Medical Informatics, 155
Yale-New Haven Hospital, 228
Y-Me National Breast Cancer
  Organization, 194, 252

Z

Zollinger-Ellison Syndrome, 483

℞ ONLY

TAXOL®
(paclitaxel) Injection

Brief Summary of Prescribing Information, 10/99. For complete prescribing information, please consult official package circular.

WARNING

TAXOL® (paclitaxel) Injection should be administered under the supervision of a physician experienced in the use of cancer chemotherapeutic agents. Appropriate management of complications is possible only when adequate diagnostic and treatment facilities are readily available.

Anaphylaxis and severe hypersensitivity reactions characterized by dyspnea and hypotension requiring treatment, angioedema, and generalized urticaria have occurred in 2%-4% of patients receiving TAXOL in clinical trials. Fatal reactions have occurred in patients despite premedication. All patients should be pretreated with corticosteroids, diphenhydramine, and H_2 antagonists. (See **DOSAGE AND ADMINISTRATION** section.) Patients who experience severe hypersensitivity reactions to TAXOL should not be rechallenged with the drug.

TAXOL therapy should not be given to patients with solid tumors who have baseline neutrophil counts of less than 1,500 cells/mm³ and should not be given to patients with AIDS-related Kaposi's sarcoma if the baseline neutrophil count is less than 1000 cells/mm³. In order to monitor the occurrence of bone marrow suppression, primarily neutropenia, which may be severe and result in infection, it is recommended that frequent peripheral blood cell counts be performed on all patients receiving TAXOL.

INDICATIONS

TAXOL is indicated as first-line and subsequent therapy for the treatment of advanced carcinoma of the ovary. As first-line therapy, TAXOL is indicated in combination with cisplatin.

TAXOL is indicated for the adjuvant treatment of node-positive breast cancer administered sequentially to standard doxorubicin-containing combination chemotherapy. In the clinical trial, there was an overall favorable effect on disease-free and overall survival in the total population of patients with receptor-positive and receptor-negative tumors, but the benefit has been specifically demonstrated by available data (median follow-up 30 months) only in the patients with estrogen and progesterone receptor-negative tumors. (See **CLINICAL STUDIES: Breast Carcinoma** section in full prescribing information.)

TAXOL is indicated for the treatment of breast cancer after failure of combination chemotherapy for metastatic disease or relapse within 6 months of adjuvant chemotherapy. Prior therapy should have included an anthracycline unless clinically contraindicated.

TAXOL, in combination with cisplatin, is indicated for the first-line treatment of non-small cell lung cancer in patients who are not candidates for potentially curative surgery and/or radiation therapy.

TAXOL is indicated for the second-line treatment of AIDS-related Kaposi's sarcoma.

CONTRAINDICATIONS

TAXOL is contraindicated in patients who have a history of hypersensitivity reactions to TAXOL or other drugs formulated in Cremophor® EL (polyoxyethylated castor oil).

TAXOL should not be used in patients with solid tumors who have baseline neutrophil counts of < 1500 cells/mm³ or in patients with AIDS-related Kaposi's sarcoma with baseline neutrophil counts of <1000 cells/mm³.

WARNINGS

Anaphylaxis and severe hypersensitivity reactions characterized by dyspnea and hypotension requiring treatment, angioedema, and generalized urticaria have occurred in 2%-4% of patients receiving TAXOL in clinical trials. Fatal reactions have occurred in patients despite premedication. All patients should be pretreated with corticosteroids, diphenhydramine, and H_2 antagonists. (See **DOSAGE AND ADMINISTRATION** section.) Patients who experience severe hypersensitivity reactions to TAXOL should not be rechallenged with the drug.

Bone marrow suppression (primarily neutropenia) is dose-dependent and is the dose-limiting toxicity. Neutrophil nadirs occurred at a median of 11 days. TAXOL should not be administered to patients with baseline neutrophil counts of less than 1500 cells/mm³ (<1000 cells/mm³ for patients with KS). Frequent monitoring of blood counts should be instituted during TAXOL treatment. Patients should not be re-treated with subsequent cycles of TAXOL until neutrophils recover to a level >1500 cells/mm³ (>1000 cells/mm³ for patients with KS) and platelets recover to a level >100,000 cells/mm³.

Severe conduction abnormalities have been documented in < 1% of patients during TAXOL therapy and in some cases requiring pacemaker placement. If patients develop significant conduction abnormalities during TAXOL infusion, appropriate therapy should be administered and continuous cardiac monitoring should be performed during subsequent therapy with TAXOL.

Pregnancy: TAXOL can cause fetal harm when administered to a pregnant woman. Administration of paclitaxel during the period of organogenesis to rabbits at doses of 3.0 mg/kg/day (about 0.2 the daily maximum recommended human dose on a mg/m² basis) caused embryo- and fetotoxicity, as indicated by intrauterine mortality, increased resorptions and increased fetal deaths. Maternal toxicity was also observed at this dose. No teratogenic effects were observed at 1.0 mg/kg/day (about 1/15 the daily maximum recommended human dose on a mg/m² basis); teratogenic potential could not be assessed at higher doses due to extensive fetal mortality.

There are no adequate and well-controlled studies in pregnant women. If TAXOL is used during pregnancy, or if the patient becomes pregnant while receiving this drug, the patient should be apprised of the potential hazard to the fetus. Women of childbearing potential should be advised to avoid becoming pregnant.

PRECAUTIONS

Contact of the undiluted concentrate with plasticized polyvinyl chloride (PVC) equipment or devices used to prepare solutions for infusion is not recommended. In order to minimize patient exposure to the plasticizer DEHP [di-(2-ethylhexyl)phthalate], which may be leached from PVC infusion bags or sets, diluted TAXOL solutions should preferably be stored in bottles (glass, polypropylene) or plastic bags (polypropylene, polyolefin) and administered through polyethylene-lined administration sets.

TAXOL should be administered through an in-line filter with a microporous membrane not greater than 0.22 microns. Use of filter devices such as IVEX-2® filters which incorporate short inlet and outlet PVC-coated tubing has not resulted in significant leaching of DEHP.

Drug Interactions: In a Phase I trial using escalating doses of TAXOL (110-200 mg/m²) and cisplatin (50 or 75 mg/m²) given as sequential infusions, myelosuppression was more profound when TAXOL (paclitaxel) Injection was given after cisplatin than with the alternate sequence (i.e., TAXOL before cisplatin). Pharmacokinetic data from these patients demonstrated a decrease in paclitaxel clearance of approximately 33% when TAXOL was administered following cisplatin.

The metabolism of TAXOL is catalyzed by cytochrome P450 isoenzymes CYP2C8 and CYP3A4. In the absence of formal clinical drug interaction studies, caution should be exercised when administering TAXOL concomitantly with known substrates or inhibitors of the cytochrome P450 isoenzymes CYP2C8 and CYP3A4. (See **CLINICAL PHARMACOLOGY** section in full prescribing information.)

Potential interactions between TAXOL, a substrate of CYP3A4 and protease inhibitors (ritonavir, saquinavir, indinavir, and nelfinavir), which are substrates and/or inhibitors of CYP3A4 have not been evaluated in clinical trials.

Reports in the literature suggest that plasma levels of doxorubicin (and its active metabolite doxorubicinol) may be increased when paclitaxel and doxorubicin are used in combination.

Hematology: TAXOL therapy should not be administered to patients with baseline neutrophil counts of less than 1,500 cells/mm³. In order to monitor the occurrence of myelotoxicity, it is recommended that frequent peripheral blood cell counts be performed on all patients receiving TAXOL. Patients should not be re-treated with subsequent cycles of TAXOL until neutrophils recover to a level >1500 cells/mm³ and platelets recover to a level >100,000 cells/mm³. In the case of severe neutropenia (<500 cells/mm³ for seven days or more) during a course of TAXOL therapy, a 20% reduction in dose for subsequent courses of therapy is recommended.

For patients with advanced HIV disease and poor-risk AIDS-related Kaposi's sarcoma, TAXOL, at the recommended dose for this disease, can be initiated and repeated if the neutrophil count is at least 1000 cells/mm³.

Hypersensitivity Reactions: Patients with a history of severe hypersensitivity reactions to products containing Cremophor® EL (e.g., cyclosporin for injection concentrate and teniposide for injection concentrate) should not be treated with TAXOL. In order to avoid the occurrence of severe hypersensitivity reactions, all patients treated with TAXOL should be premedicated with corticosteroids (such as dexamethasone), diphenhydramine and H_2 antagonists (such as cimetidine or ranitidine). Minor symptoms such as flushing, skin reactions, dyspnea, hypotension or tachycardia do not require interruption of therapy. However, severe reactions, such as hypotension requiring treatment, dyspnea requiring bronchodilators, angioedema or generalized urticaria require immediate discontinuation of TAXOL and aggressive symptomatic therapy. Patients who have developed severe hypersensitivity reactions should not be rechallenged with TAXOL.

Cardiovascular: Hypotension, bradycardia, and hypertension have been observed during administration of TAXOL, but generally do not require treatment. Occasionally TAXOL infusions must be interrupted or discontinued because of initial or recurrent hypertension. Frequent vital sign monitoring, particularly during the first hour of TAXOL infusion, is recommended. Continuous cardiac monitoring is not required except for patients with serious conduction abnormalities. (See **WARNINGS** section.)

Nervous System: Although, the occurrence of peripheral neuropathy is frequent, the development of severe symptomatology is unusual and requires a dose reduction of 20% for all subsequent courses of TAXOL.

TAXOL contains dehydrated alcohol USP, 396 mg/mL; consideration should be given to possible CNS and other effects of alcohol. (See **PRECAUTIONS: Pediatric Use** section.)

Hepatic: There is evidence that the toxicity of TAXOL is enhanced in patients with elevated liver enzymes. Caution should be exercised when administering TAXOL to patients with moderate to severe hepatic impairment and dose adjustments should be considered.

Injection Site Reaction: Injection site reactions, including reactions secondary to extravasation, were usually mild and consisted of erythema, tenderness, skin discoloration, or swelling at the injection site. These reactions have been observed more frequently with the 24-hour infusion than with the 3-hour infusion. Recurrence of skin reactions at a site of previous extravasation following administration of TAXOL at a different site, i.e., "recall", has been reported rarely.

Rare reports of more severe events such as phlebitis, cellulitis, induration, skin exfoliation, necrosis and fibrosis have been received as part of the continuing surveillance of TAXOL safety. In some cases the onset of the injection site reaction either occurred during a prolonged infusion or was delayed by a week to ten days.

A specific treatment for extravasation reactions is unknown at this time. Given the possibility of extravasation, it is advisable to closely monitor the infusion site for possible infiltration during drug administration.

Carcinogenesis, Mutagenesis, Impairment of Fertility: The carcinogenic potential of TAXOL has not been studied.

Paclitaxel has been shown to be clastogenic *in vitro* (chromosome aberrations in human lymphocytes) and *in vivo* (micronucleus test in mice). Paclitaxel was not mutagenic in the Ames test or the CHO/HGPRT gene mutation assay.

Administration of paclitaxel prior to and during mating produced impairment of fertility in male and female rats at doses equal to or greater than 1 mg/kg/day (about 0.04 the daily maximum recommended human dose on a mg/m² basis). At this dose, paclitaxel caused reduced fertility and reproductive indices, and increased embryo- and fetotoxicity. (See **WARNINGS** section.)

Pregnancy: Pregnancy "Category D". (See **WARNINGS** section.)

Nursing Mothers: It is not known whether the drug is excreted in human milk. Following intravenous administration of carbon-14 labeled TAXOL to rats on days 9 to 10 postpartum, concentrations of radioactivity in milk were higher than in plasma and declined in parallel with the plasma concentrations. Because many drugs are excreted in human milk and because of the potential for serious adverse reactions in nursing infants, it is recommended that nursing be discontinued when receiving TAXOL therapy.

Pediatric Use: The safety and effectiveness of TAXOL in pediatric patients have not been established.

There have been reports of central nervous system (CNS) toxicity (rarely associated with death) in a clinical trial in pediatric patients in which TAXOL was infused intravenously over 3 hours at doses ranging from 350 mg/m² to 420 mg/m². The toxicity is most likely attributable to the high dose of the ethanol component of the TAXOL vehicle given over a short infusion time. The use of concomitant antihistamines may intensify this effect. Although a direct effect of the paclitaxel itself cannot be discounted, the high doses used in this study (over twice the recommended adult dosage) must be considered in assessing the safety of TAXOL for use in this population.

ADVERSE REACTIONS

Pooled Analysis of Adverse Event Experiences from Single-Agent Studies: The following data is an adverse event summary (see full prescribing information, Table 9) based on the experience of 812 patients (493 with ovarian carcinoma and 319 with breast carcinoma) enrolled in 10 studies who received single-agent TAXOL (paclitaxel) Injection. Two hundred and seventy-five patients were treated in eight Phase 2 studies with TAXOL doses ranging from 135 to 300 mg/m^2 administered over 24 hours (in four of these studies, G-CSF was administered as hematopoietic support). Three hundred and one patients were treated in the randomized Phase 3 ovarian carcinoma study which compared two doses (135 or 175 mg/m^2) and two schedules (3 or 24 hours) of TAXOL. Two hundred and thirty-six patients with breast carcinoma received TAXOL (135 or 175 mg/m^2) administered over 3 hours in a controlled study.

The following is an adverse event summary of percent incidence in 812 patients receiving TAXOL: **Bone Marrow-** Neutropenia (<2000/mm^3) 90 and (<500/mm^3) 52; Leukopenia (<4000/mm^3) 90 and (<1,000/mm^3) 17; Thrombocytopenia (<100,000/mm^3) 20 and (<50,000/mm^3) 7; Anemia (<11 g/dL) 78 and (<8 g/dL) 16; Infections 30; Bleeding 14; Red Cell Transfusions 25; Platelet Transfusions 2; **Hypersensitivity Reaction** (with premedication)- All 41; Severe (Grade III/IV) 2; **Cardiovascular-** Vital Sign Changes (during first 3 hours of infusion) Bradycardia (N=537) 3 and Hypotension (N=532) 12; Significant Cardiovascular Events 1; **Abnormal ECG-** All Patients 23; Patients with normal baseline (N=559) 14; **Peripheral Neuropathy-** Any 60; Severe (III/IV) 3; **Myalgia/Arthralgia-** Any 60; Severe (Grade III/IV) 8; **Gastrointestinal-** Nausea and vomiting 52; Diarrhea 38; Mucositis 31; **Alopecia-** 87; **Hepatic** (Patients with normal baseline)- Bilirubin elevations (N=765) 7; Akaline phosphatase elevations (N=575) 22; AST (SGOT) elevations (N=591) 19; **Injection Site Reaction-** 13. None of the observed toxicities were clearly influenced by age.

Disease-Specific Adverse Event Experiences First-Line Ovary in Combination: The following (see full prescribing information, Table 10) shows the frequency (based on worst course analysis) of important adverse events (as percent of patients) in the 409 patients with Phase 3 first-line Ovarian Cancer treated with TAXOL (i.e., 135 mg/m^2/Cisplatin (75 mg/m^2) vs Cyclophosphamide 750 mg/m^2/Cisplatin (75 mg/m^2). **Bone Marrow-** Neutropenia (<2,000/mm^3) 96 vs 92 and (<500/mm^3) 81 ($p<0.05$) vs 58 ($p<0.05$); Thrombocytopenia (<100,000/mm^3) 26 vs 30 and (<50,000/mm^3)10 vs 9; Anemia (<11 g/dL) 88 vs 86 and (<8 g/dL) 13 vs 9; Infections 21 vs 15; Febrile Neutropenia 15 ($p<0.05$) vs 4 ($p<0.05$). **Hypersensitivity Reaction** (with premedication)- All 8 ($p<0.05$) vs 1 ($p<0.05$); Severe (grade III/IV) 3 ($p<0.05$) vs no reported cases ($p<0.05$). **Peripheral Neuropathy-** Any 25 vs 20; Severe (grade III/IV) 3 vs no reported cases ($p<0.05$). **Nausea and Vomiting-** Any 65 vs 69; Severe (grade III/IV) 10 vs 11. **Myalgia/Arthralgia-** Any 9 ($p<0.05$) vs 2 ($p<0.05$); Severe (grade III/IV) 1 vs no reported cases. **Diarrhea-** Any 16 ($p<0.05$) vs 8 ($p<0.05$); Severe (grade III/IV) 4 vs 1. **Asthenia-** Any 17 ($p<0.05$) vs 10 ($p<0.05$); Severe (grade III/IV) 1 vs 1; **Alopecia-** Any ($p<0.05$) 55 vs 37 ($p<0.05$); Severe (grade III/IV) 6 vs 8.

Second-Line Ovary: For the 403 patients who received single-agent TAXOL in the Phase 3 second-line ovarian carcinoma study, the following shows the incidence of important adverse events. The following (see full prescribing information, Table 11) shows the frequency (based on worst course analysis) of important adverse events (as percent of patients) in the 403 patients with Phase 3 second-line Ovarian Cancer treated with four different TAXOL regimens (i.e., 175 mg/m^2/3 vs 175 mg/m^2/24 vs 135 mg/m^2/3 vs 135 mg/m^2/24. **Bone Marrow-** Neutropenia (<2,000/mm^3) 78 vs 98 vs 78 vs 98 and (<500/mm^3) 27 vs 75 vs 14 vs 67; Thrombocytopenia (<100,000/mm^3) 4 vs 18 vs 8 vs 6 and (<50,000/mm^3)1 vs 7 vs 2 vs 1; Anemia (<11g/dL) 84 vs 90 vs 68 vs 88 and (<8 g/dL) 11 vs 12 vs 6 vs 10; Infections 26 vs 29 vs 20 vs 18. **Hypersensitivity Reaction** (with premedication)- All 41 vs 45 vs 38 vs 45; Severe (grade III/IV) 2 vs 0 vs 2 vs 1. **Peripheral Neuropathy-** Any 63 vs 60 vs 55 vs 42; Severe (grade III/IV) 1 vs 2 vs 0 vs 0. **Mucositis-** Any 17 vs 35 vs 21 vs 25; Severe (grade III/IV) 0 vs 3 vs 0 vs 2.

Myelosuppression was dose and schedule related, with the schedule effect being more prominent. The development of severe hypersensitivity reactions (HSRs) was rare; 1% of the patients and 0.2% of the courses overall. There was no apparent dose or schedule effect seen for the HSRs. Peripheral neuropathy was clearly dose-related, but schedule did not appear to affect the incidence.

Adjuvant Breast: For the Phase 3 adjuvant breast carcinoma study, the following table shows the incidence of important severe adverse events for the 3121 patients (total population) who were evaluable for safety as well as for a group of 325 patients (early population) who, per the study protocol, were monitored more intensively than other patients.

Table 12: Frequency[a] of Important Severe[b] Adverse Events in the Phase 3 Adjuvant Breast Carcinoma Study

	Percent of Patients			
	Early Population		Total Population	
	AC[c] (n=166)	AC[c] followed by T[d] (n=159)	AC[c] (n=1551)	AC[c] followed by T[d] (n=1570)
• Bone Marrow[e]				
- Neutropenia				
< 500/mm^3	79	76	48	50
- Thrombocytopenia				
< 50,000/mm^3	27	25	11	11
- Anemia				
< 8 g/dL	17	21	8	8
- Infections	6	14	5	6
- Fever without Infection	–	3	<1	1
• Hypersensitivity Reaction[f]	1	4	1	2
• Cardiovascular Events	1	2	1	2
• Neuromotor Toxicity	1	1	<1	1
• Neurosensory Toxicity	–	3	<1	3
• Myalgia/Arthralgia	–	2	<1	2
• Nausea/Vomiting	13	18	8	9
• Mucositis	13	4	6	5

[a] Based on worst course analysis.
[b] Severe events are defined as at least Grade III toxicity.
[c] Patients received 600 mg/m^2 cyclophosphamide and doxorubicin at doses of either 60 mg/m^2, 75 mg/m^2, or 90 mg/m^2 (with prophylactic G-CSF support and ciprofloxacin), every 3 weeks for four courses.
[d] TAXOL following four courses of AC at a dose of 175 mg/m^2/3 hours every 3 weeks for four courses.
[e] The incidence of febrile neutropenia was not reported in this study.
[f] All patients were to receive premedication.

The incidence of an adverse event for the total population likely represents an underestimation of the actual incidence given that safety data were collected differently based on enrollment cohort. However, since safety data were collected consistently across regimens, the safety of the sequential addition of TAXOL (paclitaxel) Injection following AC therapy may be compared with AC therapy alone. Compared to patients who received AC alone, patients who received AC followed by TAXOL experienced more Grade III/IV neurosensory toxicity, more Grade III/IV myalgia/arthralgia, more Grade III/IV neurologic pain (5% vs 1%), more Grade III/IV flu-like symptoms (5% vs 3%), and more Grade III/IV hyperglycemia (3% vs 1%). During the additional four courses of treatment with TAXOL, two deaths (0.1%) were attributed to treatment. During TAXOL treatment, Grade IV neutropenia was reported for 15% of patients, Grade II/III neurosensory toxicity for 15%, Grade II/III myalgias for 23%, and alopecia for 46%.

The incidences of severe hematologic toxicities, infections, mucositis, and cardiovascular events increased with higher doses of doxorubicin.

Breast Cancer After Failure of Initial Chemotherapy: For the 458 patients who received single-agent TAXOL in the Phase 3 breast carcinoma study, the following table shows the incidence of important adverse events by treatment arm (each arm was administered by a 3-hour infusion).

Table 13: Frequency[a] of Important Adverse Events in the Phase 3 Study of Breast Cancer After Failure of Initial Chemotherapy or within 6 months of Adjuvant Chemotherapy

		Percent of Patients	
		175/3[b] (n=229)	135/3[b] (n=229)
• Bone Marrow			
- Neutropenia	< 2,000/mm^3	90	81
	< 500/mm^3	28	19
- Thrombocytopenia	< 100,000/mm^3	11	7
	< 50,000/mm^3	3	2
- Anemia	< 11 g/dL	55	47
	< 8 g/dL	4	2
- Infections		23	15
- Febrile Neutropenia		2	2
• Hypersensitivity Reaction[c]			
- All		36	31
- Severe[†]		0	<1
• Peripheral Neuropathy			
- Any symptoms		70	46
- Severe symptoms[†]		7	3
• Mucositis			
- Any symptoms		23	17
- Severe symptoms[†]		3	<1

[a] Based on worst course analysis.
[b] TAXOL dose in mg/m^2/infusion duration in hours.
[c] All patients received premedication.
[†] Severe events are defined as at least Grade III toxicity.

Myelosuppression and peripheral neuropathy were dose related. There was one severe hypersensitivity reaction (HSR) observed at the dose of 135 mg/m^2.

First-Line NSCLC in Combination: In the study conducted by the Eastern Cooperative Oncology Group (ECOG), patients were randomized to either TAXOL (T) 135 mg/m^2 as a 24-hour infusion in combination with cisplatin (c) 75 mg/m^2, TAXOL (T) 250 mg/m^2 as a 24-hour infusion in combination with cisplatin (c) 75 mg/m^2 with G-CSF support, or cisplatin (c) 75 mg/m^2 on day 1, followed by etoposide (VP) 100 mg/m^2 on days 1, 2 and 3 (control). The following (see full prescribing information, Table 14) shows the frequency (based on worst course analysis) of important adverse events (percent of patients) in the phase 3 study for first-line NSCLC. **Bone Marrow-** Neutropenia (<2,000/mm^3) 89 vs 86 vs 84 and (<500/mm^3) 74 ($p<0.05$) vs 65 vs 55; Thrombocytopenia (normal) 48 vs 68 vs 62 and (<50,000/mm^3) 6 vs 12 vs 16; Anemia (normal) 94 vs 96 vs 95 and (<8 g/dL) 22 vs 19 vs 28; Infections 38 vs 31 vs 35. **Hypersensitivity Reaction** (with premedication)- All 16 vs 27 vs 13; Severe (grade III/IV) 1 vs 4 ($p<0.05$) vs 1. **Arthralgia/Myalgia-** Any 21 ($p<0.05$) vs 42 ($p<0.05$) vs 9; Severe (grade III/IV) 3 vs 11 vs 1. **Nausea and Vomiting-** Any 85 vs 87 vs 81; Severe (grade III/IV) 27 vs 29 vs 22. **Mucositis-** Any 18 vs 28 vs 16; Severe (grade III/IV) 1 vs 4 vs 2. **Neuromotor Toxicity-** Any 37 vs 47 vs 44; Severe (grade III/IV) 6 vs 12 vs 7. **Neurosensory Toxicity-** Any 48 vs 61 vs 25; Severe (grade III/IV) 13 vs 28 ($p<0.05$) vs 8. **Cardiovascular Events-** Any 33 vs 39 vs 24; Severe (grade III/IV) 13 vs 12 vs 8.

Toxicity was generally more severe in the high-dose TAXOL treatment arm (T250/c75) than in the low-dose TAXOL arm (T135/c75). Compared to the cisplatin/etoposide arm, patients in the low-dose TAXOL arm experienced more arthralgia/myalgia of any grade and more severe neutropenia. The incidence of febrile neutropenia was not reported in this study.

Kaposi's Sarcoma: The following shows the frequency (based on worst course analysis) of important adverse events (as percent of patients) in the 85 patients with KS treated with two different single-agent TAXOL regimens (i.e., 135 mg/m^2 q3wk vs 100 mg/m^2 q2wk): **Bone Marrow-** Neutropenia (<2000/mm^3) 100 vs 95; (<500/mm^3) 76 vs 35; Thrombocytopenia (<100,000/mm^3) 52 vs 27 and (50,000/mm^3) 17 vs 5; Anemia (<11 g/dL) 86 vs 73 and (<8g/dL) 34 vs 25; Febrile Neutropenia 55 vs 9. **Opportunistic Infection-** Any 76 vs 54; Cytomegalovirus 45 vs 27; Herpes Simplex 38 vs 11; *Pneumocystis carinii* 14 vs 21; *M. avium intracellulare* 24 vs 4; Candidiasis, esophageal 7 vs 9; Cryptosporidiosis 7 vs 7; Cryptococcal meningitis 3 vs 2; Leukoencephalopathy -no reported events vs 2. **Hypersensitivity Reaction** (with premedication)- All 14 vs. 9. **Cardiovascular-** Hypotension 17 vs 9; Bradycardia 3 vs no reported events. **Peripheral Neuropathy-** Any 79 vs 46; Severe (III/IV) 10 vs 2. **Myalgia/Arthralgia-**Any 93 vs 48; Severe (III/IV) 14 vs 16. **Gastrointestinal-** Nausea and vomiting 69 vs 70; Diarrhea 90 vs 73; Mucositis 45 vs 20. **Renal (creatinine elevation)-** Any 34 vs 18; Severe (grade III/IV) 7 vs 5. **Discontinuation for drug toxicity-** 7 vs 16.

As demonstrated above, toxicity was more pronounced in the study utilizing TAXOL at a dose of 135 mg/m^2 every 3 weeks than in the study utilizing TAXOL at a dose of 100 mg/m^2 every 2 weeks. Notably, severe neutropenia (76% versus 35%), febrile neutropenia (55% versus 9%), and opportunistic infections (76% versus 54%) were more common with the former dose and schedule. The differences between the two studies with respect to dose escalation and use of hematopoietic growth factors, as described above, should be taken into account. (See **CLINICAL STUDIES: AIDS-Related Kaposi's Sarcoma** section in full prescribing information.) Note also that only 26% of the 85 patients in these studies received concomitant treatment with protease inhibitors, whose effect on paclitaxel metabolism has not yet been studied.

Adverse Event Experiences by Body System: Unless otherwise noted, the following discussion refers to the overall safety database of 812 patients with solid tumors treated with single-agent TAXOL (paclitaxel) Injection in clinical studies. Toxicities that occurred with greater severity or frequency in previously untreated patients with ovarian carcinoma or NSCLC who received TAXOL in combination with cisplatin or in patients with breast cancer who received TAXOL after doxorubicin/cyclophosphamide in the adjuvant setting and that occurred with a difference that was clinically significant in these populations are also described. The frequency and severity of important adverse events for the Phase 3 ovarian carcinoma, breast carcinoma, NSCLC, and the Phase 2 Kaposi's sarcoma studies are presented above by treatment arm. In addition, rare events have been reported from postmarketing experience or from other clinical studies. The frequency and severity of adverse events have been generally similar for patients receiving TAXOL for the treatment of ovarian, breast, or lung carcinoma or Kaposi's sarcoma, but patients with AIDS-related Kaposi's sarcoma may have more frequent and severe hematologic toxicity, infections, and febrile neutropenia. These patients require a lower dose intensity and supportive care. (See **CLINICAL STUDIES: AIDS-Related Kaposi's Sarcoma** section in full prescribing information.) Toxicities that were observed only in or were noted to have occurred with greater severity in the population with Kaposi's sarcoma and that occurred with a difference that was clinically significant in this population are described.

Hematologic: Bone marrow suppression was the major dose-limiting toxicity of TAXOL. Neutropenia, the most important hematologic toxicity, was dose and schedule dependent and was generally rapidly reversible. Among patients treated in the Phase 3 second-line ovarian study with a 3-hour infusion, neutrophil counts declined below 500 cells/mm^3 in 14% of the patients treated with a dose of 135 mg/m^2 compared to 27% at a dose of 175 mg/m^2 (p=0.05). In the same study, severe neutropenia (<500 cells/mm^3) was more frequent with the 24-hour than with the 3-hour infusion; infusion duration had a greater impact on myelosuppression than dose. Neutropenia did not appear to increase with cumulative exposure and did not appear to be more frequent nor more severe for patients previously treated with radiation therapy.

In the study where TAXOL was administered to patients with ovarian carcinoma at a dose of 135 mg/m^2/24 hours in combination with cisplatin versus the control arm of cyclosphosphamide plus cisplatin, the incidences of grade IV neutropenia and of febrile neutropenia were significantly greater in the TAXOL plus cisplatin arm than in the control arm. Grade IV neutropenia occurred in 81% on the TAXOL plus cisplatin arm versus 58% on the cyclophosphamide plus cisplatin arm, and febrile neutropenia occurred in 15% and 4% respectively. On the TAXOL/cisplatin arm, there were 35/1074 (3%) courses with fever in which Grade IV neutropenia was reported at some time during the course. When TAXOL followed by cisplatin was administered to patients with advanced NSCLC in the ECOG study, the incidences of Grade IV neutropenia were 74% (TAXOL 135 mg/m^2/24 hours followed by cisplatin) and 65% (TAXOL 250 mg/m^2/24 hours followed by cisplatin and G-CSF) compared with 55% in patients who received cisplatin/etoposide.

Fever was frequent (12% of all treatment courses). Infectious episodes occurred in 30% of all patients and 9% of all courses; these episodes were fatal in 1% of all patients, and included sepsis, pneumonia and peritonitis. In the Phase 3 second-line ovarian study, infectious episodes were reported in 20% and 26% of the patients treated with a dose of 135 mg/m^2 or 175 mg/m^2 given as 3-hour infusions, respectively. Urinary tract infections and upper respiratory tract infections were the most frequently reported infectious complications. In the immunosuppressed patient population with advanced HIV disease and poor-risk AIDS-related Kaposi's sarcoma, 61% of the patients reported at least one opportunistic infection. (See **CLINICAL STUDIES: AIDS-Related Kaposi's Sarcoma** section in full prescribing information.) The use of supportive therapy, including G-CSF, is recommended for patients who have experienced severe neutropenia. (See **DOSAGE AND ADMINISTRATION** section.)

Thrombocytopenia was uncommon, and almost never severe (<50,000 cells/mm^3). Twenty percent of the patients experienced a drop in their platelet count below 100,000 cells/mm^3 at least once while on treatment; 7% had a platelet count <50,000 cells/mm^3 at the time of their worst nadir. Bleeding episodes were reported in 4% of all courses and by 14% of all patients but most of the hemorrhagic episodes were localized and the frequency of these events was unrelated to the TAXOL dose and schedule. In the Phase 3 second-line ovarian study, bleeding episodes were reported in 10% of the patients; no patients treated with the 3-hour infusion received platelet transfusions. In the adjuvant breast carcinoma trial, the incidence of severe thrombocytopenia and platelet transfusions increased with higher doses of doxorubicin.

Anemia (Hb <11 g/dL) was observed in 78% of all patients and was severe (Hb <8 g/dL) in 16% of the cases. No consistent relationship between dose or schedule and the frequency of anemia was observed. Among all patients with normal baseline hemoglobin, 69% became anemic on study but only 7% had severe anemia. Red cell transfusions were required in 25% of all patients and in 12% of those with normal baseline hemoglobin levels.

Hypersensitivity Reactions (HSRs): All patients received premedication prior to TAXOL (see **WARNINGS** and **PRECAUTIONS: Hypersensitivity Reactions** sections). The frequency and severity of HSRs were not affected by the dose or schedule of TAXOL administration. In the Phase 3 second-line ovarian study, the 3-hour infusion was not associated with a greater increase in HSRs when compared to the 24-hour infusion. Hypersensitivity reactions were observed in 20% of all courses and in 41% of all patients. These reactions were severe in less than 2% of the patients and 1% of the courses. No severe reactions were observed after course 3 and severe symptoms occurred generally within the first hour of TAXOL infusion. The most frequent symptoms observed during these severe reactions were dyspnea, flushing, chest pain and tachycardia.

The minor hypersensitivity reactions consisted mostly of flushing (28%), rash (12%), hypotension (4%), dyspnea (2%), tachycardia (2%) and hypertension (1%). The frequency of hypersensitivity reactions remained relatively stable during the entire treatment period.

Rare reports of chills and reports of back pain in association with hypersensitivity reactions have been received as part of the continuing surveillance of TAXOL safety.

Cardiovascular: Hypotension, during the first 3 hours of infusion, occurred in 12% of all patients and 3% of all courses administered. Bradycardia, during the first 3 hours of infusion, occurred in 3% of all patients and 1% of all courses. In the Phase 3 second-line ovarian study, neither dose nor schedule had an effect on the frequency of hypotension and bradycardia. These vital sign changes most often caused no symptoms and required neither specific therapy nor treatment discontinuation. The frequency of hypotension and bradycardia were not influenced by prior anthracycline therapy.

Significant cardiovascular events possibly related to single-agent TAXOL (paclitaxel) Injection occurred in approximately 1% of all patients. These events included syncope, rhythm abnormalities, hypertension and venous thrombosis. One of the patients with syncope treated with TAXOL at 175 mg/m^2 over 24 hours had progressive hypotension and died. The arrhythmias included asymptomatic ventricular tachycardia, bigeminy and complete AV block requiring pacemaker placement. Among patients with NSCLC treated with TAXOL in combination with cisplatin in the Phase 3 study, significant cardiovascular events occurred in 12%-13%. This apparent increase in cardiovascular events is possibly due to an increase in cardiovascular risk factors in patients with lung cancer.

Electrocardiogram (ECG) abnormalities were common among patients at baseline. ECG abnormalities on study did not usually result in symptoms, were not dose-limiting, and required no intervention. ECG abnormalities were noted in 23% of all patients. Among patients with a normal ECG prior to study entry, 14% of all patients developed an abnormal tracing while on study. The most frequently reported ECG modifications were non-specific repolarization abnormalities, sinus bradycardia, sinus tachycardia and premature beats. Among patients with normal ECGs at baseline, prior therapy with anthracyclines did not influence the frequency of ECG abnormalities.

Cases of myocardial infarction have been reported rarely. Congestive heart failure has been reported typically in patients who have received other chemotherapy, notably anthracyclines. (See **PRECAUTIONS: Drug Interactions** section.)

Rare reports of atrial fibrillation and supraventricular tachycardia have been received as part of the continuing surveillance of TAXOL safety.

Respiratory: Rare reports of interstitial pneumonia, lung fibrosis and pulmonary embolism have been received as part of the continuing surveillance of TAXOL safety. Rare reports of radiation pneumonitis have been received in patients receiving concurrent radiotherapy.

Neurologic: The frequency and severity of neurologic manifestations were dose-dependent, but were not influenced by infusion duration. Peripheral neuropathy was observed in 60% of all patients (3% severe) and in 52% (2% severe) of the patients without pre-existing neuropathy.

The frequency of peripheral neuropathy increased with cumulative dose. Neurologic symptoms were observed in 27% of the patients after the first course of treatment and in 34%-51% from course 2 to 10.

Peripheral neuropathy was the cause of TAXOL discontinuation in 1% of all patients. Sensory symptoms have usually improved or resolved within several months of TAXOL discontinuation. The incidence of neurologic symptoms did not increase in the subset of patients previously treated with cisplatin. Pre-existing neuropathies resulting from prior therapies are not a contraindication for TAXOL therapy. In patients with NSCLC, administration of TAXOL followed by cisplatin resulted in greater incidence of severe neurotoxicity compared to the incidence in patients with ovarian or breast cancer treated with single-agent TAXOL. Severe neurosensory symptoms were noted in 13% of NSCLC patients receiving TAXOL 135 mg/m^2 by 24-hour infusion followed by cisplatin 75 mg/m^2 and 8% of NSCLC patients receiving cisplatin/etoposide (see **ADVERSE REACTIONS: First-Line NSCLC in Combination** section.)

Other than peripheral neuropathy, serious neurologic events following TAXOL administration have been rare (<1%) and have included grand mal seizures, syncope, ataxia and neuroencephalopathy.

Rare reports of autonomic neuropathy resulting in paralytic ileus have been received as part of the continuing surveillance of TAXOL safety. Optic nerve and/or visual disturbances (scintillating scotomata) have also been reported, particularly in patients who have received higher doses than those recommended. These effects generally have been reversible. However, rare reports in the literature of abnormal visual evoked potentials in patients have suggested persistent optic nerve damage.

Arthralgia/Myalgia: There was no consistent relationship between dose or schedule of TAXOL and the frequency or severity of arthralgia/myalgia. Sixty percent of all patients treated experienced arthralgia/myalgia; 8% experienced severe symptoms. The symptoms were usually transient, occurred two or three days after TAXOL administration, and resolved within a few days. The frequency and severity of musculoskeletal symptoms remained unchanged throughout the treatment period.

Hepatic: No relationship was observed between liver function abnormalities and either dose or schedule of TAXOL administration. Among patients with normal baseline liver function 7%, 22% and 19% had elevations in bilirubin, alkaline phosphatase and AST (SGOT), respectively. Prolonged exposure to TAXOL was not associated with cumulative hepatic toxicity.

Rare reports of hepatic necrosis and hepatic encephalopathy leading to death have been received as part of the continuing surveillance of TAXOL safety.

Renal: Among the patients treated for Kaposi's sarcoma with TAXOL, five patients had renal toxicity of grade III or IV severity. One patient with suspected HIV nephropathy of grade IV severity had to discontinue therapy. The other four patients had renal insufficiency with reversible elevations of serum creatinine.

Gastrointestinal (GI): Nausea/vomiting, diarrhea and mucositis were reported by 52%, 38% and 31% of all patients, respectively. These manifestations were usually mild to moderate. Mucositis was schedule dependent and occurred more frequently with the 24-hour than with the 3-hour infusion.

In patients with poor-risk AIDS-related Kaposi's sarcoma, nausea/vomiting, diarrhea, and mucositis were reported by 69%, 79%, and 28% of patients, respectively. One third of patients with Kaposi's sarcoma complained of diarrhea prior to study start. (See **CLINICAL STUDIES: AIDS-Related Kaposi's Sarcoma** section in full prescribing information.)

In the first-line Phase 3 ovarian carcinoma study, the incidence of nausea and vomiting when TAXOL was administered in combination with cisplatin appeared to be greater compared with the database for single-agent TAXOL in ovarian and breast carcinoma. In the same study, diarrhea of any grade was reported more frequently (16%) compared to the control arm (8%) (p=0.008), but there was no difference for severe diarrhea.

Rare reports of intestinal obstruction, intestinal perforation, pancreatitis, ischemic colitis, and dehydration have been received as part of the continuing surveillance of TAXOL safety. Rare reports of neutropenic enterocolitis (typhlitis), despite the coadministration of G-CSF, were observed in patients treated with TAXOL alone and in combination with other chemotherapeutic agents.

Injection Site Reaction: Injection site reactions, including reactions secondary to extravasation, were usually mild and consisted of erythema, tenderness, skin discoloration, or swelling at the injection site. These reactions have been observed more frequently with the 24-hour infusion than with the 3-hour infusion. Recurrence of skin reactions at a site of previous extravasation following administration of TAXOL at a different site, i.e., "recall", has been reported rarely.

Rare reports of more severe events such as phlebitis, cellulitis, induration, skin exfoliation, necrosis and fibrosis have been received as part of the continuing surveillance of

TAXOL (paclitaxel) Injection safety. In some cases the onset of the injection site reaction either occurred during a prolonged infusion or was delayed by a week to ten days.

A specific treatment for extravasation reactions is unknown at this time. Given the possibility of extravasation, it is advisable to closely monitor the infusion site for possible infiltration during drug administration.

Other Clinical Events: Alopecia was observed in almost all (87%) of the patients. Transient skin changes due to TAXOL-related hypersensitivity reactions have been observed, but no other skin toxicities were significantly associated with TAXOL administration. Nail changes (changes in pigmentation or discoloration of nail bed) were uncommon (2%). Edema was reported in 21% of all patients (17% of those without baseline edema); only 1% had severe edema and none of these patients required treatment discontinuation. Edema was most commonly focal and disease-related. Edema was observed in 5% of all courses for patients with normal baseline and did not increase with time on study.

Rare reports of skin abnormalities related to radiation recall as well as reports of maculopapular rash and pruritus have been received as part of the continuing surveillance of TAXOL safety.

Reports of asthenia and malaise have been received as part of the continuing surveillance of TAXOL safety. In the Phase 3 trial of TAXOL 135 mg/m² over 24 hours in combination with cisplatin as first-line therapy of ovarian cancer, asthenia was reported in 17% of the patients, significantly greater than the 10% incidence observed in the control arm of cyclophosphamide/cisplatin.

Accidental Exposure: Upon inhalation, dyspnea, chest pain, burning eyes, sore throat and nausea have been reported. Following topical exposure, events have included tingling, burning and redness.

OVERDOSAGE

There is no known antidote for TAXOL overdosage. The primary anticipated complications of overdosage would consist of bone marrow suppression, peripheral neurotoxicity and mucositis. Overdoses in pediatric patients may be associated with acute ethanol toxicity (see **PRECAUTIONS: Pediatric Use** section).

DOSAGE AND ADMINISTRATION

Note: Contact of the undiluted concentrate with plasticized PVC equipment or devices used to prepare solutions for infusion is not recommended. In order to minimize patient exposure to the plasticizer DEHP [di-(2-ethylhexyl)phthalate], which may be leached from PVC infusion bags or sets, diluted TAXOL solutions should be stored in bottles (glass, polypropylene) or plastic bags (polypropylene, polyolefin) and administered through polyethylene-lined administration sets.

All patients should be premedicated prior to TAXOL administration in order to prevent severe hypersensitivity reactions. Such premedication may consist of dexamethasone 20 mg PO administered approximately 12 and 6 hours before TAXOL, diphenhydramine (or its equivalent) 50 mg I.V. 30 to 60 minutes prior to TAXOL, and cimetidine (300 mg) or ranitidine (50 mg) I.V. 30 to 60 minutes before TAXOL.

For patients with **carcinoma of the ovary**, the following regimens are recommended:

1) For previously untreated patients with carcinoma of the ovary, the recommended regimen, given every 3 weeks, is TAXOL administered intravenously over 24 hours at a dose of 135 mg/m² followed by cisplatin at a dose of 75 mg/m².

2) In patients previously treated with chemotherapy for carcinoma of the ovary, TAXOL has been used at several doses and schedules; however, the optimal regimen is not yet clear (see **CLINICAL STUDIES: Ovarian Carcinoma** section in full prescribing information). The recommended regimen is TAXOL 135 mg/m² or 175 mg/m² administered intravenously over 3 hours every 3 weeks.

For patients with **carcinoma of the breast**, the following regimens are recommended (see **CLINICAL STUDIES: Breast Carcinoma** section in full prescribing information):

1) For the adjuvant treatment of node-positive breast cancer, the recommended regimen is TAXOL, at a dose of 175 mg/m² intravenously over 3 hours every 3 weeks for four courses administered sequentially to doxorubicin-containing combination chemotherapy. The clinical trial used four courses of doxorubicin and cyclophosphamide (See **CLINICAL STUDIES: Breast Carcinoma** section in full prescribing information).

2) After failure of initial chemotherapy for metastatic disease or relapse within 6 months of adjuvant chemotherapy, TAXOL at a dose of 175 mg/m² administered intravenously over 3 hours every 3 weeks has been shown to be effective.

For patients with **non-small cell lung carcinoma**, the recommended regimen, given every 3 weeks, is TAXOL administered intravenously over 24 hours at a dose of 135 mg/m² followed by cisplatin, 75 mg/m².

For patients with **AIDS-related Kaposi's sarcoma**, TAXOL administered at a dose of 135 mg/m² given intravenously over 3 hours every 3 weeks or at a dose of 100 mg/m² given intravenously over 3 hours every 2 weeks is recommended (dose intensity 45-50 mg/m²/week). In the two clinical trials evaluating these schedules (see **CLINICAL STUDIES: AIDS-Related Kaposi's Sarcoma** section in full prescribing information), the former schedule (135 mg/m² every 3 weeks) was more toxic than the latter. In addition, all patients with low performance status were treated with the latter schedule (100 mg/m² every 2 weeks).

Based upon the immunosuppression in patients with advanced HIV disease, the following modifications are recommended in these patients:

1) Reduce the dose of dexamethasone as one of the three premedication drugs to 10 mg PO (instead of 20 mg PO);

2) Initiate or repeat treatment with TAXOL only if the neutrophil count is at least 1000 cells/mm³;

3) Reduce the dose of subsequent courses of TAXOL by 20% for patients who experience severe neutropenia (neutrophil <500 cells/mm³ for a week or longer); and

4) Initiate concomitant hematopoietic growth factor (G-CSF) as clinically indicated.

For the therapy of patients with solid tumors (ovary, breast, and NSCLC), courses of TAXOL should not be repeated until the neutrophil count is at least 1,500 cells/mm³ and the platelet count is at least 100,000 cells/mm³. TAXOL should not be given to patients with AIDS-related Kaposi's sarcoma if the baseline or subsequent neutrophil count is less than 1000 cells/mm³. Patients who experience severe neutropenia (neutrophil <500 cells/mm³ for a week or longer) or severe peripheral neuropathy during TAXOL therapy should have dosage reduced by 20% for subsequent courses of TAXOL. The incidence of neurotoxicity and the severity of neutropenia increase with dose.

Preparation and Administration Precautions: TAXOL is a cytotoxic anticancer drug and, as with other potentially toxic compounds, caution should be exercised in handling TAXOL. The use of gloves is recommended. If TAXOL solution contacts the skin, wash the skin immediately and thoroughly with soap and water. Following topical exposure, events have included tingling, burning and redness. If TAXOL contacts mucous membranes, the membranes should be flushed thoroughly with water. Upon inhalation, dyspnea, chest pain, burning eyes, sore throat, and nausea have been reported.

Given the possibility of extravasation, it is advisable to closely monitor the infusion site for possible infiltration during drug administration. (See **PRECAUTIONS: Injection Site Reaction** section.)

Preparation for Intravenous Administration: TAXOL (paclitaxel) Injection must be diluted prior to infusion. TAXOL should be diluted in 0.9% Sodium Chloride Injection, USP; 5% Dextrose Injection, USP; 5% Dextrose and 0.9% Sodium Chloride Injection, USP or 5% Dextrose in Ringer's Injection to a final concentration of 0.3 to 1.2 mg/mL. The solutions are physically and chemically stable for up to 27 hours at ambient temperature (approximately 25°C) and room lighting conditions. Parenteral drug products should be inspected visually for particulate matter and discoloration prior to administration whenever solution and container permit.

Upon preparation, solutions may show haziness, which is attributed to the formulation vehicle. No significant losses in potency have been noted following simulated delivery of the solution through I.V. tubing containing an in-line (0.22 micron) filter.

Data collected for the presence of the extractable plasticizer DEHP [di-(2-ethylhexyl)phthalate] show that levels increase with time and concentration when dilutions are prepared in PVC containers. Consequently, the use of plasticized PVC containers and administration sets is not recommended. TAXOL solutions should be prepared and stored in glass, polypropylene, or polyolefin containers. Non-PVC containing administration sets, such as those which are polyethylene-lined, should be used.

TAXOL should be administered through an in-line filter with a microporous membrane not greater than 0.22 microns. Use of filter devices such as IVEX-2® filters which incorporate short inlet and outlet PVC-coated tubing has not resulted in significant leaching of DEHP.

The Chemo Dispensing Pin™ device or similar devices with spikes should not be used with vials of TAXOL since they can cause the stopper to collapse resulting in loss of sterile integrity of the TAXOL solution.

Stability: Unopened vials of TAXOL Injection are stable until the date indicated on the package when stored between 20°-25°C (68°-77°F), in the original package. Neither freezing nor refrigeration adversely affects the stability of the product. Upon refrigeration, components in the TAXOL vial may precipitate, but will redissolve upon reaching room temperature with little or no agitation. There is no impact on product quality under these circumstances. If the solution remains cloudy or if an insoluble precipitate is noted, the vial should be discarded. Solutions for infusion prepared as recommended are stable at ambient temperature (approximately 25°C) and lighting conditions for up to 27 hours.

HOW SUPPLIED

NDC 0015-3475-30 30 mg/5 mL multidose vial individually packaged in a carton.
NDC 0015-3476-30 100 mg/16.7 mL multidose vial individually packaged in a carton.
NDC 0015-3479-11 300 mg/50 mL multidose vial individually packaged in a carton.

Storage: Store the vials in original cartons between 20°-25°C (68°-77°F). Retain in the original package to protect from light.

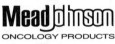

ONCOLOGY PRODUCTS

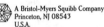

A Bristol-Myers Squibb Company
Princeton, NJ 08543
U.S.A.

K4-B001A-11-99

Adapted from: 347630DIM-07
Revised October 1999

IVEX-2® is the registered trademark of the Millipore Corporation.
Chemo Dispensing Pin™ is a trademark of B. Braun Medical Incorporated.

℞ ONLY

PARAPLATIN®

(carboplatin for injection)

Brief Summary of Prescribing Information, 4/99. For complete prescribing information, please consult official package circular.

WARNING
PARAPLATIN® (carboplatin for injection) should be administered under the supervision of a qualified physician experienced in the use of cancer chemotherapeutic agents. Appropriate management of therapy and complications is possible only when adequate treatment facilities are readily available.

Bone marrow suppression is dose related and may be severe, resulting in infection and/or bleeding. Anemia may be cumulative and may require transfusion support. Vomiting is another frequent drug-related side effect.

Anaphylactic-like reactions to PARAPLATIN have been reported and may occur within minutes of PARAPLATIN administration. Epinephrine, corticosteroids, and antihistamines have been employed to alleviate symptoms.

INDICATIONS
Initial Treatment of Advanced Ovarian Carcinoma: PARAPLATIN is indicated for the initial treatment of advanced ovarian carcinoma in established combination with other approved chemotherapeutic agents. One established combination regimen consists of PARAPLATIN and cyclophosphamide (CYTOXAN®). Two randomized controlled studies conducted by the NCIC and SWOG with PARAPLATIN vs. cisplatin, both in combination with cyclophosphamide, have demonstrated equivalent overall survival between the two groups (see **CLINICAL STUDIES** section).

There is limited statistical power to demonstrate equivalence in overall pathologic complete response rates and long term survival (≥ 3 years) because of the small number of patients with these outcomes: the small number of patients with residual tumor < 2 cm after initial surgery also limits the statistical power to demonstrate equivalence in this subgroup.

Secondary Treatment of Advanced Ovarian Carcinoma: PARAPLATIN is indicated for the palliative treatment of patients with ovarian carcinoma recurrent after prior chemotherapy, including patients who have been previously treated with cisplatin.

Within the group of patients previously treated with cisplatin, those who have developed progressive disease while receiving cisplatin therapy may have a decreased response rate.

CONTRAINDICATIONS
PARAPLATIN is contraindicated in patients with a history of severe allergic reactions to cisplatin or other platinum-containing compounds, or mannitol.

PARAPLATIN should not be employed in patients with severe bone marrow depression or significant bleeding.

WARNINGS
Bone marrow suppression (leukopenia, neutropenia, and thrombocytopenia) is dose-dependent and is also the dose-limiting toxicity. Peripheral blood counts should be frequently monitored during PARAPLATIN treatment and, when appropriate, until recovery is achieved. Median nadir occurs at day 21 in patients receiving single-agent PARAPLATIN. In general, single intermittent courses of PARAPLATIN should not be repeated until leukocyte, neutrophil, and platelet counts have recovered.

Since anemia is cumulative, transfusions may be needed during treatment with PARAPLATIN, particularly in patients receiving prolonged therapy.

Bone marrow suppression is increased in patients who have received prior therapy, especially regimens including cisplatin. Marrow suppression is also increased in patients with impaired kidney function. Initial PARAPLATIN dosages in these patients should be appropriately reduced (see **DOSAGE AND ADMINISTRATION** section) and blood counts should be carefully monitored between courses. The use of PARAPLATIN in combination with other bone marrow suppressing therapies must be carefully managed with respect to dosage and timing in order to minimize additive effects.

PARAPLATIN has limited nephrotoxic potential, but concomitant treatment with aminoglycosides has resulted in increased renal and/or audiologic toxicity, and caution must be exercised when a patient receives both drugs. Clinically significant hearing loss has been reported to occur in pediatric patients when PARAPLATIN was administered at higher than recommended doses in combination with other ototoxic agents.

PARAPLATIN can induce emesis, which can be more severe in patients previously receiving emetogenic therapy. The incidence and intensity of emesis have been reduced by using premedication with antiemetics. Although no conclusive efficacy data exist with the following schedules of PARAPLATIN, lengthening the duration of single intravenous administration to 24 hours or dividing the total dose over five consecutive daily pulse doses has resulted in reduced emesis.

Although peripheral neurotoxicity is infrequent, its incidence is increased in patients older than 65 years and in patients previously treated with cisplatin. Pre-existing cisplatin-induced neurotoxicity does not worsen in about 70% of the patients receiving PARAPLATIN as secondary treatment.

Loss of vision, which can be complete for light and colors, has been reported after the use of PARAPLATIN with doses higher than those recommended in the package insert. Vision appears to recover totally or to a significant extent within weeks of stopping these high doses.

As in the case of other platinum coordination compounds, allergic reactions to PARAPLATIN have been reported. These may occur within minutes of administration and should be managed with appropriate supportive therapy. There is increased risk of allergic reactions including anaphylaxis in patients previously exposed to platinum therapy. (See **CONTRAINDICATIONS** and **ADVERSE REACTIONS: Allergic Reactions** section.)

High dosages of PARAPLATIN (more than four times the recommended dose) have resulted in severe abnormalities of liver function tests.

PARAPLATIN may cause fetal harm when administered to a pregnant woman. PARAPLATIN has been shown to be embryotoxic and teratogenic in rats. There are no adequate and well-controlled studies in pregnant women. If this drug is used during pregnancy, or if the patient becomes pregnant while receiving this drug, the patient should be apprised of the potential hazard to the fetus. Women of childbearing potential should be advised to avoid becoming pregnant.

PRECAUTIONS
General: Needles or intravenous administration sets containing aluminum parts that may come in contact with PARAPLATIN should not be used for the preparation or administration of the drug. Aluminum can react with carboplatin causing precipitate formation and loss of potency.

Drug Interactions: The renal effects of nephrotoxic compounds may be potentiated by PARAPLATIN.

Carcinogenesis, Mutagenesis, Impairment of Fertility: The carcinogenic potential of carboplatin has not been studied, but compounds with similar mechanisms of action and mutagenicity profiles have been reported to be carcinogenic. Carboplatin has been shown to be mutagenic both *in vitro* and *in vivo*. It has also been shown to be embryotoxic and teratogenic in rats receiving the drug during organogenesis. Secondary malignancies have been reported in association with multidrug therapy.

Pregnancy: Pregnancy "Category D". (See **WARNINGS** section.)

Nursing Mothers: It is not known whether carboplatin is excreted in human milk. Because there is a possibility of toxicity in nursing infants secondary to PARAPLATIN (carboplatin for injection) treatment of the mother, it is recommended that breast-feeding be discontinued if the mother is treated with PARAPLATIN.

Pediatric Use: Safety and effectiveness in pediatric patients have not been established (see **WARNINGS, Audiologic Toxicity** section).

ADVERSE REACTIONS
For a comparison of toxicities when carboplatin or cisplatin was given in combination with cyclophosphamide, see the **COMPARATIVE TOXICITY** subsection of the **CLINICAL STUDIES** section in the full prescribing information.

ADVERSE EXPERIENCES IN PATIENTS WITH OVARIAN CANCER

		First Line Combination Therapy* Percent	Second Line Single Agent Therapy** Percent
Bone Marrow			
Thrombocytopenia	< 100,000/mm³	66	62
	< 50,000/mm³	33	35
Neutropenia	< 2,000 cells/mm³	96	67
	< 1,000 cells/mm³	82	21
Leukopenia	< 4,000 cells/mm³	97	85
	< 2,000 cells/mm³	71	26
Anemia	< 11 g/dL	90	90
	< 8 g/dL	14	21
Infections		16	5
Bleeding		8	5
Transfusions		35	44
Gastrointestinal			
Nausea and vomiting		93	92
Vomiting		83	81
Other GI side effects		46	21
Neurologic			
Peripheral neuropathies		15	6
Ototoxicity		12	1
Other sensory side effects		5	1
Central neurotoxicity		26	5
Renal			
Serum creatinine elevations		6	10
Blood urea elevations		17	22
Hepatic			
Bilirubin elevations		5	5
SGOT elevations		20	19
Alkaline phosphatase elevations		29	37
Electrolytes loss			
Sodium		10	47
Potassium		16	28
Calcium		16	31
Magnesium		61	43
Other side effects			
Pain		44	23
Asthenia		41	11
Cardiovascular		19	6
Respiratory		10	6
Allergic		11	2
Genitourinary		10	2
Alopecia		49	2
Mucositis		8	1

***Use with cyclophosphamide for initial treatment of ovarian cancer:** Data are based on the experience of 393 patients with ovarian cancer (regardless of baseline status) who received initial combination therapy with PARAPLATIN and cyclophosphamide in two randomized controlled studies conducted by SWOG and NCIC (see **CLINICAL STUDIES** section in the full prescribing information).

Combination with cyclophosphamide as well as duration of treatment may be responsible for the differences that can be noted in the adverse experience table.

****Single agent use for the secondary treatment of ovarian cancer:** Data are based on the experience of 553 patients with previously treated ovarian carcinoma (regardless of baseline status) who received single-agent PARAPLATIN.

In the narrative section that follows, the incidences of adverse events are based on data from 1,893 patients with various types of tumors who received PARAPLATIN as single-agent therapy.

Hematologic Toxicity: Bone marrow suppression is the dose-limiting toxicity of PARAPLATIN. Thrombocytopenia with platelet counts below 50,000/mm³ occurs in 25% of the patients (35% of pretreated ovarian cancer patients); neutropenia with granulocyte counts below 1,000/mm³ occurs in 16% of the patients (21% of pretreated ovarian cancer patients); leukopenia with WBC counts below 2,000/mm³ occurs in 15% of the patients (26% of pretreated ovarian cancer patients). The nadir usually occurs about day 21 in patients receiving single-agent therapy. By day 28, 90% of patients have platelet counts above 100,000/mm³; 74% have neutrophil counts above 2,000/mm³; 67% have leukocyte counts above 4,000/mm³.

Marrow suppression is usually more severe in patients with impaired kidney function. Patients with poor performance status have also experienced a higher incidence of severe leukopenia and thrombocytopenia.

The hematologic effects, although usually reversible, have resulted in infectious or hemorrhagic complications in 5% of the patients treated with PARAPLATIN, with drug related death occurring in less than 1% of the patients. Fever has also been reported in patients with neutropenia.

Anemia with hemoglobin less than 11 g/dL has been observed in 71% of the patients who started therapy with a baseline above that value. The incidence of anemia increases with increasing exposure to PARAPLATIN. Transfusions have been administered to 26% of the patients treated with PARAPLATIN (44% of previously treated ovarian cancer patients).

Bone marrow depression may be more severe when PARAPLATIN is combined with other bone marrow suppressing drugs or with radiotherapy.

Gastrointestinal Toxicity: Vomiting occurs in 65% of the patients (81% of previously treated ovarian cancer patients) and in about one-third of these patients it is severe. Carboplatin, as a single agent or in combination, is significantly less emetogenic than cisplatin; however, patients previously treated with emetogenic agents, especially cisplatin, appear to be more prone to vomiting. Nausea alone occurs in an additional 10% to 15% of patients. Both nausea and vomiting usually cease within 24 hours of treatment and are often responsive to antiemetic measures. Although no conclusive efficacy data exist with the following schedules, prolonged administration of PARAPLATIN (carboplatin for injection), either by continuous 24-hour infusion or by daily pulse doses given for five consecutive days, was associated with less severe vomiting than the single dose intermittent schedule. Emesis was increased when PARAPLATIN was used in combination with other emetogenic compounds. Other gastrointestinal effects observed frequently were pain, in 17% of the patients; diarrhea, in 6%; and constipation, also in 6%.

Neurologic Toxicity: Peripheral neuropathies have been observed in 4% of the patients receiving PARAPLATIN (6% of pretreated ovarian cancer patients) with mild paresthesias occurring most frequently. Carboplatin therapy produces significantly fewer and less severe neurologic side effects than does therapy with cisplatin. However, patients older than 65 years and/or previously treated with cisplatin appear to have an increased risk (10%) for peripheral neuropathies. In 70% of the patients with pre-existing cisplatin-induced peripheral neurotoxicity, there was no worsening of symptoms during therapy with PARAPLATIN. Clinical ototoxicity and other sensory abnormalities such as visual disturbances and change in taste have been reported in only 1% of the patients. Central nervous system symptoms have been reported in 5% of the patients and appear to be most often related to the use of antiemetics.

Although the overall incidence of peripheral neurologic side effects induced by PARAPLATIN is low, prolonged treatment, particularly in cisplatin pretreated patients, may result in cumulative neurotoxicity.

Nephrotoxicity: Development of abnormal renal function test results is uncommon, despite the fact that carboplatin, unlike cisplatin, has usually been administered without high-volume fluid hydration and/or forced diuresis. The incidences of abnormal renal function tests reported are 6% for serum creatinine and 14% for blood urea nitrogen (10% and 22%, respectively, in pretreated ovarian cancer patients). Most of these reported abnormalities have been mild and about one-half of them were reversible.

Creatinine clearance has proven to be the most sensitive measure of kidney function in patients receiving PARAPLATIN, and it appears to be the most useful test for correlating drug clearance and bone marrow suppression. Twenty-seven percent of the patients who had a baseline value of 60 mL/min or more demonstrated a reduction below this value during PARAPLATIN therapy.

Hepatic Toxicity: The incidences of abnormal liver function tests in patients with normal baseline values were reported as follows: total bilirubin, 5%; SGOT, 15%; and alkaline phosphatase, 24%; (5%, 19%, and 37%, respectively, in pretreated ovarian cancer patients). These abnormalities have generally been mild and reversible in about one-half of the cases, although the role of metastatic tumor in the liver may complicate the assessment in many patients. In a limited series of patients receiving very high dosages of PARAPLATIN and autologous bone marrow transplantation, severe abnormalities of liver function tests were reported.

Electrolyte Changes: The incidences of abnormally decreased serum electrolyte values reported were as follows: sodium, 29%; potassium, 20%; calcium, 22%; and magnesium, 29%; (47%, 28%, 31%, and 43%, respectively, in pretreated ovarian cancer patients). Electrolyte supplementation was not routinely administered concomitantly with PARAPLATIN, and these electrolyte abnormalities were rarely associated with symptoms.

Allergic Reactions: Hypersensitivity to PARAPLATIN has been reported in 2% of the patients. These allergic reactions have been similar in nature and severity to those reported with other platinum-containing compounds, i.e., rash, urticaria, erythema, pruritus, and rarely bronchospasm and hypotension. Anaphylactic reactions have been reported as part of postmarketing surveillance (see **WARNINGS** section). These reactions have been successfully managed with standard epinephrine, corticosteroid, and antihistamine therapy.

Other Events: Pain and asthenia were the most frequently reported miscellaneous adverse effects; their relationship to the tumor and to anemia was likely. Alopecia was reported (3%). Cardiovascular, respiratory, genitourinary, and mucosal side effects have occurred in 6% or less of the patients. Cardiovascular events (cardiac failure, embolism, cerebrovascular accidents) were fatal in less than 1% of the patients and did not appear to be related to chemotherapy. Cancer-associated hemolytic uremic syndrome has been reported rarely.

Malaise, anorexia and hypertension have been reported as part of postmarketing surveillance.

OVERDOSAGE

There is no known antidote for PARAPLATIN overdosage. The anticipated complications of overdosage would be secondary to bone marrow suppression and/or hepatic toxicity.

DOSAGE AND ADMINISTRATION

NOTE: Aluminum reacts with carboplatin causing precipitate formation and loss of potency, therefore, needles or intravenous sets containing aluminum parts that may come in contact with the drug must not be used for the preparation or administration of PARAPLATIN.

Single Agent Therapy: PARAPLATIN, as a single agent, has been shown to be effective in patients with recurrent ovarian carcinoma at a dosage of 360 mg/m² I.V. on day 1 every 4 weeks (alternatively see **Formula Dosing**). In general, however, single intermittent courses of PARAPLATIN should not be repeated until the neutrophil count is at least 2,000 and the platelet count is at least 100,000.

Combination Therapy with Cyclophosphamide: In the chemotherapy of advanced ovarian cancer, an effective combination for previously untreated patients consists of:

PARAPLATIN—300 mg/m² I.V. on day 1 every 4 weeks for six cycles (alternatively see **Formula Dosing**).

Cyclophosphamide (CYTOXAN®)—600 mg/m² I.V. on day 1 every 4 weeks for six cycles. For directions regarding the use and administration of cyclophosphamide (CYTOXAN®), please refer to its package insert. (See **CLINICAL STUDIES** section.)

Intermittent courses of PARAPLATIN in combination with cyclophosphamide should not be repeated until the neutrophil count is at least 2,000 and the platelet count is at least 100,000.

Dose Adjustment Recommendations: Pretreatment platelet count and performance status are important prognostic factors for severity of myelosuppression in previously treated patients.

The suggested dose adjustments for single agent or combination therapy shown in the table below are modified from controlled trials in previously treated and untreated patients with ovarian carcinoma. Blood counts were done weekly, and the recommendations are based on the lowest post-treatment platelet or neutrophil value.

Platelets	Neutrophils	Adjusted Dose* (From Prior Course)
> 100,000	> 2,000	125%
50-100,000	500-2,000	No Adjustment
< 50,000	< 500	75%

*Percentages apply to PARAPLATIN as a single agent or to both PARAPLATIN and cyclophosphamide in combination. In the controlled studies, dosages were also adjusted at a lower level (50% to 60%) for severe myelosuppression. Escalations above 125% were not recommended for these studies.

PARAPLATIN is usually administered by an infusion lasting 15 minutes or longer. No pre- or post-treatment hydration or forced diuresis is required.

Patients with Impaired Kidney Function: Patients with creatinine clearance values below 60 mL/min are at increased risk of severe bone marrow suppression. In renally-impaired patients who received single agent PARAPLATIN therapy, the incidence of severe leukopenia, neutropenia, or thrombocytopenia has been about 25% when the dosage modifications in the table below have been used.

Baseline Creatinine Clearance	Recommended Dose on Day 1
41-59 mL/min	250 mg/m²
16-40 mL/min	200 mg/m²

The data available for patients with severely impaired kidney function (creatinine clearance below 15 mL/min) are too limited to permit a recommendation for treatment.[1,2]

These dosing recommendations apply to the initial course of treatment. Subsequent dosages should be adjusted according to the patient's tolerance based on the degree of bone marrow suppression.

Formula Dosing: Another approach for determining the initial dose of PARAPLATIN (carboplatin for injection) is the use of mathematical formulae, which are based on a patient's pre-existing renal function[3-5] or renal function and desired platelet nadir.[6] Renal excretion is the major route of elimination for carboplatin. (See **CLINICAL PHARMACOLOGY** section.) The use of dosing formulae, as compared to empirical dose calculation based on body surface area, allows compensation for patient variations in pretreatment renal function that might otherwise result in either underdosing (in patients with above average renal function) or overdosing (in patients with impaired renal function).

A simple formula for calculating dosage, based upon a patient's glomerular filtration rate (GFR in mL/min) and PARAPLATIN target area under the concentration versus time curve (AUC in mg/mL• min), has been proposed by Calvert.[3-5] In these studies, GFR was measured by ^{51}Cr-EDTA clearance.[7]

CALVERT FORMULA FOR CARBOPLATIN DOSING

Total Dose (mg)=(target AUC) x (GFR + 25)

Note: With the Calvert formula, the total dose of PARAPLATIN is calculated in mg, <u>not</u> mg/m².

The target AUC of 4-6 mg/mL• min using single agent PARAPLATIN appears to provide the most appropriate dose range in previously treated patients.[4] This study also showed a trend between the AUC of single agent PARAPLATIN administered to previously treated patients and the likelihood of developing toxicity.[1]

	% Actual Toxicity in Previously Treated Patients	
AUC (mg/mL•min)	Gr 3 or Gr 4 Thrombocytopenia	Gr 3 or Gr 4 Leukopenia
4 to 5	16%	13%
6 to 7	33%	34%

HOW SUPPLIED

PARAPLATIN® (carboplatin for injection)

NDC 0015-3213-30 — **50 mg** vials, individually cartoned, shelf packs of 10 cartons, 10 shelf packs per case. (Yellow flip-off seals)

NDC 0015-3214-30 — **150 mg** vials, individually cartoned, shelf packs of 10 cartons, 10 shelf packs per case. (Violet flip-off seals)

NDC 0015-3215-30 — **450 mg** vials, individually cartoned, shelf packs of 6 cartons, 10 shelf packs per case. (Blue flip-off seals)

REFERENCES

1. Egorin MJ, et al: Pharmacokinetics and Dosage Reduction of Cis-diammine(1,1-cyclobutanedicarboxylato) Platinum in Patients with Impaired Renal Function. *Cancer Res* 1984; 44:5432–5438.
2. Carboplatin, Etoposide, and Bleomycin for Treatment of Stage IIC Seminoma Complicated by Acute Renal Failure. Cancer Treatment Reports November 1987; Vol. 71,11:1123-1124.
3. Calvert AH, et al: Carboplatin Dosage: Prospective Evaluation of a Simple Formula Based on Renal Function. *J Clin Oncol* 1989; 7:1748-1756.
4. Jodrell DI, et al: Relationships Between Carboplatin Exposure and Tumor Response and Toxicity in Patients with Ovarian Cancer. *J Clin Oncol* 1992; 10:520-528.
5. Sorensen BT, et al: Dose-Toxicity Relationship of Carboplatin in Combination with Cyclophosphamide in Ovarian Cancer Patients. *Cancer Chemother Pharmacol* 1991; 28:397-401.
6. Egorin MJ, et al: Prospective Validation of a Pharmacologically Based Dosing Scheme for the Cis-diamminedichloroplatinum (II) Analogue Diamminecyclobutanedicarboxylatoplatinum. *Cancer Res* 1985; 45:6502-6506.
7. Daugaard G, et al: Effects of Cisplatin on Different Measures of Glomerular Function in the Human Kidney with Special Emphasis on High-Dose. *Cancer Chemother Pharmacol* 1988; 21:163-167.

U.S. Patent Nos. 4,140,707
4,657,927

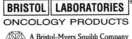

BRISTOL LABORATORIES®
ONCOLOGY PRODUCTS
A Bristol-Myers Squibb Company
Princeton, NJ 08543
U.S.A.

K2-B001A-9-99
1080187A1

Adapted from: 3213DIM-11
Revised April 1999

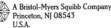